In vitro fertilization
Second edition

This comprehensively updated and expanded new edition builds on its successful and popular predecessor, retaining the practical features which made the first edition such an essential guide to IVF. The new edition describes the most recent additions to the range of current ART clinical treatments, including the use of testicular and epididymal sperm, blastocyst stage transfer, new perspectives in cryobiology and cryopreservation techniques, and has an additional chapter on preimplantation genetic diagnosis. By incorporating the very latest laboratory techniques and protocols with an even greater emphasis on quality control, it provides an indispensable and practical account. The introductory chapters covering the scientific background that underpins effective laboratory practice have been substantially expanded to include the most recent information available, derived from research in mammalian systems into the molecular biology of oogenesis, oocyte maturation and early embryo metabolism. This new edition distils a wealth of practical and scientific detail for the benefit of all IVF practitioners.

In vitro fertilization

SECOND EDITION

KAY ELDER

Director of Continuing Education
Bourn Hall Clinic

BRIAN DALE

Scientific Director
Centre for Reproductive Biology, Naples

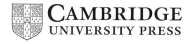

CAMBRIDGE UNIVERSITY PRESS

PUBLISHED BY THE PRESS SYNDICATE OF THE UNIVERSITY OF CAMBRIDGE
The Pitt Building, Trumpington Street, Cambridge, United Kingdom

CAMBRIDGE UNIVERSITY PRESS
The Edinburgh Building, Cambridge CB2 2RU, UK   http://www.cup.cam.ac.uk
40 West 20th Street, New York, NY 10011-4211, USA   http://www.cup.org
10 Stanford Road, Oakleigh, Melbourne 3166, Australia
Ruiz de Alarcón 13, 28014 Madrid, Spain

First published 2000

Printed in the United Kingdom at the University Press, Cambridge

Typeface Times 11/14 pt [VN]

A catalogue record for this book is available from the British Library

ISBN 0 521 77863 8 paperback

Every effort has been made in preparing this book to provide accurate and up-to-date information which is in accord with accepted standards and practice at the time of publication. Nevertheless, the authors, editors and publisher can make no warranties that the information contained
herein is totally free from error, not least because clinical standards are constantly changing
through research and regulation. The authors, editors and publisher therefore disclaim all
liability for direct or consequential damages resulting from the use of material contained in this
book. The reader is strongly advised to pay careful attention to information provided by the
manufacturer of any drugs or equipment that they plan to use.

To Robbie, Bethany, Daniela, Peter, Roberta, and Rebecca

Contents

Preface

Several hundred thousand IVF children have been born worldwide since the birth of Louise Brown in 1978. Technology in assisted human reproduction is striding ahead, from the first births using frozen embryos in the early 1980s to sex-selection of embryos and the microinjection of spermatozoa for the treatment of male sterility at the beginning of the 1990s. However, research on human gametes and embryos, for various political and ethical reasons, has not followed suit. Although the clinical embryologist must be trained in standard cell culture technology, we believe it is equally important to be aware of the basic biology of these highly specialized cells, the gametes. Most of our information on gametes and early embryos has come from studies on invertebrates, less so from mammals, and therefore we have presented a general overview of gamete biology, followed by more specific descriptions of mammalian and, where possible, human gamete biology.

The first section of this book explores how gametes are produced, how they interact and the first steps of embryo development. The middle section is dedicated to the technologies used in animal ART and advanced laboratory technologies, whilst the latter section of the book describes a compilation of protocols used at Bourn Hall Clinic, Cambridge. The protocols were originally established at Bourn Hall in 1980 by Professor R.G. Edwards and Jean Purdy, following their years of research in the Cambridge University Department of Physiology and Kershaws hospital in Oldham. Over the years these protocols have been revised and adapted by many members of staff, all of whom are represented in the lists of further reading.

K.E.
B.D.

Acknowledgments

Special thanks to Mike Macnamee and Geoff Reeves for encouraging and sponsoring my career as a professional student – and to my children Robbie and Bethany who provided the inspiration, and allowed me the time and the space to continue pursuing my studies.

Kay T. Elder B.Sc.(Hons.), M.B., Ch.B., Ph.D.

I would like to dedicate this book to the late Alberto Monroy, who introduced me to the science of fertilization. Alberto's contributions were many – his strategy of applying molecular biology techniques, while maintaining a comparative approach, was visionary. Many of our present-day concepts in fertilization were conceived in the City of Naples, I hope we may be able to continue this tradition. My thanks to my family and colleagues, past and present, too numerous to mention, who have contributed to our research programme in Naples.

Brian Dale, Ph.D, D.Sc., F.I. Biol.

Sincere and grateful thanks to the colleagues who kindly contributed their expertise to the following chapters: Yves Ménézo on embryo metabolism, Robert Brittain on bovine IVF, John Morris on principles of cryobiology, Terry Leonard on setting up micromanipulators, and Joyce Harper for the chapter on preimplantation genetic diagnosis. We are also grateful to Yves Ménézo, Neal First, and Marijo Kent-First for their help in reviewing some of the material in this second edition.

1

Introduction

The 1990s witnessed a revival of interest in reproductive biology, partly due to the successful application of gamete and embryo culture to medical, veterinary and biotechnology practices, but also due to the pressing needs of today's society. In medical science, assisted reproductive technologies (ART) have been developed primarily to alleviate sterility, while in agricultural sciences the growing needs of the booming world population have provided the impetus to improve the efficiency of livestock production. The earliest documented use of ART was in 1783 when Spallazani delivered pups from an artificially inseminated bitch, but it was not until the 1900s that the Russian School of Ivanov developed artificial vaginas and insemination techniques to be used in horses, cattle and sheep. The value of artificial insemination in farm animals depends upon the fact that the male ejaculate contains many millions of spermatozoa, theoretically sufficient to inseminate hundreds of females. A major leap forward in this direction was made in the late 1940s, when the team led by Chis Polge in Cambridge, England, developed techniques to freeze and store animal spermatozoa. This same period of time also saw the development of methods to isolate and manipulate the female gamete. In vitro maturation of mammalian oocytes was first reported by Pincus over 50 years ago, when it was observed that the primary oocyte of the rabbit resumed meiosis spontaneously when liberated from its follicle and placed in a suitable culture medium. It was not, however, until 1968 that Joe Sreenan in Ireland observed nuclear maturation in vitro in bovine oocytes recovered from slaughterhouse cattle. Although experiments on animals have traditionally preceded human studies, this has not always been the case in reproductive biology, where many of the new techniques and breakthroughs have been made using human gametes in a clinical setting.

In nature, efficient reproduction relies on the synchronized behaviour of animals, the synchronized physiology of their reproductive organs and the

1

synchronized interaction of the male and female gametes. This fundamental principle of synchronization has to be respected in ART, irrespective of the technique or species involved.

Fertilization marks the creation of a new and unique individual. It ensures immortality by transferring genetic information from one generation to the next and, by creating variation, allows evolutionary forces to operate. In addition to delivering the paternal genome, the spermatozoon triggers the quiescent female gamete into metabolic activity, releasing the meiotic block so that early embryogenesis may be sustained. Many texts portray fertilization as a process of activation and penetration of a large cell by a small cell. On the contrary, fertilization is a highly specialized example of cell-to-cell interaction, where each gamete activates its partner. Thus, in order to trigger metabolic activation of the oocyte, the spermatozoon itself must encounter and respond to signals originating from the oocyte and its investments. Sperm–oocyte interaction is a complex multistep process that starts with the specific recognition of complementary receptors on the surfaces of the two gametes and terminates with syngamy, the union of the maternal and paternal chromosomes. The central event is fusion of the plasma membranes of the two cells. Both activation of the spermatozoon and activation of the oocyte are regulated by changes in intracellular messengers such as Ca^{2+}, H^+, cyclic adenosine monophosphate (cAMP), cyclic adenosine diphosphate ribose (cADPr) and inositol-1,4,5 trisphosphate (IP3).

Although gametes from a particular batch from any individual animal appear to be homogeneous, they are in fact an extremely heterogeneous population of cells. Physiological parameters, ranging from the number of ion channels expressed in the plasma membrane, to the amount of Ca^{2+} released into the cytosol during activation, may vary ten-fold from cell to cell. With respect to viability, it has been estimated that in the sea urchin, for example, only 2% of spermatozoa are actually capable of fertilization. While in vitro techniques have made it possible for us to study the fertilization process in many animals, animal studies have also given rise to many misleading concepts. To date, our knowledge of human gametes is scant, and we therefore must look for guidance by resorting to information from animal models. This may be feasible at the physiological level, where we should seek to identify unifying concepts, but care must be taken when extrapolating data at the molecular level.

The first phase in the sexual reproduction of animals is gametogenesis, a process of transformation whereby certain cells become the highly specialized sex cells: spermatogenesis in the male and oogenesis in the female. In both male and female, the primordial germ cells originate outside the gonad. In the mouse, primordial germ cells are first seen in the yolk sac; these are motile and invasive, and migrate through the dorsal mesentery of the hindgut to arrive at the gonadal ridges and colonize the indifferent gonad, a mass of mesoderm on the dorsal body wall. The indifferent gonad also contains elements of the regressing mesonephric kidney, which will differentiate into the rete testis in the male and the ovarian rete in the female.

When the primordial germ cells have completed their migration, they lose their motile characteristics and proliferate rapidly, dividing by mitosis to increase their number. This proliferation is followed by a period of cell growth, which is much more significant in the female gamete than in the male gamete. The key event of gametogenesis, in both sexes, is the halving of the number of chromosomes during meiosis (Figure 1.1). Meiosis is a specialized cell cycle consisting of two successive rounds of chromosome segregation following a single round of DNA replication, producing progeny cells with half as many chromosomes as their parents. Thus, in man, where the chromosome number of somatic cells is 46, each oocyte and each spermatozoon has only 23 chromosomes. However, the similarity between oogenesis and spermatogenesis ends at this point. In the male, each primary spermatocyte divides meiotically to produce four spermatids, each destined to become a functional spermatozoon; in the female, of the four cells produced from each primary oocyte, only one develops into a viable oocyte (Figure 1.2). An unequal distribution of cytoplasm at division results in the production of three small cells, the polar bodies, which eventually degenerate.

A further distinction between the two gametes is that the spermatozoon acquires the ability to fertilize the oocyte only following the completion of meiosis; in the majority of animals, the oocyte is capable of interacting with the spermatozoon before meiosis is complete. Meiosis in oocytes is arrested at various stages of the division cycle, depending upon the species, and is re-initiated as a result of fertilization (Figure 1.3). However, the sea urchin and some coelenterates are exceptions to this rule, in that their oocytes have completed meiosis before fertilization. Strictly speaking only in these two cases may the female gametes at the time of fertilization be described as 'ripe eggs'; in all other cases they should be considered as oocytes. The process whereby the oocyte attains the ability to interact with spermatozoa, described by Delage in 1901 as cytoplasmic maturation, seems to be independent of the nuclear division cycle. It should be noted, however, that, in oocytes that are normally fertilized before the completion of meiosis, the male nucleus remains quiescent in the cytoplasm until meiosis is completed.

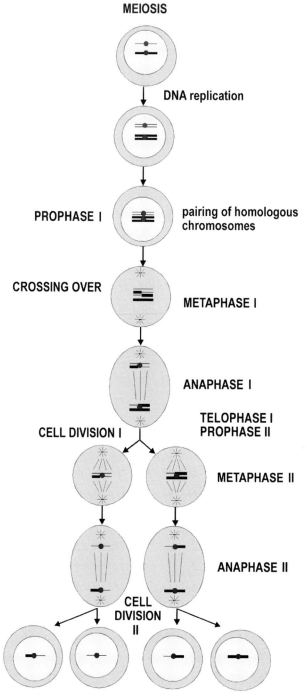

Figure 1.1   Meiosis. Four chromosomally unique haploid cells are generated from each diploid cell.

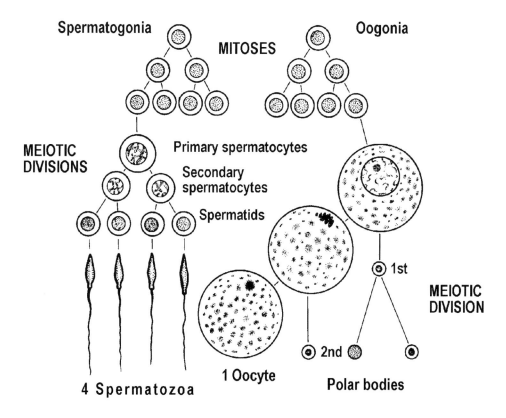

Figure 1.2   Gametogenesis in the male gives rise to four functional spermatozoa, while in the female only one of the four daughter cells becomes a functional oocyte. Modified from Dale (1983).

The volume of a spermatozoon is a mere fraction of that of the oocyte. However, spermatozoa are often extremely long cells, reaching up to 40 μm in sea urchins, 2–5 mm in some amphibia and 12 mm in some insects. There is great variation in the shape of spermatozoa, but, at the risk of oversimplifying, we may regard them morphologically and functionally to be composed of four regions:

1.   The head containing the nucleus and the acrosome
2.   The neck containing the centrioles
3.   The middle piece, containing mitochondria and
4.   The tail piece or flagellum.

Essentially the spermatozoon is a very compact cell with a few highly specializ-ed cytoplasmic structures, including the flagellum for motility, and the acros-ome, which is instrumental in sperm–oocyte binding and fusion.

Prophase of 1st division	Metaphase of 1st division	Metaphase of 2nd division	Maturation complete
Nereis (Annelid)	*Chaetopterus* (Annelid)	Amphibians	Sea urchins
Pomatoceros (Annelid)	Ascidians	Fish	Coelenterates
Spisula (Mollusc)		Mammals	

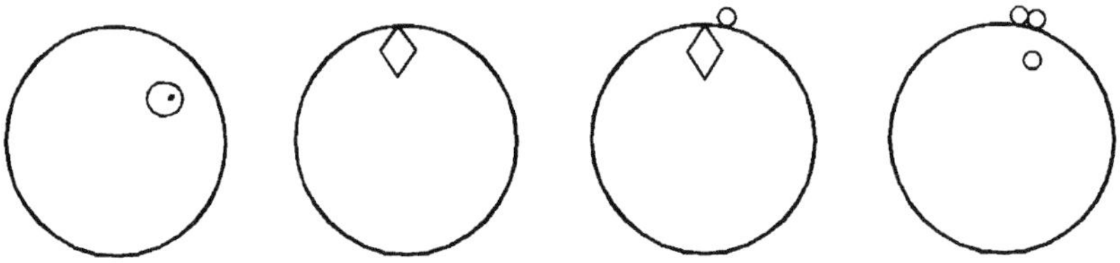

Figure 1.3   The different stages of meiotic arrest in oocytes from various species. Modified from Dale (1983).

The size of oocytes also varies widely: in marine invertebrates oocytes are about 60–150 µm in diameter, in mammals about 100 µm and in fish and amphibia about 1 mm – and we are all familiar with the dimensions of bird eggs. Despite these differences in size, some generalities about their structure are apparent.

During the growth phase of oogenesis there is an intense synthesis of RNA and, to a lesser extent, of proteins; in other words the material required to support early post-fertilization development of the embryo is formed. Typical cytoplasmic components of oocytes include yolk granules, pigment granules and mitochondria; cortical granules, a layer of membrane-bound vesicles located immediately beneath the plasma membrane, are common to many oocytes. Most oocytes are surrounded by several extracellular coats. The innermost layer is a fibrous glycoprotein sheet which plays a crucial role in sperm–oocyte interaction: this is known as the vitelline coat in echinoderms and amphibians, the chorion in ascidians and the zona pellucida in mammals. A variety of structures lie external to this: the jelly layer in sea urchins and amphibians, the follicle cells in ascidians and the cumulus oophorus (which also consists of follicle cells) in mammals. Finally, in birds and reptiles we find the tough, outer, inorganic shells, which are deposited around the oocyte after fertilization. All the extracellular components, apart from the inorganic shells, are present at fertilization, and therefore, in order to fuse with the oocyte plasma membrane, the spermatozoon has to interact with and traverse these outer layers.

Further reading

Austin, C.R. (1965) *Fertilization.* Prentice-Hall, New Jersey.

Austin, C.R. & Short, R.V. (1972) *Germ Cells and Fertilization.* Cambridge University Press, Cambridge.

Balinsky, B.I. (1965) *An Introduction to Embryology.* Saunders, London.

Bodmer, C.W. (1968) *Modern Embryology.* Holt, Rinehart and Winston, New York.

Dale, B. (1983) *Fertilization in Animals.* Edward Arnold, London.

Hirshfield, A.N. (1991) Development of follicles in the mammalian ovary. *International Review of Cytology* **234**:43–55.

Longo, F. (1987) *Fertilization.* Academic Press, New York.

Metz, C. & Monroy, A. (1985) *Biology of Fertilization.* Academic Press, New York.

Wassarman, P. (1987) The biology and chemistry of fertilization, *Science* **235**:553–60.

2

Producing gametes

Oocyte growth

The growth of oocytes usually takes place over a long period, and the increase in size is often dramatic: the frog oocyte is an extreme example of this. The young oocyte, with a diameter of less than 50 µm, grows over a period of three years to reach a final diameter of 1500 µm – this represents an increase in size by a factor of over 20 000. Mammalian oocytes are much smaller, with a time scale of weeks rather than years in their growth period. However the increase in size is also considerable. For example, the mouse oocyte grows from some 20 µm to a final diameter of 70 µm, an increase in size by a factor of 40. All oocytes are large: certainly larger than the average somatic cell, which is usually about 10 µm in diameter. The size of the full-grown oocyte depends principally on the amount of stored foodstuffs in the cytoplasm, although the nucleus also enlarges to some extent. The characteristic nucleus of the immature oocyte is called the germinal vesicle. Yolk is the major food storage product, although large quantities of lipid and glycogen granules are also found in some oocytes. The chemical composition of yolk varies from species to species according to its protein:fat ratio. In invertebrates and lower vertebrates, yolk is usually found in the form of small granules, evenly distributed throughout the cytoplasm and contributing around 20–30% of the total oocyte volume. Amphibian yolk, by contrast, contributes up to 80% of the oocyte volume and is organized into large flattened platelets. These platelets vary in size and are unequally distributed throughout the cytoplasm, the majority of the yolk lying at one pole: the vegetal pole. In teleost fish, birds and reptiles the yolk forms a compact central mass surrounded by a thin surface layer of cytoplasm with the nucleus in a thickened cytoplasmic cap at one end of the oocyte: the animal pole. Insect oocytes are similar but, in addition to the peripheral layer of cytoplasm, there is an internal mass of cytoplasm that

8

contains the nucleus. In many animals, the material stored in the oocyte during growth appears to be synthesized in parts of the body distinct from the ovary and carried to the ovary in soluble form via the blood stream. For example, in vertebrates yolk proteins and phospholipids are produced in the liver. Once inside the oocyte, the Golgi apparatus processes these soluble yolk precursors into insoluble yolk granules. During the evolution of mammalian species, the number of eggs produced has reduced, with a decrease in the amount of their stored nutrition (yolk). This may have evolved because the eggs of higher mammals develop within the reproductive tract, a protected environment that can provide a source of nutrition. The growth of human oocytes is a very slow process, taking many months to complete. The primordial oocyte undergoes a 100-fold increase in volume by the time it is mature, from 35 to 120 μm in diameter, over a period of around 85 days. The process of maturation involves the co-ordination of integrated, but independent nuclear and cytoplasmic events: the nucleus undergoes germinal vesicle breakdown, resumption of meiosis, and completion of the first meiotic division. Cytoplasmic maturation requires relocation of cytoplasmic organelles and establishment of oocyte polarity, with an increase in the number of mitochondria and ribosomes. There are alterations in membrane transport systems, and the developing Golgi apparatus expands and migrates to the periphery. Organelles appear in the cytoplasm which reflect storage and export of materials: membrane-bound vesicles, multivesicular and crystalline bodies, fat droplets and glycogen granules.

In mouse oocytes, the centrosome/microtubule complex is modified during growth. Growing oocytes show an interphase array of long microtubules, which then organize into 1–5 microtubule organizing centres (MTOC) around the nucleus. Certain classes of mRNA are selectively sequestered and processed into ribonucleoprotein particles for storage in the cytoplasm until recruited for translation by special signals generated during maturation or early development.

Follicle development

During growth and maturation, oocytes are surrounded by a layer, or layers of specialized somatic cells called follicle cells, assembled from precursor cell populations established during mammalian embryogenesis. The somatic components of the follicle (granulosa, theca, endothelial cells and supporting connective tissue) are derived from the embryonic indifferent gonad. Each primordial follicle consists of a single small oocyte surrounded by a few flattened somatic 'pregranulosa' cells, enclosed within its own complete base-ment membrane. In humans, the first primordial follicles can be seen during the fourth month of fetal gestation. As the primordial follicles are established, their pregranulosa cells enter a period of quiescence, and cell proliferation will not resume until the primordial follicle begins to grow, often months or years after it was formed. During the growth phase, the follicle develops morphologi-cally, acquiring a theca interna containing steroidogenic cells, and a theca externa of connective tissue cells forming its outer layers. The basement membrane around it must either expand or be remodelled to adjust to its increasing size, and it becomes a dynamic system that nurtures the oocyte, responding to endogenous and exogenous influences via autocrine and para-crine effects. Very small follicles have no independent blood supply, but an anastomotic network of arterioles appears just outside the basement mem-brane in medium-sized follicles. This network becomes more extensive as the follicle grows, and each ripe preovulatory follicle has its own rich blood supply. Changes in hormone levels during folliculogenesis affect the composition of the follicular fluid, which is probably the source of energy substrates for the developing oocyte. The oocyte plays a fundamental role in follicle develop-ment, and controls the differentiation of follicular granulosa cells. Granulosa cell–oocyte communication is necessary for the acquisition of oocyte develop-mental competence.

The cumulus oophorus, the mass of granulosa cells associated with the oocyte from the antral follicle stage until after fertilization, is a complex tissue unique to eutherian mammals. Cumulus cells contribute to the intrafollicular environment of the developing oocyte, and the oocyte and its surrounding cells are in close association (Figure 2.1): studies with the electron microscope reveal the presence of gap junctions between the apposing membranes. These inter-cellular junctions, common also to many somatic tissues, serve as com-municating devices through which ions and small molecules may pass. In later stages of growth, the oocyte develops numerous microvilli, possibly in order to maintain a functional surface area:volume ratio. A dense fibrillar material appears between the oocyte and its follicle cells, apparently secreted by the oocyte itself, which becomes the primary envelope – the vitelline coat, or zona pellucida in mammals (Figure 2.2). At this stage the follicle cells remain in contact with the oocyte by means of long microvilli interdigitating with the microvilli of the oocyte. Under the light microscope, this microvillous zone has the appearance of a radially striated layer and has long been known in mammals as the zona radiata. In some animals, for example echinoderms and mammals, the microvilli are withdrawn to some extent shortly before ovula-

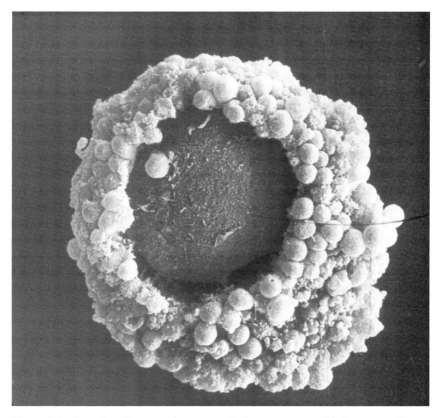

Figure 2.1   Scanning electron microscopy of a human oocyte with its surrounding corona; cumulus cells have been removed. By courtesy of Professor P.F. Kraicer, Tel Aviv University, and D. Philips, Population council, New York.

tion, resulting in a continuous vitelline coat; in others, such as bivalve molluscs, the vitelline coat remains perforated by the microvilli. The follicle cells serve to transfer materials used in oocyte growth and also provide signals to trigger the oocyte into maturation.

Cumulus cells express the ganglioside GM3 which has been implicated in cell recognition, differentiation and signalling. Blocking the gap junctions interferes with transmission or action of molecules such as 2-deoxyglucose, TGF alpha and mitogenic agents on the oocyte. In many species, denuding the oocyte of cumulus can interrupt its maturation so that it is unable to resume meiosis. Signalling between oocyte and cumulus occurs in both directions, and cumulus cells express growth factor receptors and the mRNA for a number of growth factors. They also are a source of prostaglandins, and express angiogenic factors (vascular endothelial growth factor, VEGF) which may have a role in neovascularization of follicles and angiogenesis at the implantation site

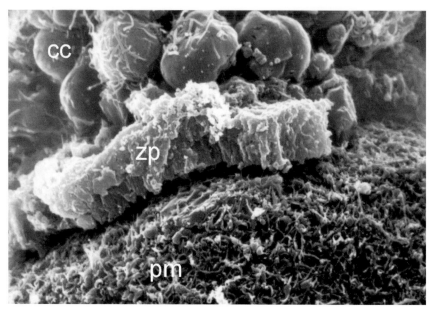

Figure 2.2   Scanning electron micrograph of the surface of an unfertilized metaphase II human oocyte, with the zona pellucida (zp) and cumulus cells (cc) partially dissected to demonstrate the microvillar organization of the plasma membrane (pm).

of the embryo. Maturation of the oocyte is associated with polarization of the cumulus cells, and secretion of a hyaluronic acid extracellular matrix. Cumulus cells express complement-binding proteins in vitro, which might help to protect the embryo from complement in tubal and uterine fluid. Their significant steroidogenic activity may contribute to local steroid levels in the luteal phase and early pregnancy.

Storing information

In order to become fully competent for further development, the oocyte must complete prematuration changes during its growth. This involves accumulation of specific RNA macromolecules which are required later in the control of embryogenesis. In animal cells, there are three main classes of RNA, designated messenger RNA (mRNA), transfer RNA (tRNA) and ribosomal RNA (rRNA); all three are involved in the synthesis of protein, and the relative amounts of the three types of RNA present varies from species to species. In the amphibian *Xenopus*, there is considerable synthesis of rRNA during oogenesis, which falls off during maturation and is then undetectable until the beginning of gastrulation. This means that the ribosomes in the oocyte are present in sufficient quantity to support protein synthesis in an embryo containing many thousands of cells. How does the oocyte manage to synthesize such a huge amount of rRNA, corresponding to the total synthesis of some 200 000 liver cells? In amphibians, this is achieved by a process called gene amplification: the rRNA genes are replicated many times over, forming several hundred copies. The germinal vesicle of the *Xenopus* oocyte contains many nucleoli; each nucleolus contains rRNA genes and is a site of rRNA synthesis. This mechanism of producing large amounts of rRNA in a relatively short period is by no means universally adopted, although gene amplification has also been detected in some invertebrate oocytes. In some insects, e.g. *Drosophila*, the nurse cells actively synthesize RNA which is then transferred to the oocyte via the cytoplasmic connections.

In the giant silk worm *Antheraea*, the DNA of the oocyte does not participate in RNA synthesis, and the nurse cells synthesize all of the RNA stored in the oocyte. This nurse cell–oocyte co-operation is certainly of great interest – but we should not forget that these two cell types are of common origin. Not all oocytes store large quantities of RNA. Mammalian oocytes contain a lesser amount of stored RNA, and new RNA is synthesized after activation of the zygotic genome during the early cleavage stages of the embryo. In the immature oocytes of some vertebrates and invertebrates, the diplotene chromosomes are extremely elongated with thin loops extending from the main axis – these are known as lampbrush chromosomes. The loops of lampbrush chromosomes are sites of intense RNA and protein synthesis and the RNA:DNA ratio is over 100 times the RNA:DNA ratio found in liver chromatin. The base content of loop RNA is not comparable to that of rRNA, but resembles DNA, suggesting that it is in fact messenger RNA. What is the significance of this large quantity of mRNA? In species such as *Xenopus* and *Drosophila*, it appears that the embryo retains the vast majority of mRNA until the blastula stage to direct protein synthesis later in development.

In mammalian oocytes, transcription increases as the follicle starts to grow; there is a dramatic increase in the size of the nucleolus as RNA accumulates in the nucleus, including a significant proportion of translatable polyadenylated mRNA. Nucleosomes contain DNA packaged within chromatin, which also contains structural proteins such as histones, and expression of particular genes at specific times involves careful regulation of transcriptional machinery. DNA methylation turns off transcription, and demethylation occurs when a gene is going to be expressed. In addition, high levels of histone acetylation correlate with gene activity, and reduced levels with gene silencing. Patterns of demethylation and acetylation are always correlated, and both are necessary for DNA transcription. It seems that the genes that undergo methylation are promoter/enhancer genes, regulating expression/transcription, rather than structural genes. The amino-terminal tails of core histones are targets for acetylation, which reduces the affinity of the histone tail for DNA. Transcription depends on the binding of sequence-specific transcription factors to the DNA, and histone acetylation causes a change in nucleosome organization which allow contact between acetylated tails and transcription factors. The nucleosome undergoes a conformational change, analogous to uncoiling a spring. Acetylation and deacetylation of core histones appears to be involved in the mechanism of signal transduction.

When the oocyte is fully grown, following germinal vesicle breakdown, transcription of new RNA stops almost completely until the time of zygotic genome activation (ZGA) when the new embryonic genome takes over. During the period prior to ZGA, the oocyte is dependent upon its pool of stored mRNA, which has been processed with elegant mechanisms that control its expression. The stability of mRNA is related to the length of its polyA tail: a long polyA tail is required for translation, but this long tail also makes the message vulnerable to degradation. It has been demonstrated that there are at least two different mechanisms of mRNA adenylation in oocyte cytoplasm – the genes are transcribed with long polyA tails, but some messengers are trancribed and translated during growth, whereas others are 'masked' by deadenylation, reducing the tail to less than 40 'A' residues to make them translationally inactive. The short polyA tail also protects these messages from degradation. In later stages of maturation, the masked genes can then be activated by selective polyadenylation when their products are required. Both gene types contain a highly conserved specific sequence in their 3' untranslatable regions (UTR) which signals polyadenylation. The mRNA for the masked transcripts also contains a further sequence 5' to the polyadenylation signal, known as the cytoplasmic polyadenylation element (CPE) or the adenylation control element (ACE). It seems that this sequence controls the expression of stored mRNAs: ACE-containing mRNAs are masked and protected from degradation, whilst non-ACE containing mRNAs, available for immediate translation have long and relatively stable polyA tails.

Another control mechanism which may be involved this complex regulation of transcription and translation during oocyte development is the packaging of the mRNAs in association with ribonucleoprotein particles. This packaging probably plays a part in controlling the access of ribosomes to regulatory elements within the mRNA.

In mammals, maternal mRNA rapidly disappears after the major activation of the genome, i.e. at the 2-cell stage in the mouse, 4–6 cell in humans, and 8-cell in sheep and cattle. However, a small amount is needed almost until the blastocyst stage, because the increase in zygotic gene expression takes place gradually. There is some evidence to suggest that stores of maternal RNA in the oocytes of older women may be depleted, perhaps due to dysfunction or disruption of the mechanisms which control its storage.

Thus the growing oocyte contains a large amount of information that is masked, but the rest of the protein synthesizing machinery is functional. This problem was approached by injecting foreign mRNA into oocytes. When rabbit haemoglobin mRNA was injected into amphibian oocytes, the oocytes synthesized rabbit haemoglobin; the more rabbit mRNA injected, the more haemoglobin was produced. The conclusion from this experiment is that the oocyte has the capacity to synthesize much more protein than it actually carries out, and that the amount of translatable mRNA is the limiting factor in protein synthesis. In addition, many proteins are synthesized during oogenesis but are set aside in the oocyte cytoplasm for use later on in development. For example, the enzymes necessary for DNA synthesis are present in the growing oocyte and yet DNA replication is switched off.

Recent experiments with interspecies nuclear transfer using nuclei from fibroblast cells transferred into bovine, sheep and monkey enucleated oocytes revealed that the first two cell division cycles were regulated by the oocyte cytoplasm; thereafter, the donor nucleus assumed regulatory control, but development arrested after a limited number of cleavage divisions. This again demonstrates that the oocyte itself has a large reserve of functional activity, sufficient to sustain initial cell division cycles, but differentiation events in both cytoplasmic and nuclear compartments are essential for continued development.

The regional organization of the oocyte: polarization

Polarization represents a differential distribution of morphological, biochemical, physiological and functional parameters in the cell. The appearance of polarization signals the triggering of the developmental programme. The growing oocyte does not have a homogeneous structure; in particular, many cytoplasmic organelles become segregated to various regions of the oocyte and this regional organization determines some of the basic properties of the embryo. In all animal oocytes, the pole where the nuclear divisions occur, resulting in the formation of the polar bodies, is called the animal pole. The opposite pole, which often contains a high concentration of nutrient reserves, is called the vegetal pole. Many cytoplasmic inclusions and organelles are distributed according to this animal–vegetal (A–V) axis: yolk is usually more dense at the vegetal pole than at the animal pole, and in some animals, particularly amphibians, there is a density gradient of pigment granules. The familiar unpigmented region of the frog oocyte is, in fact, the vegetal hemisphere. In cases where the heterogeneous organization of the cytoplasm cannot be detected, either by light or electron microscopy, it can usually be inferred from developmental studies. During the 1930s, the Swedish zoologist S. Horstadius carried out classical experiments on the sea urchin oocyte, in which one species of Mediterranean sea urchin, *Paracentrotus lividus*, was found to have a band of red pigment just below the equator towards the vegetal pole. This was the marker used to orientate the oocyte. When this oocyte was cut with a fine glass needle along the animal vegetal axis (which is the plane of the first cleavage division) the two halves rounded up forming two small cells. Both halves could be fertilized, and potentially gave rise to two normal plutei larvae. However, when the cut was equatorial, dividing the oocyte into animal and vegetal halves which were then fertilized, only the vegetal half gave rise to a complete pluteus. The animal half gave rise to a ciliated blastula-like sphere, which was incapable of gastrulation.

The conclusion from these experiments was that in the unfertilized sea urchin oocyte there is an uneven distribution of factors along the A–V axis, which are essential for normal development. But what are these factors – are they related to the regional organization of large cytoplasmic organelles, or are they freely diffusible molecules organized along an A–V gradient? Centrifugation of unfertilized oocytes yielded further information: the cytoplasmic components can be shifted by centrifugation at $3000\,g$ to form layers according to their relative densities. From the centripetal pole a lipid layer, a layer of clear cytoplasm containing the nucleus, a layer of mitochondria, then yolk and finally pigment granules are found. The plane of the cytoplasmic stratification is randomly oriented with respect to the A–V axis and yet such centrifuged oocytes always develop into normal plutei. More convincingly, by increasing the centrifugal force to $10\,000\,g$ the oocytes actually break, first into halves, then quarters. Each quarter may be fertilized and will develop into a perfect larva. It seems likely therefore that those cytoplasmic organelles that may be displaced by centrifugation do not determine the A–V polarity of the oocyte. What are the alternatives? One possibility is that the oocyte cortex, including the plasma membrane, may be the determining factor. Generally speaking the cortex is rigid and granules within it, such as the cortical granules, cannot be displaced by centrifugation. This would explain the normal development of oocytes following the dramatic displacement of cytoplasmic organelles. All oocytes have a polarized organization and the embryo maintains this A–V axis throughout development. However, the axis is not always rigidly determined as in the sea urchin. For example, the unfertilized ascidian oocyte may be cut into two halves along any plane and yet both halves when fertilized will give rise to normal larvae. This indicates that the fragments are capable of reorganizing themselves and developing a new A–V axis. How does polarity originate? Unfortunately little information is available. In the molluscs *Dentalium* and *Lymnaea*, the process seems to be epigenetic; the area of contact between the oocyte and the ovary wall becomes the vegetal pole. Finally, in addition to A–V polarity, many oocytes express a bilateral symmetry either before fertilization, as in insects, or shortly afterwards, as in ascidian oocytes.

Scanning electron microscopy shows that mouse oocytes have a microvillus-free area on the plasma membrane, adjacent to the first polar body and overlying the meiotic spindle. Human oocytes show no polarity in the distribution and length of the microvilli, either in the animal or the vegetal pole. Studies with flurorescent lectins reveal no signs of polarization in membrane sugar distribution. However, Antczak and Van Blerkom (1997) found that two regulatory proteins involved in signal transduction and transcription activation (leptin and STAT3) are polarized in mouse and human oocytes and preimplantation embryos. They suggest that a subpopulation of follicle cells may be partly responsible for the polarized distribution of these proteins in the oocyte, and that they may be involved in determining its animal pole, and in the establishment of the inner cell mass and trophoblast in the preimplantation embryo.

The intracellular location of mRNAs and protein translation machinery is related to cell cytoskeleton regulation. Several lines of evidence suggest that mammalian ooplasm redistributes after sperm entry during fertilization (Edwards & Beard, 1997).

Oogenesis in the human

The mitotic phase of germ cell proliferation in the human female terminates before birth, and by the fifth month of fetal life all oogonia have entered their first meiotic division to become primary oocytes. During the first meiotic prophase primordial follicles are formed, oocytes surrounded by mesenchymal ovarian cells. The oocytes arrest in diplotene with a characteristic large nucleus, the germinal vesicle, and can remain viable in this arrested state for up to 50 years (Figures 2.3 and 2.4). A total of about 200 000 germ cells are available

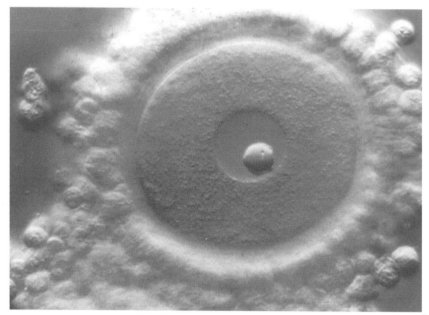

Figure 2.3   Rat oocyte at the germinal vesicle stage. By courtesy of Professor P.F. Kraicer, Tel Aviv University, and D. Philips, Population Council, New York.

for the reproductive life span at puberty, when recruitment of some of these primordial follicles begins. The recruited follicle grows from 20 μm to several hundred μm, and the oocyte itself grows from 10 μm to about 100 μm. The growth phase essentially involves synthesis and storage of large amounts of proteins, metabolic substrates, and polyadenylated mRNA. During this growth period, the surrounding granulosa cells divide mitotically, and the zona pellucida, a glycoprotein coat synthesized by the oocyte, is secreted between the oocyte and the cells. Gap junctions allow transfer of substrates and developmental information between the oocyte and the cytoplasmic projections of the accessory cells that penetrate the zona pellucida. As a follicle enters its final phase of growth, fluid-filled spaces appear between the granulosa cells – these are called pre-antral follicles, many of which will undergo atresia.

One of the most intriguing mysteries in ovarian physiology is what factors determine whether one follicle remains quiescent, another begins to develop but later becomes atretic, while still a third matures and ovulates. Over 99% of follicles are destined to die rather than ovulate; the degenerative process by which these cells are irrevocably committed to undergo cell death is termed atresia. Atretic oocytes show germinal vesicle breakdown, followed by frag-

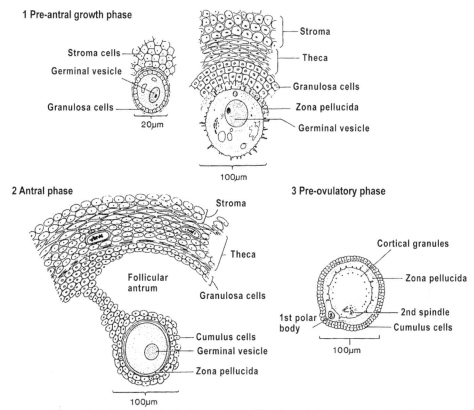

Figure 2.4 Oogenesis in the human. Modified from Johnson & Everitt (1990).

mentation and disruption of the oocyte–cumulus complex – granulosa cells from an aspirated atretic follicle show clear signs of fragmentation. Despite its critical role during the recruitment of follicles for ovulation, the mechanisms underlying the onset and progression of atresia remain poorly understood. There are four degenerative stages during ovarian development which result in a massive loss of ovarian cells:

1. During migration of primordial germ cells from the yolk sac to the genital ridge – many of these cells undergo degeneration.
2. At the time of entry into the first meiotic stage, some germ cells undergo attrition before follicles are formed.
3. In the later stages of development, early antral follicles either differentiate or undergo atresia.
4. If ovulatory signals are absent, the mature follicle also may undergo degeneration. After ovulation, the corpora lutea have a finite life span and undergo luteolysis.

Under the influence of circulating gonadotrophins, fluid spaces in pre-antral follicles coalesce into a single large antral cavity in antral (Graafian) follicles. The pre-antral phase lasts for 8–12 days in women, and during this phase the accumulated follicular fluid suspends the oocyte with its surrounding cumulus cells. The fluid appears to be formed by filtration of thecal blood through a molecular sieve which blocks some molecules of MW 250 000, and is impermeable to proteins above MW 850 000. Its composition differs considerably from plasma, with lower glucose and lipid concentrations, different amino acid concentrations, and the presence of steroid binding proteins. Follicular fluid also contains chondroitin-like material and heparan sulphate.

At the preovulatory stage, gap junctions between the cumulus cells create a compact tissue mass around the oocyte. Granulosa and theca cells of the fully mature follicle are highly differentiated, with tissue-specific functional features. Granulosa cells in a mature follicle show receptors for LH and FSH, as well as IGF-1 receptors and GnRH binding sites. They have steroidogenic enzyme systems, and synthesize a heat-shock protein (hsp90) and anti-Mullerian hormone. Theca cells of the mature follicle are the major source of androgens, and also synthesize renin, relaxin, prostaglandin and angiogenic factors. In response to the LH surge, the cumulus oophorus expands almost 40-fold, due to the accumulation of a voluminous extracellular matrix. Simultaneously, the gap junctions between cumulus cells, and between cumulus and granulosa cells disappear, with the deposition of a large, mucified extracellular matrix. This extracellular matrix results from massive *de novo* synthesis of hyaluronic acid by the cumulus cells after the LH surge.

When LH receptors appear on granulosa cells, the follicles can respond to exogenous gonadotropins and be stimulated to ovulate. Under natural conditions, the endogenous LH surge will induce final maturation within the next 24–36 hours. This surge of LH causes a rapid further accumulation of fluid in the pre-ovulatory oocyte over a period of approximately 36 hours, leading to a follicle of around 25 mm diameter (in the human) which then ovulates. Fimbria of the oviduct are thought to sweep the ovulated oocyte into the oviductal ampulla where fertilization will occur. In this final maturation stage of oogenesis, the nuclear membrane breaks down, meiosis is reinitiated and the first polar body is extruded. The female cell is now in the stage of second metaphase. Concomitantly, a process of cytoplasmic maturation is initiated, which includes a decrease in potassium conductance, a depolarization of the plasma membrane and migration of cortical granules to the surface of the oocyte.

The later phases of follicular growth prior to the LH surge (the 'follicular phase') probably represent a period of prematuration development, and oocytes are exposed to significant increases in gonadotropin, growth factor and oestrogen. The preovulatory follicle is heavily dependent on gonadotropins for its hour-to-hour survival. If deprived of hormonal support, it quickly degenerates, and its ability to ovulate in response to hCG is compromised as early as 3 hours after hormonal withdrawal in the rat – by 12 hours all follicles are incapable of ovulating.

Just before ovulation, most of the volume of the follicle consists of follicular fluid, and the cumulus oocyte complex is attached to the wall of the follicle by the stigma, which faces outwards so that the oocyte is always released rather than being trapped in the follicle. The basement membrane becomes increasingly permeable, and eventually breaks down completely. Theca cells that had previously been excluded from the follicle now begin to invade, forming tracts of 'paraluteal' cells, which grow into the follicle to form the nascent corpus luteum. Some bleeding occurs, and a small scar forms on the surface of the ovary. Steroidogenesis rapidly switches to progesterone synthesis after the LH surge.

In vitro culture of whole follicles opens up new opportunities to investigate folliculogenesis, and to unravel the regulatory mechanisms responsible for normal follicle development and ovulation. This has been successful in rodents (mouse, rat and hamster), but is more difficult in domestic species: the ovaries are fibrous and difficult to dissect, and there are resulting restrictions in nutrient, gas and waste exchange. Whereas the follicles of rats and mice grow relatively fast, and require only a short period of 14–16 days in culture, those of domestic species require a period of several months. Human primordial follicles take approximately 10 weeks to reach the antral stage. Culture systems for cow and pig follicles are at an early stage of development, and are being used to define the characteristics of pre-antral follicle growth. These preliminary studies will lay the basis for the development of more refined culture systems, which may eventually be used to produce meiotically competent oocytes. Practical application of small pre-antral follicle culture for in vitro production of mature oocytes is still far away, but it is a goal to be eventually reached.

Meiotic arrest and resumption of meiosis

Maturation is the third and final phase of oogenesis, during which several changes occur in the oocyte, preparing it for ovulation and its imminent interaction with a spermatozoon. The endpoint in vivo is the release from the follicle of a metaphase II oocyte with the potential to support normal embryonic development, and maturation involves nuclear, meiotic and cytoplasmic events, including changes in the organization of the plasma membrane as a part of cytoplasmic maturation.

Oocytes normally arrest twice during meiosis:

1. Throughout the growth period, the diffused chromosomes are surrounded by an intact nuclear membrane, the large oocyte nucleus or Germinal Vesicle, GV. The cell cycle is blocked in the G2 phase, at prophase of the first meiotic division. This first arrest in the prophase I (P-I:G2 phase) stage may be long, ranging from weeks in lower animals to decades in higher vertebrates. Reinitiation of meiosis in fully grown oocytes (after puberty in mammals) is the first indication of oocyte maturation. This represents transition from G2 to M phase, and involves condensation of interphase chromatin, breakdown of the nuclear membrane resulting in the mixture of nucleoplasm and cytoplasm, spindle formation and chromosome segregation. The semicontracted chromosomes, now in the cytoplasm, migrate to the periphery of the oocyte where they become arranged on the spindle. Mammalian oocytes complete the first meiotic division by extruding half of their chromosomes in the first polar body. In most animals, the meiotic cycle does not proceed to completion, but is arrested a second time, usually at metaphase of the first or second division (see Figure 1.3).

2. As a general scheme, hormones trigger the release from this first meiotic block, driving the oocyte to a second arrest at metaphase II (M-II) in vertebrates, or metaphase I (M-I) in many invertebrates, including ascidians, molluscs and insects. The spermatozoon triggers release from the second meiotic block.

There are exceptions to this rule: at one extreme, in some worms and molluscs, fertilization triggers release from the first meiotic block. At the other extreme, in sea urchins and coelenterates the second meiotic block is at the pronucleus stage, G1 of the first mitotic division, and the spermatozoon enters the oocyte at this late stage (see Figure 1.3). In starfish oocytes, the second meiotic block is not obvious. The hormone 1-methyladenine triggers the P-I blocked oocytes to undergo germinal vesicle breakdown and the spermatozoon usually enters the oocyte shortly thereafter, but, in any case, before metaphase I. In ascidians, fertilization drives the oocytes through the first and second meiotic divisions. In all oocytes that are normally fertilized before the completion of meiosis, the sperm nucleus remains inactive in the cytoplasm until the oocyte ejects both polar bodies.

Progression from the first to the second meiotic arrest is usually referred to as oocyte maturation, and the oocyte is now ready to be ovulated, i.e. expelled from the ovary. Shortly after ovulation, fertilization occurs; removal of the second meiotic block at fertilization is called oocyte activation.

Meiosis differs from mitosis in terms of

1. Checkpoints controls
2. DNA replication
3. Dependence on external stimuli
4. Regulation of cell cycle control proteins

Cell cycle checkpoints control the order and timing of cell cycle transition, ensuring that critical events such as DNA replication and chromosome separation are completed correctly – one process must be completed before another starts. During meiotic division, recombination must be completed before the beginning of cell division so that a correct segregation of homologous chromosomes is obtained. Several genes have been identified in yeast that are responsible for causing a meiotic block when double strand DNA breaks are not repaired. A checkpoint specific to meiotic cells ensures that anaphase I does not begin until paired chromosomes are correctly attached to the spindle. This control resembles the spindle-assembly checkpoint of mitotic cells.

J. Fulka et al. (1998) carried out a series of experiments to test DNA-responsive cell cycle checkpoints in bovine and mouse oocytes, using UV irradiation to induce DNA damage or chemical treatment to prevent chromosome condensation. Their results suggest that replication-dependent checkpoints may be either inactive or highly attenuated in fully grown mammalian oocytes; this should be borne in mind when considering the effects of endocrine or in vitro manipulations carried out during assisted reproduction cycles, or the in vitro maturation of oocytes. Although resumption of meiosis apparently has no cell cycle checkpoint, the first cell cycle does, as does each embryonic cell cycle.

Micromanipulation experiments in spermatocytes show that tension on the spindle generated by attached homologues acts as a checkpoint. If this tension is eliminated by experimental manipulation, anaphase is prevented. A major difference between the mitotic and meiotic cell cycles lies in the fact that during meiosis the oocyte can be blocked at precise phases of the cell cycle, until a specific stimulus (e.g. hormone or sperm) removes the block. In somatic cells, a state of quiescence, or cell cycle block in response to a specific physiological state of the cell is described as the G0 phase of the cell cycle. However, G0 differs from meiotic blocks in terms of cell cycle regulation and the activity of the key kinases that maintain the arrest.

Resumption of meiosis

In preantral follicles during mammalian oogenesis, the oocytes are incapable of activating the molecular machinery for completing meiosis. At the time of antrum formation, the oocyte becomes intrinsically capable of resuming maturation, but maturation arrest is maintained by the integrity of the follicle wall. Minor alterations in the architecture of the follicle wall, the cells surrounding the oocyte or the connections between the cumulus oocyte complex and the mural granulosa trigger meiosis. The preovulatory LH surge removes the inhibitory influence of the follicle wall, and replaces it with a stimulating one that reactivates meiotic progression with a complex cascade of events leading to maturation and ovulation. LH receptors are present only on the somatic cells of the follicle, not on the oolemma – and therefore the somatic cells must send a second message signal to the oocyte; a variety of messages are produced which are transmitted to the oocyte in a specific sequential order. Before the LH surge, the oocytes are 'on standby', in meiotic arrest which is maintained by the diffusion of cAMP from the cumulus to the oocyte. LH alters gap junctions, and the flux of inhibitory signals to the oocyte is interrupted. Within a few seconds, a calcium rise decreases membrane conductance to K^+ causing cumulus–corona cells to depolarize. A rapid increase in intracellular calcium is transmitted to the oocyte, diffusing from the cortical region to the centre of the cell. Calcium elevations are transient in the cumulus cells, and long lasting in the oocyte.

Two protein complexes, M-phase promoting factor (MPF) and cytostatic factor (CSF) are involved in regulating progression through meiosis. It has been hypothesised that meiotic arrest is mediated by a cAMP-dependent protein kinase substrate, which undergoes dephosphorylation when cAMP levels decrease. Although the exact substrates have not been identified, it is generally accepted that progression through the meiotic cell cycle is regulated by a series of protein kinases and phosphatases.

In the early 1970s, oocyte cytoplasmic transfer experiments led Masui and colleagues to discover that maturing amphibian oocytes produce a factor that causes them to resume meiosis. This factor was termed 'Maturation Promoting Factor', or MPF. MPF is now used to represent M-phase promoting factor, reflecting its involvement in both meiosis and mitosis. Two main components of MPF have been identified:

1. A 34kD catalytic subunit derived from the cdk family of tyrosine kinases, serine/threonine kinase p34^{cdc2} (cdk1).
2. A 45kD regulatory subunit, cyclin B2.

Both components, cdk1 and cyclin B are functionally and structurally conserved through evolution – MPF has been shown to be a universal cell cycle regulator of both mitosis and meiosis. Cyclin undergoes periodic synthesis and degradation, while the levels of cdk1 remain constant throughout the cell cycle. Association with cyclin is essential for cdk1 kinase activity, which shows a strong preference for histone H1 as substrate: MPF activity can be measured by phosphorylation of histone H1.

Cdk1 activity is regulated by phosphorylation and dephosphorylation of specific tyrosine residues, as well as by physical binding with cyclins (B- and A-types). Cyclin B is regulated by its synthesis and degradation, and possibly also by phosphorylation. MPF activity oscillates with the meiotic cycles: it is generally low in P-I oocytes, increases after GVBD, reaches a high level during M-I, and disappears transiently at the time of first polar body extrusion. Activity reappears at M-II, and remains at an elevated level until fertilization, then decreases at exit from M-II. A large amount of data concerning MPF regulation during fertilization was gathered from the amphibians *Rana* and *Xenopus*, but the same pattern of activation has been described in all vertebrates and invertebrates studied so far. Although the precise mechanisms involved are not identical in different mammalian species, MPF has been shown to be present in maturing oocytes of the pig, mouse, rabbit and cow. In ascidian oocytes, MPF activity oscillates between two maximal levels at M-I and M-II, and two very low levels, at the metaphase–anaphase transition of both meiotic divisions.

A complex sequence of events initiated by the LH surge increases MPF activity at the exit of the first meiotic block, and it may be maintained at a high level during the second meiotic block by a second factor, CSF. Cytostatic Factor (CSF) was also discovered by Masui and colleagues in 1971: cytoplasm from an unfertilized amphibian oocyte injected into a blastomere of a two-cell embryo caused metaphase arrest of the cell. Although the biological activity of CSF has been largely characterized, its biochemical components and mechanism of action remain elusive. It is generally accepted that the main components of CSF include the product of the proto-oncogene *c-mos*, mitogen associated protein kinase (MAPK), and possibly cdk2 kinase.

The *c-mos* proto-oncogene product, Mos protein, expressed in female germ cells, has a specific role in the meiotic cell cycle. Mos is a serine/threonine kinase, and, in *Xenopus* oocytes, it is required for MPF activation, increases at the time of GVBD, and remains high until M-II. In meiosis II, Mos maintains MPF at a high level of activity by preventing cyclin degradation, and subsequent inactivation of MPF seems to induce its proteolysis. However, in mouse oocytes, Mos kinase is only necessary for metaphase arrest at meiosis II before fertilization. Mos is a potent activator of the MAP kinase pathway, and MAPK may phosphorylate some of the substrates modified by the active MPF, preventing the oocyte from entering interphase between metaphase I and II. It appears to maintain chromosome condensation and is involved in reorganization of microtubules that leads to spindle formation at metaphase I, contributing to the stabilization of the spindle at metaphase II. It therefore mediates a spindle assembly checkpoint.

Studies by Cho et al. (1974) suggested that cAMP could serve as the physiological inhibitor involved in the maintenance of meiotic arrest; post-ovulatory mature oocytes contain lower levels of cAMP than follicular im-mature oocytes. Early fusion studies with *Xenopus* oocytes demonstrated that cAMP inhibits MPF activation. Once MPF has been activated, its ability to induce the transition of nuclei to metaphase is no longer sensitive to cAMP, and more recent studies suggest that cAMP regulates posttranslational modi-fication of the kinase protein in meiotic prophase. However, it has also been shown that the maturation-associated decrease in intracellular cAMP is essen-tial, but not sufficient, for reinitiation of meiosis, and an activated cAMP-dependent protein kinase (PKA) mediates the negative action of cAMP on resumption of meiosis. The biological activity of MPF seems to be that of histone H1 phosphorylation; it is postulated that a phosphorylated histone H1 alters nucleosome packing, and may contribute to chromosome condensation. In addition, further experiments with the purified kinase subunit suggest a possible role in metaphase on transcription or translation regulation, micro-filament rearrangement, reorganization of the intermediate filament network, and nuclear disassembly.

Mammalian ovulation and maturation is under the control of pituitary hormones, in particular follicle stimulating hormone (FSH) and luteinizing hormone (LH), but the situation is complex, and involves the additional interplay of ovarian hormones, oestrogen and progesterone. The preovulatory surge of LH provides the physiological trigger for resumption of meiosis; however, when oocytes are removed from follicles and placed in culture, meiotic maturation occurs in the absence of gonadotrophins. The ability to resume meiosis in vitro is not shared by all isolated oocytes, and, in assisted conception treatment cycles, the processes of nuclear and cytoplasmic matura-tion can be uncoupled by ovarian stimulation or by attempts to mature oocytes in vitro. The rate of follicular development may be accelerated by external endocrine manipulation, but this does not necessarily assure equival-ent acceleration of oocyte development/maturation, and may compromise the quality, or developmental competence, of the eggs. Oocyte competence is related to the storage of protein factors and stable mRNA, and meiotic incompetence may be related to deficiencies in the MPF subunits, or in some of the regulatory elements responsible for MPF kinase activation. Changes in microtubular morphology or activity may also play an important role in the acquisition of meiotic competence, and these may be regulated in part by MAP kinase. A failure in MAP kinase activity may, in turn, be related to a deficiency in Mos protein.

In summary, the production of a viable oocyte depends on three key processes:

1. The fully grown oocyte must recognize regulatory signals generated by follicular cells.
2. Extensive reprogramming within the oocyte must be induced – this involves activation of appropriate signal transduction mechanisms.
3. Individual molecular changes must be integrated to drive the two parallel but distinct processes involved in meiotic progression and the acquisition of developmental competence.

The oocyte depends on the follicular compartment for direct nutrient support, and for regulatory signals. After the LH surge, new steroid, peptide and protein signals are generated, and alterations to preovulatory steroid profiles can selectively disrupt protein reprogramming and individual components of the fertilization process. Localized short- and long-lived maternal mRNAs regulate the initial stages of development and differentiation in the early embryo.

There is no doubt that the process of oocyte growth and maturation is a highly complex process, involving a three-dimensional series and sequence of regulatory elements at several different molecular levels. The final evolution of a mature oocyte which has the potential for fertilization and further development is dependent upon the correct completion and synchronization of all processes involved: although an overview is emerging, many aspects still remain to be elucidated. Thus it is impossible to assess and gauge the consequences of manipulations during assisted reproduction practice, and it is essential to maintain an awareness of the complexity and sensitivity of this delicate and highly elegant biological system. Our in vitro attempts to mimic Nature will only succeed if they are carried out within this frame of reference.

Spermatogenesis in mammals

The process of spermatogenesis can be divided into three phases: proliferation, reduction division (meiosis) and differentiation. These are associated with specific germ cell types – spermatogonia, spermatocytes, and spermatids, respectively. In the male, interphase germ cells start to proliferate by mitoses at puberty. This is followed by meiosis and a gradual reorganization of cellular components, characterized by a loss of cytoplasm. In the adult mammal, it has been estimated that about 500 spermatozoa per second are produced per gram of testis. The stem cells, or A0 spermatogonia, are located in the intratubular compartment, at the base of the seminiferous epithelium. At intervals, A-1 spermatogonia emerge from this population and undergo a fixed number of mitotic divisions to form a clone of daughter cells; they produce stem cells that remain along the base, as well as cells that are committed to the formation of spermatozoa. After the final mitotic division (B spermatogonia) the primary spermatocytes move into the adluminal compartment and enter into meiosis. In this compartment, they undergo two meiotic divisions to form, first two daughter secondary spermatocytes, and eventually four early spermatids. Although spermatid nuclei contain haploid sets of chromosomes, the autosomes continue to synthesize low levels of ribosomal and messenger RNA and proteins, and they enter into a prolonged phase of terminal differentiation known as spermiogenesis. Round spermatids undergo a morphological transformation from a small round cell into an elongated structure with a condensed nucleus and a flagellum, with a species-specific shape. This differentiation process takes approximately 2 weeks in most species, and follows 16-18 well-defined stages. The spermatid DNA becomes highly condensed, and somatic histones are replaced with protamines. Cytoplasmic re-organization gives rise to the tail and the midpiece containing the mitochondria and associated control mechanisms necessary for motility, the acrosome is constructed from Golgi membranes, and a residual body casts off excess cytoplasm. Sperm modelling is probably regulated by the Sertoli cells, and the cells are moved to the centre of the tubular lumen as spermatogenesis proceeds. In man, spermatogenesis is complete in 64 days. The rate of progression of cells through spermatogenesis is constant and unaffected by external factors such as hormones (Figure 2.5). A major point of control is the timing of translation of stored mRNAs: for example, the protamine1 gene is transcribed in round spermatids, and the mRNA is stored for up to 1 week before it is translated in elongating spermatids. Other mRNAs are stored for only hours or a few days, indicating that there must be a defined temporal programme of translational control.

The seminiferous tubules form the bulk of the volume of the testis. The round tubules are separated from each other by a small amount of connective tissue that contains, in addition to blood vessels, a few lymphocytes, plasma

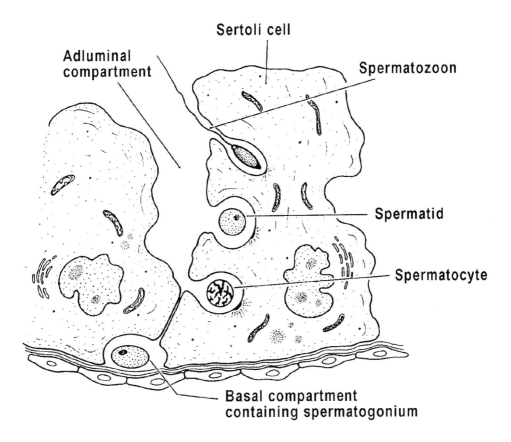

Figure 2.5   Spermatogenesis in the mammal. Maturation and modelling of the male gamete is regulated by the Sertoli cell. Modified after Johnson & Everitt (1990).

cells and clumps of interstitial Leydig cells. The tubules are lined by spermatogenic epithelium, which is made up of gametogenic cells at different stages of maturation – a cross-section of any normal seminiferous tubule reveals 4 or 5 distinct generations of germ cells. The younger generation cells are at the basement membrane, and the more differentiated cells approach the lumen of the tubule. This growth pattern has a wavelike cycle with intermingling of different stages in close approximation – any single cross-section of the tubule does not always reveal all generations of spermatogenesis. The tubules rest on a delicate anuclear basement membrane that in turn rests upon a connective tissue layer, the tunica propria. The supporting Sertoli cells, which are believed to nourish the germ cells, form a continuous layer connected by tight junctions. They are large cells with large pale nuclei, polymorphous in shape. The abundant cytoplasm extends from the periphery of the tubule to the lumen, stretching through the layers of developing germ cells. Mature spermatozoa can be seen attached to and surrounding the Sertoli cells prior to their release.

A number of different aetiologies can disrupt the orderly pattern of spermatogenesis, and immature forms, especially spermatocytes, slough into the lumina of the tubules in the presence of testicular pathology. Less frequently, maturation may proceed to the spermatid stage and be arrested there.

Mammalian spermatozoa leaving the testis are not capable of fertilizing oocytes. They gain this ability while passing down the epididymis, a process known as epididymal maturation. The spermatozoal head acquires the ability to adhere to the zona pellucida, with an increase in net negative charge. Many antigens with a demonstrable role in egg binding and fusion are synthesized in the testis as precursors, and then activated at some point in the epididymis either through direct biochemical modification, by changing their cellular localization, or both. Examples of such antigen processing include a membrane-bound hyaluronidase (PH20/2B1), fertilin, proacrosin, 1,4-galactosyl-transferase (GalTase) and putative zona ligands sp56 and p95. Changes in lectin binding ability of the sperm plasma membrane during epididymal maturation indicate alterations to the terminal saccharide residues of glycoproteins, and membrane lipids also undergo changes in their physical and chemical composition.

Although all the necessary morphological structures for flagellar activity are assembled during spermiogenesis, testicular spermatozoa are essentially motionless, even when washed and placed in a physiological solution. Sperm from the caput epididymis begin to display motility, and by the time they reach the cauda they are capable of full progressive forward motility. The ability to move is probably regulated at the level of the plasma membrane, since demembranation and exposure to ATP, cAMP and Mg^{2+} triggers movement. Transfer of a forward motility protein and carnitin from the epididymal fluid are believed to be important for the development of sperm motility. Since the osmolality and chemical composition of the epididymal fluid varies from one segment to the next, it may be that the sperm plasma membrane is altered stepwise as it progresses down the duct, and motility is controlled by the interplay between cAMP, cytosolic Ca^{2+}, and pH. During maturation, the spermatozoa use up endogenous reserves of metabolic substrates, becoming dependent on exogenous sources such as fructose; at which point they shed their cytoplasmic droplet.

In man, spermatozoa released into the seminiferous tubular lumen pass via the rete testis through the ductuli efferentia into the caput epididymis. They traverse the epididymis in 2–14 days, and are stored in the cauda, vas, seminal vesicles and ampullae prior to ejaculation.

The epididymis is divided into different regions: the caput is the upper third, formed by ductuli efferentia which are lined by pseudostratified columnar ciliated epithelium – such as is found in nasal and bronchial passages. Patients with upper epididymal obstruction often have associated nasal or respiratory problems (Young's syndrome) or mucoviscidosis. The vasa efferentia tubules unite to form the single coiled tubule of the corpus, with flatter, non-ciliated epithelium, and microvilli on the luminal surface. It starts to form a muscular wall towards the cauda, where the lumen is wider, and spermatozoa can be stored prior to ejaculation.

The process of spermatogenesis is controlled by the hypothalamic–pituitary axis, with release of gonadotropin releasing hormones. Sertoli cells respond to pituitary FSH, and secrete androgen binding proteins (ABP). Pituitary LH stimulates the interstitial cells of Leydig to produce testosterone, which combines with ABP in the seminiferous tubules, and testosterone controls LH secretion by negative feedback to the hypothalamus, maintaining the high intratesticular testosterone appropriate for normal spermatogenesis. Sertoli cells also produce inhibin, which exerts a negative feedback effect on pituitary FSH secretion. It probably also has a minor controlling influence on the secretion of LH. Injury to the seminiferous epithelium which damages Sertoli cells, and thus inhibin production, will cause serum FSH to rise, with resulting effects on spermatogenesis.

The epithelium of the tubules is very sensitive to toxins or to ischaemia. Damage may result in partial, focal or total obliteration of the spermatogenic epithelium, including the Sertoli cells, while the Leydig cells remain functionally normal. Any lesion which arrests maturation to a stage preceding spermiogenesis will result in azoospermia. A generalized maturation arrest will cause azoospermia, as will a mixture of maturation arrest and atrophy. In cases of severe injury, the tubules may be totally destroyed and become hyalinized, or may be replaced by fibrous tissue. As the whole tubule is destroyed, this disorder is associated with a much reduced testis size, with absence of Sertoli cells resulting in raised serum FSH. Lesions can be focal, resulting in oligospermia of varying severity, and patients with focal lesions may have normal levels of FSH in their serum.

Further reading

Antczak, M. & Van Blerkom, J. (1997) Oocyte influences on early development: the regulatory proteins leptin and STAT3 are polarized in mouse and human oocytes and differentially distributed within the cells of the preimplantation stage embryo. *Molecular Human Reproduction* **3**:1067–86.

Bellve, A. & O'Brien, D. (1983) In: *Mechanism and Control of Animal Fertilization*. Academic Press, New York.

Briggs, D., Miller, D., & Gosden, R. (1999) Molecular biology of female gametogensis. In: *Molecular Biology in Reproductive Medicine*. Parthenon Press, pp. 251–67.

Byskov, A.G., Andersen, C.Y., Nordholm, L., Thorgersen, H., Xia, G., Wassman, O., Andersen, J.V., Guddal, E. & Roed, T. (1995) Chemical structure of sterols that activate oocyte meiosis. *Nature* **374**:559–62.

Canipari, R., Epifano, O., Siracusa, G. & Salustri, A. (1995) Mouse oocytes inhibit plasminogen activator production by ovarian cumulus and granulosa cells. *Developmental Biology* **167**:371–8.

Cho, W.K., Stern, S. & Biggers, J.D. (1974) Inhibitory effect of dibutyryl cAMP on mouse oocyte maturation in vitro. *Journal of Experimental Zoology* **187**:383–6.

Choo, Y,K,, Chiba, K., Tai, T., Ogiso, M. & Hoshi, M. (1995) Differential distribution of gangliosides in adult rat ovary during the oestrous cycle. *Glycobiology* **5**:299–309.

Dale, B. (1996) In: (Greger, R. & Windhorst, U. eds.) '*Comprehensive Human Physiology*'. Springer Verlag.

Dekel, N. (1996) Protein phosphorylation/dephosphorylation in the meiotic cell cycle of mammalian oocytes. *Reviews of Reproduction* **1**:82–8.

Edwards, R.G. & Beard, H. (1997) Oocyte polarity and cell determination in early mammalian embryos. *Molecular Human Reproduction* **3**:868–905.

Elder, K. & Elliott, T. (eds.) (1998) The use of epidydimal and testicular sperm in IVF. *Worldwide Conferences in Reproductive Biology* **2**, Ladybrook Publications, Australia

Fulka, J. Jr, First, N. & Moor, R.M. (1998) Nuclear and cytoplasmic determinants involved in the regulation of mammalian oocyte maturation. *Molecular Human Reproduction* **4(1)**:41–9.

Gosden, T.G., Boland, N.I., Spears, N., Murray, A.A., Chapman, M.,Wade, J.C., Zhody, N. & Brown, N. (1993) The biology and technology of follicular oocyte development in vitro. *Reproductive Medicine Reviews* **2**:129–52.

Gregory, L. & Leese, H.J. (1996) *Journal of the British Fertility Society* **1(2)** *Human Reproduction* **11**, Natl Suppl.:96–102.

Gurdon, J.B. (1967) On the origin and persistence of a cytoplasmic state inducing nuclear DNA synthesis in frog's eggs *Proceedings of the National Academy of Science of, USA* **58**, 545–52.

Hess, R.A. (1999) Spermatogenesis, overview. *Encyclopedia of Reproduction* vol. 4, pp. 539–45. Academic Press, New York.

Johnson, M. & Everitt, B. (1990) *Essential Reproduction*. Blackwell Scientific Publications, Oxford.

Jones, R. (1998) Spermiogenesis and sperm maturation in relation to development of fertilizing capacity. In: (A. Lauria et al., eds.), *Gametes: Development and Function*. Serono Symposia, Rome, pp. 205–18.

Masui, Y. (1985) In: (Metz C.B. & Monroy, A. eds.), *Biology of Fertilization*. Academic Press, pp. 189–219.

Moore, H.D.M. (1996) The influence of the epididymis on human and animal sperm maturation and storage. *Human Reproduction* **11**, Natl, Suppl.:103–10.

Nurse, P. (1990) Universal control mechanisms resulting in the onset of M-phase. *Nature* **344**:503–8.

Sagata, N. (1996) Meiotic metaphase arrest in animal oocytes: its mechanisms and biological significance.*Trends in Cell Biology* **6**:22–8.

Spears, N., Boland, N.I., Murray, A.A. & Gosden, R.G. (1994) Mouse oocytes derived from in vitro grown primary ovarian follicles are fertile. *Human Reproduction* **9**:527–32.

Sutovsky, P., Flechon, J.E., Flechon, B., Motlik, J., Peynot, N., Chesne, P., & Heyman, Y. (1993) Dynamic changes of gap junctions and cytoskeleton in in vitro culture of cattle oocyte cumulus complexes. *Biology of Reproductions* **49**:1277–87.

Taylor, C.T. & Johnson, P.M. (1996) Complement-binding proteins are strongly expressed by human preimplantation blastocysts and cumulus cells as well as gametes. *Molecular Human Reproduction* **2**:52–9.

Telfer, E.E. (1996) The development of methods for isolation and culture of preantral follicles from bovine and porcine ovaries. *Theriogenology* **45**:101–10.

Van Blerkom, J. & Motta, P. (1979) *The Cellular basis of Mammalian Reproduction.* Urban and Schwarzenberg.

Yanagamachi, R. (1994) Mammalian Fertilization. In: (E. Knobil & J. Neill eds.), *The Physiology of Reproduction* New York, Raven Press, pp. 189–317.

3

Sperm–oocyte interaction

The acrosome and the vitelline coat

In Nature, fertilization is a complex process of cell–cell interaction which starts with the specific recognition and binding of spermatozoa to oocytes and ultimately leads to the fusion of the male and female pronuclei. The initial stages of fertilization depend principally on two structures: the acrosome of the spermatozoon (Figure 3.1) and the vitelline coat or zona pellucida of the oocyte. For convenience, we may consider three major events in sperm–oocyte interaction:

1. Attachment of the spermatozoon to the vitelline coat (zona pellucida).
2. The spermatozoon undergoes the acrosome reaction, as a result of which digestive enzymes are released and the inner acrosomal membrane is exposed.
3. This highly fusogenic sperm membrane makes contact with the oocyte plasma membrane and the two membranes fuse together.

The vitelline coat is composed of protein and carbohydrates in the form of glycoprotein units which are probably stabilized by disulphide bonds. The principal carbohydrate appears to be fucose and the glycoprotein units are synthesized by the oocyte itself. The form of the vitelline coat varies greatly from species to species. For example, in the sea urchin the vitelline coat is very thin and adheres tightly to the oocyte surface following the contours of the surface microvilli, whereas in the starfish it is much thicker and is perforated by the microvilli. The situation in mammals and ascidians is quite different: the vitelline coat is extremely thick and, in fact, it may be removed manually using fine steel needles. In the ascidians, the vitelline coat is actually separated from the oocyte surface by a layer of cells called test cells. How does the spermatozoon attach to the vitelline coat and what is the molecular basis for this interaction? There are complementary molecules on the surface of the spermatozoal head and on the vitelline coat. Plant lectins such as concanavalin A

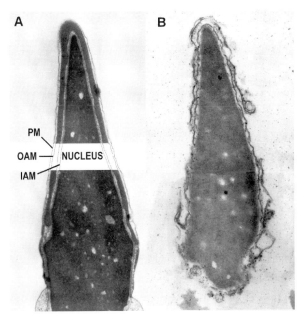

Figure 3.1   Transmission electron microscope (TEM) section through a human spermatozoon showing the plasma membrane (pm) and outer (oam) and inner (iam) acrosomal membranes. To the right is a TEM of a human spermatozoon after exposure to the calcium ionophore A23187 has triggered the acrosome reaction.

and fucose binding protein, which are proteins that bind specifically to certain carbohydrates, bind both to the surface of the egg and to the head of the spermatozoon in ascidians. Fucose is an important molecule in the process of gamete binding, as evidenced by the fact that addition of this sugar to a mixture of spermatozoa and oocytes inhibits fertilization – i.e., fucose competitively inhibits sperm–oocyte interaction. Whatever the nature of the complementary structures, binding of the spermatozoon to the vitelline coat induces the acrosome reaction.

Turning now to the spermatozoon, consider the structure of the apically situated acrosome. Although again there is considerable variation between species, the acrosome of *Saccoglossus*, a hemichordate, is considered to be relatively typical. The membrane bound acrosomal granule, which contains lytic agents such as proteases, sulphatases and glycosidases is bound within the plasma membrane of the spermatozoon. When the spermatozoon attaches to the vitelline coat, the permeability of the sperm plasma membrane is altered causing a transient change in the concentration of several intracellular ions, as a result of which the acrosome reaction is triggered. Using *Saccoglossus* as an example, four stages in the reaction may be considered:

1. The acrosome membrane fuses with the sperm plasma membrane at the tip of the acrosome.
2. The acrosomal granule breaks down releasing lysins. These enzymes either 'dissolve' a pathway through the vitelline coat or alter it in such a way as to allow the penetration of the acrosomal tubule.
3. This tubule is formed by the extension of the inner acrosomal membrane, by polymerization of actin or actin-like fibres located in the subacrosomal region.
4. When the tip of the acrosomal tubule contacts the oocyte plasma membrane, the two membranes fuse.

In some animals, an insoluble protein component of the acrosomal granule known as 'bindin' remains attached to the extended tubule during growth and is thought to be involved in the 'adhesion' of gametes. It is technically difficult to study the time sequence of these events, but the first two are thought to occur within 1 second, whilst completion of the reaction (i.e. up to fusion of the two gametes) may take 7–9 seconds (e.g. in the annelid *Hydroides* and the hemichordate *Saccoglossus*).

Cytological investigations have revealed that the acrosome is of Golgi origin. The Golgi body in an early spermatid consists of a series of concentrically arranged membranes around an aggregation of small vesicles. One of the vesicles increases in size and fills with particulate material, and vesicle growth may come about as the result of fusion of several smaller vesicles. When the vesicle containing the future acrosomal granule reaches a certain size, it migrates towards the nucleus. Shortly afterwards, the nucleus starts to elongate, the vesicle loses much of its fluid content and the vesicle membrane wraps around the front of the nucleus forming the typical acrosome. This generalized picture of sperm–oocyte interaction, where the spermatozoon attaches to the vitelline coat with its acrosome intact and an acrosomal tubule is produced as part of the process, is not universal. In starfish and sea cucumbers, the acrosome reaction occurs when the spermatozoon contacts the outer surface of the jelly layer. Here the acrosomal tubule is extremely long, reaching 20 µm in the starfish, and extends across the width of the jelly layer to make contact with the oocyte surface. In sea urchins, where the acrosome reaction occurs upon contact with the vitelline coat, the acrosomal tubule is very short, usually less than 1 µm – not surprising, considering the close apposition of the vitelline coat and the plasma membrane in these oocytes. In mammals and ascidians, the vitelline coat is very thick and, in the latter case, distant from the oocyte surface. Here the acrosome reaction also occurs upon contact of the spermatozoon with the vitelline coat, but an acrosomal tubule is not formed as part of the process. Finally, in bony fish, where the oocyte is covered by a thick chorion and the spermatozoon makes contact with the oocyte surface by way of a micropyle, the spermatozoon lacks an acrosome.

Sperm–oocyte fusion

Although the oocyte is an extremely large cell, it is by no means freely accessible to the spermatozoon. The extracellular coats, and, in some cases, the heterogenous organization of the oocyte itself, limit the number of spermatozoa which are able to reach the oocyte surface. Before interacting with the vitelline coat the spermatozoa must traverse and interact with the outer oocyte investments, which in sea urchins, ascidians and mammals are the jelly layer, the follicle cells and the cumulus cells respectively (Figure 3.2). All of these layers drastically reduce the number of spermatozoa which reach the underlying vitelline coat. In the sea urchin, the jelly layer itself, which is tough and compact after spawning, apparently induces a premature acrosome reaction and thereby reduces the number of viable sperm which reach the vitelline coat by up to 90%. In ascidians, spermatozoa can only react with restricted areas of the vitelline coat which are not covered by the follicle cells. Having traversed the outer investments, the spermatozoa must bind to and then penetrate the vitelline coat. It appears that not all of the bound sperm are able to do this, and many are not triggered into an acrosome reaction. This may be due to the heterogeneity of the glycoproteins in the vitelline coat. It is well accepted that the integral glycoproteins of cell membranes display a certain degree of micro-heterogeneity due to differential glycosylation, i.e. the sugar side chains of these molecules vary slightly. In order for sperm to attach to the vitelline coat, a specific molecular fit may be required to induce the acrosome reaction.

An additional factor limiting sperm-oocyte fusion is the organization of the oocyte plasma membrane. In some oocytes, sperm fusion is restricted to a limited area of the oocyte surface. In ascidians, this occurs in a region of about 30 degrees at the vegetal pole, and can be demonstrated in live oocytes deprived of their vitelline coat. In amphibians, the site of spermatozoal entry is restricted to the animal hemisphere. The most striking case is that of *Discoglossus* in which the site of interaction is limited to a small dimple at the animal pole. The fine structural organization of these sites is different from that of the rest of the egg surface. In *Xenopus* and *Rana* spermatozoa can be 'forced' to

(a)

(b)

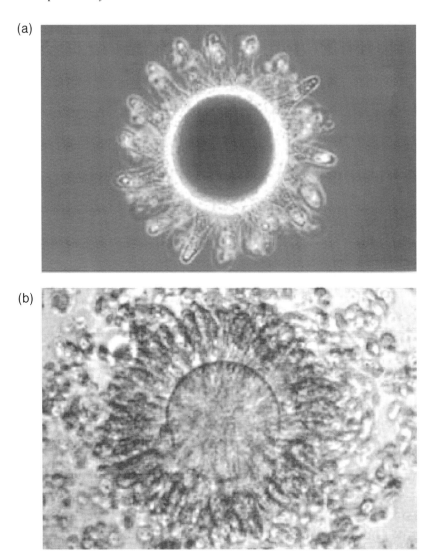

Figure 3.2   (a) Metaphase I oocyte of the ascidian *Ciona intestinalis* with its
surrounding chorion and star-shaped follicle cells. (b) Metaphase II human oocyte
with its corona–cumulus complex.

penetrate the vegetal pole, although such sperm are unable to develop into
pronuclei. The restriction in area available for sperm penetration is, of course,
most obvious in the case of oocytes with micropyles (i.e. fish, insects, squid).
The diameter of the micropyle is usually the same as the head of the spermatozoon and, as mentioned previously, the spermatozoa lack an acrosome. In
trout and other salmonids, when a spermatozoon reaches the oocyte plasma

membrane the cortical alveoli begin to open and their contents form a plug in the micropyle. Thus only one spermatozoon is allowed to reach the oocyte surface.

In the course of evolution, it seems that no method has been devised which allows the union of one spermatozoon with one oocyte without great wastage of spermatozoa. In most animals, spermatozoa are produced in huge excess, irrespective of whether fertilization occurs externally in the sea or internally in the female tract. In man, the sperm–oocyte ratio can be as high as 10^9:1 and in the sea urchin 10^4:1. Despite these high ratios, behavioural adaptations are also necessary to ensure fertilization: in the case of echinoderms and some polychaetes, this takes the form of aggregation of mature animals and the simultaneous spawning of the sexes. In mammals, spermatozoa are deposited in the female tract, with a synchrony of mating. In aquatic animals, dilution of gametes in the surrounding medium and loss to predators greatly reduces the probability of fertilization. In mammals, of the millions of spermatozoa ejaculated only a few reach the site of fertilization, which in most species is the ampulla of the fallopian tube. In a study of fertilization in the mouse in vivo a 1:1 sperm–oocyte ratio was discovered in the ampullae – supernumerary spermatozoa were never observed.

In other animals, notably insects and nematodes, sperm utilization is much more efficient. In *Drosophila*, there is a 1:1 relationship between the progeny recovered and the number of spermatozoa counted in the seminal receptacles. In hermaphrodite fertilization of the nematode *Caenorhabditis elegans*, every spermatozoon fertilizes an oocyte – however, in this case not all oocytes are fertilized because the oocytes are produced in excess. The high efficiency of sperm utilization in insects and nematodes with internal fertilization may be an important adaptation as it enables volume to be minimized, and allows provision of nutrients for the stored spermatozoa. It seems, therefore, that in most animals, although great quantities of spermatozoa are produced, very few reach the oocyte. Those that do then encounter the problem of penetrating the extracellular coats and fusing with the oocyte plasma membrane. Polyspermy, a lethal condition where several spermatozoa enter the oocyte, is probably rare in nature.

Activation of the spermatozoon

The majority of reports on sperm–oocyte interaction emphasize the activation of the oocyte by the spermatozoon; however, prior activation of the spermatozoon is a prerequisite for successful fertilization. Activation of the male gamete involves several behavioural, physiological and structural changes, some of which are induced at shedding by exposure to environmental signals, and others are induced whilst the spermatozoon is interacting with the oocyte and its extracellular investments. All of these changes are essential for successful fertilization, including changes in motility, capacitation, acrosome reaction, penetration, binding and fusion.

Motility

Spermatozoa are maintained in the testis in a quiescent state. Many factors may be responsible for this metabolic suppression, such as physical restraint, low pH and low oxygen tension of the seminal fluid. In most marine invertebrates, shedding of the spermatozoa into the sea induces motility, presumably by the reversal of the restraining conditions of the testes. Once released they are fervently active, and if they do not encounter an oocyte they rapidly deplete their energy supply and die. Their lifespan depends on their activity; generally speaking the less active they are the longer they live. In teleost fish, motility is also induced when the spermatozoa are shed into the aquatic environment; the triggering factor here is the tonicity of the new environment. In fresh-water fish, the external medium is hypotonic with respect to the seminal plasma whereas in marine fish it is hypertonic; therefore in the former species a hypotonic shock induces motility, and in the latter species a hypertonic shock is responsible. In salmonid fish, the seminal plasma has a high K^+ content of about 80 mM which suppresses motility; when spermatozoa are shed, the K^+ is diluted and sperm start to move about vigorously.

Chemotaxis

Once motile, the spermatozoon must encounter an oocyte before its energy reserves are depleted. Many mechanisms have evolved to facilitate gamete encounter, including the synchronization of gamete production and release, copulatory devices and the production of chemical attractants by the ovary or oocytes. The phenomenon of chemotaxis in fertilization (the oriented movement of spermatozoa in a chemical gradient), although an intuitively attractive mechanism, has only been demonstrated in a few animals, for example cnidarians and tunicates. For example, the spermatozoa of the hydrozoan *Campanularia* orientate and swim towards the female gonangium, or alternatively follow a gradient of female gonangial extract. In the siphonophoran *Muggiaea*, the chemical attractant is produced by an extracellular structure of the oocyte

called the cupule. In both cases, the nature of the chemo-attractants is unknown, although they appear to be low molecular weight proteins. In all other
cases, the encounter of gametes apparently occurs randomly. Rothschild and
Swann in the early 1950s calculated the theoretical collision rate of sea urchin
oocytes and spermatozoa by treating the fertilization reaction as a first-order
chemical reaction. That is, they estimated the probability of a sperm–oocyte
collision using parameters such as sperm density, speed of the spermatozoon
and oocyte radius. The actual successful collision rate at a particular density
may be determined by kinetic experiments. This method involves dropping
oocytes into a freshly prepared suspension of spermatozoa and then taking
aliquots at fixed time intervals, i.e. 5 s, 10 s, 30 s, 60 s, etc. A small amount of
detergent, such as sodium lauryl sulphate, is added to each aliquot to immediately stop the 'fertilization reaction'. Effectively all oocytes which have already
interacted with a spermatozoon continue to develop, while the fertilizing
capacity of all remaining free spermatozoa is abolished.

Capacitation

Although sperm–oocyte interaction in most species, particularly those practis-
ing external fertilization, appears to be a random event, spermatozoa from
many animals exhibit behavioural changes when they contact the oocyte
surface or female tissues. These behavioural changes, which have been termed
capacitation, are essential for successful fertilization. In amphibians, spermatozoa attain the ability to fertilize following exposure to the jelly layers surrounding the oocyte, which are a product of the female reproductive tract. The frog
Discoglossus provides an interesting example: ejaculated spermatozoa of this
anuran are immotile and organized into bundles. Upon contact with the
outermost jelly layer of the oocyte, individual spermatozoa start moving,
escape from the bundle and penetrate the gelatinous animal plug. Sperm
motility in some teleost fish also seems to be enhanced when they contact the
surface of the chorion, while sperm of the hydroid *Campanularia* must interact
with a surface component of the gonangium epithelial cells before attaining
fertilizability.

    Capacitation of mammalian spermatozoa, which takes place in the female
genital tract, is more fully understood. The time required for capacitation
varies from species to species and ranges from less than 1 hour in the mouse to
6 hours in the human (Table 3.1). Two changes seem to occur: first the
epididymal and seminal plasma proteins coating the spermatozoa are removed, followed by an alteration in the glycoproteins of the sperm plasma

Table 3.1. *Survival parameters of mammalian gametes in vivo.*

	Time required for capacitation (h)	Duration of sperm Motility (h)	Fertility (h)	Fertilizable life of oocytes (h)
Mouse	< 1	13	6	15
Sheep	1–5	48	30–48	12–15
Rat	2–3	17	14	12
Hamster	2–4	—	—	9–12
Pig	3–6	50	24–48	10
Rabbit	5	43–50	28–36	6–8
Rhesus monkey	5–6	—	—	23
Man	5–6	48–60	24–48	6–24
Dog	—	268	134	24

From Gwatkin (1974).

membranes. Capacitation may take place within the uterus or oviducts, or in vitro by contact with the cumulus oophorus. In the latter case, the spermatozoa become intimately attached to the cumulus cells for 2–3 hours, during which time these cells, by secreting glycosidases, alter the sperm surface components. Follicular fluid can also promote capacitation in vitro. A low molecular weight motility factor found in follicular fluid, ovary, uterus and oviduct may increase sperm metabolism (and hence motility) by lowering ATP and increasing cyclic AMP levels within the sperm. Table 3.1 demonstrates the duration of fertility and motility of mammalian spermatozoa within the oviduct, together with the fertilizable life of oocytes.

Acrosome reaction

The acrosome reaction is the final prerequisite step in the activation of the spermatozoon before gamete fusion is possible. First, there is an absolute Ca^{2+} requirement – the acrosome reaction only occurs in the presence of Ca^{2+}. The reaction may also be induced artificially by adding the ionophore A23187, a chemical which carries Ca^{2+} across cell membranes (Figure 3.1), to the sperm medium, or simply by increasing the environmental concentration of Ca^{2+}. An artificially high pH of about 9–9.5 will also induce this reaction, and it is also well known that invertebrate spermatozoa release H^+ when activated. Finally, the polymerization of subacrosomal actin which causes the extension of the acrosomal tubule depends on the influx of cations, particularly Mg^{2+} and K^+. Although the minute size of the male gamete hinders experimentation, it

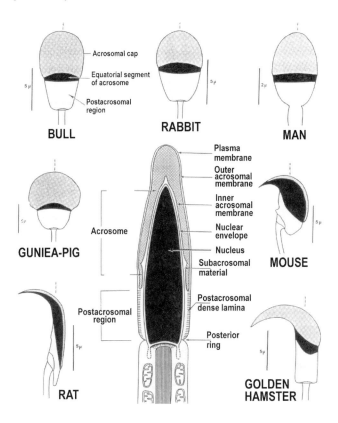

Figure 3.3   Variation in shape of mammalian spermatozoa with, at the centre, a schematic representation showing the layout of the several membranes. Modified from Yanagimachi (1994).

appears that the physiological events leading to the acrosome reaction parallel those leading to activation of the oocyte. These include changes in the ion permeability of the plasma membrane, alterations in the intracellular level of free Ca^+ and an alkalinization of the cytoplasm. The influx of calcium triggers the fusion of the acrosomal membranes and the exocytosis of the acrosomal contents.

Sperm–oocyte interaction in mammals

In mammals, fertilization is internal and the male gametes must be introduced into the female tract at coitus. Coitus itself ranges from minutes in man to hours in camels, but is accompanied by many physiological changes. Penile erection in man may be elicited by tactile and psychogenic stimuli such as visual cues. A decrease in resistance and consequently dilatation in the arteries supplying the penis with closure of the arterio-venous shunts and venous bleed valves causes erection. The testes may increase their volume by as much as 50% owing to vasocongestion. Ejaculation of semen is achieved by contraction of the smooth muscles of the urethra and the striated muscles in the penis. Muscle contraction is sequential and results in the mixing of the prostatic liquid rich in acid phosphatase, the vas deferens fraction containing spermatozoa, and the seminal vesicle fraction containing fructose.

In the woman, tactile stimulation of the glans clitoris and vaginal wall leads to engorgement of the vagina and labia majora and an increase in vaginal dimension. At orgasm, frequent vaginal contractions occur, and uterine contractions begin in the fundus and spread to the lower uterine segment. In man, rabbit, sheep, cow and cat, the semen is ejaculated into the vagina. In the pig, dog and horse, it is deposited directly into the cervix and uterus. In many species, the semen coagulates rapidly after deposition in the female tract, as a result of interaction with an enzyme of prostatic origin. The coagulation may serve to retain spermatozoa in the vagina or to protect them from the acid environment. In the human, this coagulation is dissolved within one hour by progressive action of a second proenzyme, also of prostatic origin. Within minutes of mating, spermatozoa may be detected in the cervix or uterus. In the human, 99% of the spermatozoa are lost from the vagina. The few that enter the tract may survive for many hours in the cervical crypts of mucus. In the absence of progesterone, cervical mucus permits sperm penetration into the upper female tract. Although data are inconclusive, it appears that activity of the musculature of the female tract is not required for sperm transport. Prostaglandins present in the semen are not required for sperm transport, since these are removed in artificial insemination. It is probable that the spermatozoa move through the uterus under their own propulsion and are transported in currents set up by the action of uterine cilia. The cervical crypts may serve as a reservoir regulating flow of spermatozoa into the tract, while the utero–tubal junction may act as a sphincter. The earliest appearance of spermatozoa in the oviducts is 4–7 hours in hamster and rabbit. Few sperm reach the ampullae and, in the mouse, sperm–oocyte ratios in the ampullae are usually 1:1.

Capacitation in mammals

Before gaining the ability to fertilize oocytes, ejaculated mammalian spermatozoa must reside a minimum period in the female reproductive tract. This relatively undefined process, called capacitation, is thought to involve the removal of glycoproteins from the sperm surface exposing receptor sites that can respond to oocyte signals and lead to the acrosome reaction. Since epididymal maturation and capacitation are unique to mammals, this may represent an evolutionary adaptation to internal fertilization. In the human, capacitation probably starts while the spermatozoa are passing through the cervix. Many enzymes and factors from the female tract have been implicated in causing capacitation, such as arylsulphatase, fucosidase and taurine; however, to date the precise mechanism remains unknown. Certainly, the factors are not species specific, and capacitation may be induced in vitro in the absence of female signals. Capacitation is temperature-dependent and only occurs at 37 to 39 °C. Sperm surface components are removed or altered during capacitation. For example, an antigen on the plasma membrane of the mouse spermatozoon, laid down during epididymal maturation, cannot be removed by repeated washing, but disappears, or is masked during capacitation.

Acrosome reaction

The acrosome is a membrane-bound cap covering the anterior portion of the sperm head, and is found in the majority of species (Figure 3.3). This structure, or its surrounding membranes, contains a large array of hydrolytic enzymes including hyaluronidase, acrosin, proacrosin, phosphatase, arylsuphatase, collagenase, phospholipase C and β-galactosidase, to mention a few. The acrosome reaction involves fusion of the outer acrosomal membrane with the overlying plasma membrane allowing the acrosomal contents to be released. In the human, fusion appears to take place initially near the border of the acrosomal cap region and the equatorial segment of the acrosome. The acrosome reaction is relatively rapid once the correct trigger signals have been received and may take from 2 to 15 minutes in vitro. Gametes collected from the ampullae of mammals after mating show that, while free-swimming spermatozoa have unreacted acrosomes, those within the cumulus mass have either reacted acrosomes, or are in the process of reacting. The majority of spermatozoa attached to the surface of the zona pellucida surface have reacted acrosomes. One of the glycoproteins of the mouse zona pellucida, ZP3, binds to the plasma membrane over the acrosomal cap and induces the acrosome reaction.

It is not clear whether the acrosome reaction is initiated whilst the spermatozoon is interacting with the cumulus mass. However, since a major component of the cumulus matrix is hyaluronic acid, and the acrosome contains hyaluronidase, it is feasible to suggest that the reaction may start in the cumulus.

Progesterone trapped in the cumulus mass may prime the sperm cell to respond to ZP3, and progesterone signals appear to be transduced by protein tyrosine kinase. The acrosome reaction may also be induced in vitro in the absence of any maternal signal. In mammalian spermatozoa, ZP3 may be considered a regulatory ligand which triggers the acrosome reaction. G-proteins are found in the plasma membrane and outer acrosomal membranes.

Although we are far from understanding the sequence of events leading to exocytosis, potential second messenger pathways involved include:

Changes in intracellular calcium
Activation of cAMP and phosphokinase A pathways
Phospholipase C generating InsP3 and diacylglycerol (DAG)
Phospholipase D generating phosphatidic acid
Activation of phospholipase A_2 generating arachidonic acid.

Completion of the acrosome reaction does not necessarily ensure the success of in vitro fertilization. In a population of spermatozoa surrounding the cumulus mass, we may expect enormous variability. Some will acrosome react too soon, others too late: in some the trigger stimulus will be inadequate, perhaps in others the transduction mechanism will fail at some point. The cumulus mass is composed of both cellular and acellular components. The acellular matrix is made up of proteins and carboyhydrates, including hyaluronic acid. In vivo, very few spermatozoa reach the site of fertilization: therefore the idea derived from in vitro fertilization studies, that large populations of spermatozoa surrounding the oocyte mass dissolve the cumulus matrix, is probably incorrect in vivo. Fertilization occurs before the dispersion of the cumulus mass, and in vivo the sperm:oocyte ratio is close to 1:1.

Sperm–oocyte fusion

The zona pellucida, a glycoprotein sheet several microns thick secreted by the growing oocyte, has a chemical composition which consists of 70% protein, 20% hexose, 3% sialic acid and 2% sulphate. Electron microscopy shows the outer surface to have a latticed appearance. There are three major glycoproteins known as ZPl, ZP2 and ZP3, whose distribution in the human zona remains unknown at present. In the mouse, ZP2 is distributed throughout the thickness of the zona. Spermatozoa penetrate the zona in 2–15 minutes, and sperm binding to the mouse zona is mediated by the ZP3 glycoprotein. The exact nature of the complementary receptor molecule on the surface of the spermatozoon is not known, and may be either protein or glycoprotein. In the

(a)

(b)

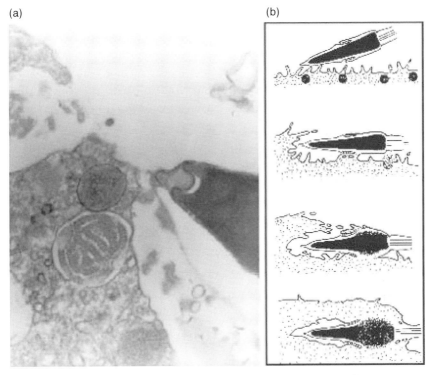

Figure 3.4   (a) Transmission electron micrograph showing the point of
sperm–oocyte fusion in the sea urchin. Sperm factor must flow through this
cytoplasmic bridge of 0.1 μm diameter. The large granule (1 μm) below the
spermatozoon is a cortical granule. (b) Stages in sperm–oocyte fusion in the
mammal. Modified from Yanagimachi (1994).

mouse, the sperm receptors appear to be on the surface of the plasma membrane of the acrosome intact spermatozoon. Receptors for ZP2, in contrast,
are located on the inner acrosomal membrane and therefore are unmasked
after the acrosome reaction. According to Wassarman and colleagues, sperm-
receptor activity resides in the O-linked oligosaccharides of ZP3. The complementary molecule of the spermatozoon may be a lectin-like protein.

It has been suggested, both in invertebrates and in mammals, that sperm
binding to its receptor on the zona is an enzyme–substrate interaction. During
penetration of the zona, the spermatozoon loses its acrosomal contents and
only the inner acrosomal membrane is in direct contact with the zona. While
passing through the zona the spermatozoon beats its tail strongly leaving a
sharp pathway behind. In eutherian mammals, the sperm-head plasma membrane of the postacrosomal region apparently fuses with the oocyte plasma
membrane (Figure 3.4). However, this region of the plasma membrane only

attains fusibility after the acrosome reaction. The surface of most oocytes, including the human, is organized into evenly spaced short microvilli. In mouse and hamster, the area overlying the metaphase spindle is microvillus-free and spermatozoa are not able to, or are less likely to, fuse with this area. The human oocyte is an exception, having no obvious surface polarity, with microvilli present over the entire surface from the animal pole to the vegetal pole.

Following gamete fusion, the sperm plasma membrane remains in the oocyte plasma membrane and indicates the point of fusion. In the rat, a fluorescently labelled conjugated antibody to a sperm plasma membrane antigen shows that immediately after fusion the sperm plasma membrane remains localized to the point of entry and, by the pronucleate stage, the antigen spreads all over the surface of the zygote. Sperm motility, although necessary for penetration of the zona, is not required for gamete fusion. Fusion is temperature, pH and Ca^{2+} dependent. Since fusion of spermatozoa to nude oocytes is not inhibited in the presence of monosaccharides or lectins, it seems that the terminal saccharides of glycoproteins are not directly involved in the process. Fusion of artificial membranes in apposition made of pure phospholipids has been observed experimentally, but in biological systems it appears to be mediated or facilitated by membrane associated proteins. In the guinea-pig, fusion is regulated by an integral membrane protein on the posterior portion of the sperm head composed of two distinct subunits.

Oocyte activation

The first event of activation in most oocytes is a depolarization of the plasma membrane. One notable exception is the hamster oocyte, which appears to undergo a series of hyperpolarizations. Close observation of the electrical response in sea urchins showed it to be biphasic, with a small steplike depolarization preceding the larger fertilization potential. Later studies showed that only successful spermatozoa gave rise to this initial event and that it also occurred in ascidian and amphibian oocytes. Since cortical granule exocytosis is not initiated until about the time of the second, larger depolarization, the fertilization potential – the period between the two events – corresponds approximately to what has been called the latent period. Single channel recordings, using the patch clamp technique, showed that the channels underlying the fertilization current had a conductance of 400 pS and were non-specific for ions. By measuring the total cell conductance at fertilization and the single channel conductance, and knowing the probability that a channel is in the open state, it was estimated that about 1000 fertilization channels were activated by the spermatozoon close to the site of fusion. Later work showed that the channels were not gated by intracellular Ca^{2+} but by ADPr (Figure 3.5). In conclusion, in invertebrate oocytes the spermatozoon induces an inward current in the oocyte plasma membrane by activating nonspecific ion channels shortly following gamete fusion.

The situation in the human is quite different: the spermatozoon induces an outward current in the oocyte plasma membrane by activating potassium channels. A second difference was found in the mechanism of fertilization channel gating, where the human potassium channel is calcium gated. In the ascidian, the channel is not calcium gated. In vitro, activation competence in oocytes is continually changing, and is not a stable, prolonged feature of ovulated eggs; therefore timing is critical in the handling of in vitro manipulations.

Releasing meiotic arrest

The universal messenger for the trigger of meiosis reinitiation in oocytes at fertilization is an increase in intracellular Ca^{2+}, released from intracellular stores in periodic waves or transients. Calcium release with similar waves may be induced parthenogenetically by a variety of physical and chemical stimuli, but the kinetics of the calcium transients are different, and do not sustain development. There are two hypotheses as to how the spermatozoon triggers intracellular Ca^{2+} release.

1. *The G-protein hypothesis*
This hypothesis for oocyte activation was extrapolated from the known events about calcium response to hormones in somatic cells. Hormone-receptor binding on the outer surface of the plasma membrane signals through a G-protein in the plasma membrane; this signal triggers the activation of Phospholipase C, leading to the formation of IP3 and hence calcium release. This model of oocyte activation suggests that the sperm behaves as an 'honorary hormone': the attachment of sperm to a sperm receptor triggers IP3 formation through a G-protein linked to this receptor.

2. *The soluble sperm factor hypothesis*
The sperm factor hypothesis, proposed by Dale and colleagues in the early 1980s, suggests that intracellular calcium release is triggered by a diffusible messenger (s) in the cytoplasm of the spermatozoon which enters the oocyte

cytoplasm after sperm–oocyte fusion. The first direct evidence for a soluble sperm factor was shown by microinjecting the soluble components from spermatozoa into sea urchin and ascidian oocytes. Several activation events were triggered, including cortical granule exocytosis and gating of plasma membrane currents. The same conclusion was reached when the experiment was repeated in mammals. The soluble sperm factor hypothesis gained further support with the advent of ICSI in the 1990s, where the events of oocyte activation follow after injection of spermatozoa into the oocyte cytoplasm.

Soluble extracts of spermatozoa can activate oocytes from different phyla as well as different species: mammalian oocytes can be partially activated by microinjecting sea urchin spermatozoa into the cytoplasm. Thus, sperm factors are not species specific, nor indeed phylum specific. Sperm extracts can also trigger calcium oscillations in somatic cells, suggesting that they are common calcium releasing agents rather than sperm-specific molecules.

It is possible that both soluble sperm factor and membrane transduction mechanisms interact to trigger oocyte activation.

Intracellular calcium release

The mode of calcium release at fertilization varies from species to species. There are three categories of calcium release mechanisms in oocytes, depending on the type of receptor located on the intracellular calcium store:

1. Inositol 1,4,5-trisphosphate (IP3)-induced calcium release (IICR)
2. Calcium-induced calcium release (CICR)
3. $NAADP^+$-induced calcium release.

IP3 is produced by the action of phospholipase C on plasma membrane lipid phosphatidylinositol bisphosphate, and IICR is triggered by the binding of IP3 to its receptor on the endoplasmic reticulum. CICR is triggered by opening the ryanodine receptor on an intracellular store, but can also be triggered in a mechanism involving the IP3 receptor. This can also be triggered by calcium itself, and appears to be modulated by cyclic ADP ribose. Cyclic ADP ribose is, in turn, produced by metabolism of nicotinamide adenine disphosphate (NAD^+) by ADP ribosyl cyclase or NAD^+ glycohydrolase. More recently, other calcium-releasing second messengers have been discovered, including cATP ribose and $NAADP^+$. Since NAD^+, NADH, $NADP^+$ and NADPH can be metabolized to calcium-releasing second messengers in sea urchin microsomes, it is possible that other calcium-releasing second messengers may be discovered in the nicotinamide nucleotide family.

In sea urchin oocytes, both IICR and CICR are triggered at fertilization. In frog oocytes, IICR appears to be uniquely activated at fertilization; however, what appears to be IICR may in fact be CICR through the IP3 receptor. The urochordate *Ciona intestinalis* also releases calcium by both IICR and CICR at fertilization, and generates repetitive calcium transients through meiosis I and II. These transients are blocked by heparin, suggesting that they may be triggered by an IP3-dependent mechanism. In mammalian oocytes there is a large increase in the sensitivity to CICR at fertilization, together with a series of repetitive calcium spikes. This again suggests that both CICR and IICR are activated at fertilization.

In conclusion, spermatozoa contain many calcium-releasing molecules, including ADPr, IP_3, nicotinamide nucleotide metabolites, calcium ions and relatively large proteins. An oligomer of 33 kDa, known as Oscillin, has been purified and considered as a candidate for soluble sperm factor; it is localized inside the plasma membrane of the equatorial segment of the sperm head, and antibodies identified homologues in human, mouse, and porcine sperm. However, the molecule was cloned and directly shown to be incapable of triggering calcium oscillations.

Oocytes, in turn, possess several calcium-release mechanisms. The active fraction in spermatozoa is not species specific, or specific to gametes: until a common activation pathway for the various calcium-release mechanisms is identified, the possibility remains that 'sperm factor' represents a collection of second messengers found in many cell types, but packaged and delivered differently in spermatozoa.

Calcium and the cell cycle proteins

In oocytes of the vertebrate *Xenopus*, fertilization calcium transients activate CaM kinase II, apparently triggering cyclin B destruction and Mos degradation leading to a decrease in MPF activity and meiosis reinitiation. However, many aspects of this pathway need to be clarified.

In invertebrate oocytes, the role of Ca^{2+}/calmodulin in M-I exit is not clear, although several lines of evidence indicate a similar mechanism to that which triggers cyclin degradation machinery. Ascidian oocytes are blocked at metaphase 1 when ovulated. Three independent events, involving distinct subcellular compartments, are triggered in the ascidian oocyte at fertilization:

1. A large inward membrane current
2. Intracellular calcium oscillations
3. Inactivation of MPF.

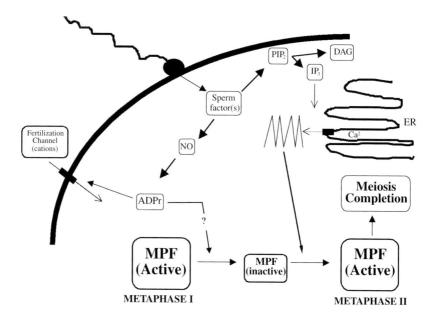

Figure 3.5   Schematic diagram to show the mechanisms involved in oocyte activation after triggering by the fertilizing sperm.

MPF activity is maximal at M-I and M-II, and decreases at exit from meiosis I and II. The fertilizing spermatozoon fuses to the plasma membrane and releases sperm factors into the oocyte (Figure 3.5). These factors stimulate both the production of IP3 and ADPr, the latter probably through the production of nitric oxide. ADPr gates the fertilization channels, and may be involved in the inactivation of MPF at meiosis I release. IP3 gates the release of intracellular calcium, which is required for the activation of MPF and the completion of meiosis II.

The cortical reaction

Oocyte structure may be modified in several ways during activation. In some oocytes there is a dramatic redistribution of cytoplasmic organelles which prepares the zygote for embryogenesis, whilst in others the cell surface contracts at one pole and expands at the other. Perhaps the first, and certainly the most obvious change comes about as a result of the cortical reaction. Cortical granules are found in the oocytes of many animals, for example echinoderms, some mammals, amphibians, annelids, fish and crustacea, although there is tremendous diversity in their form and size. In mammals, sea urchins and

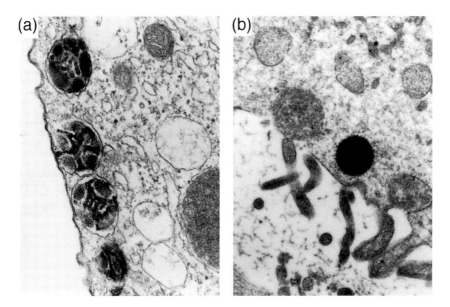

Figure 3.6   Transmission electron micrographs of the surface of unfertilized oocytes of the sea urchin (a) and human (b), showing the cortical granules.

starfish they are found immediately below the plasma membrane in a single layer, whereas in some ophiuroid echinoderms (brittle stars) they are found several layers deep (Figure 3.6). These special organelles originate as vesicles in the Golgi complex and contain, amongst other substances, enzymes and mucopolysaccharides. During activation, the granules break open releasing their contents into the perivitelline space (the gap between the oocyte plasma membrane and the vitelline coat). There are two immediate consequences of cortical granule exocytosis: the perivitelline space first increases in volume, and the vitelline coat is then transformed into a thick, hard protective structure.

Most of our information on cortical granule exocytosis has been gained from studies on the sea urchin oocyte. There are about 20 000 cortical granules per oocyte, membrane bound, about 1 μm in diameter, and their contents often look star- or spiral-shaped. The granules appear to be interconnected by thin filaments and are firmly attached to the oocyte surface. A tangential section through an oocyte clearly shows their homogeneous distribution just below the cell surface. Exocytosis starts some 10 seconds after the spermatozoon has attached to the vitelline coat. This delay is called the latent period. The granules in the immediate vicinity of the spermatozoon are the first to break down, and a wave of exocytosis then spreads slowly around the oocyte surface. Mucopolysaccharides, released from the granules into the perivitelline space, cause a rapid influx of water which distends the vitelline coat, lifting it 1–20 μm away from the oocyte surface. This wavelike progression of cortical granule exocytosis and the concomitant elevation of the vitelline coat takes approximately 20 seconds to spread around the oocyte surface. Over the next 5 minutes, the perivitelline space continues to increase and the vitelline coat hardens and thickens becoming the familiar fertilization membrane. Although it is not clear how the cortical reaction is initiated, nor how it is propagated around the oocyte, an important factor is the increase in cytoplasmic Ca^{2+}. Cortical granule exocytosis may be induced by injecting Ca^{2+} into the cytoplasm, and it can be prevented using Ca^{2+} chelating agents (molecules which bind free Ca^{2+}). Furthermore, oocytes exposed to ionophores (molecules which facilitate the passage of ions across membranes) such as amphotericin B or A23187 undergo the cortical reaction along with several other activation events. Finally, it should be pointed out that cortical granule exocytosis is essentially a process of membrane fusion, and each granule fuses with the inner aspect of the plasma membrane. In order to fuse, the granules must come into close contact with the oocyte surface, and the cytoskeleton is involved in this movement. The oocyte plasma membrane becomes a mosaic structure made up of the original membrane and the incorporated patches of cortical granules. The physiological characteristics of these inserted patches of new membrane are not known, nor is it known whether they are essential for embryogenesis; however, they do cause a considerable increase in the surface area of the oocyte.

What about the more obvious structural modifications resulting from the cortical reaction? The vitelline coat of the unfertilized oocyte is a fibrous glycoprotein structure approximately 15 nm thick. Immediately following elevation it remains thin and elastic and can easily be digested by proteolytic enzymes. During the next 5 minutes it becomes thicker, reaching approximately 90 nm, and much harder. The fertilization membrane is a laminar structure, and it is thought that the crystalline component of the cortical granules attaches to the inner aspect of the vitelline coat thereby thickening it. A trypsin-like protease also released from the granules plays an important role in this thickening and hardening – if this protease is specifically inhibited, the fertilization membrane fails to harden. A further component of the granules is a calcium-binding glycoprotein which tightly adheres to the oocyte surface forming the hyaline layer. In actual fact, a very thin hyaline layer may be present before fertilization (also of cortical granule origin) which then thickens as a result of the cortical reaction.

Teleost fish oocytes have cortical alveoli which also break down in a wavelike progression from the point of sperm entry, releasing their contents into the perivitelline space. A hyaline layer is formed, the chorion hardens and water enters into the perivitelline space causing it to increase in volume. In contrast to the situation in the sea urchin, the perivitelline space swells not by distension of the chorion (vitelline coat) but by shrinkage of the oocyte surface. The cortical alveoli of the marine worm *Nereis* also break down in a wavelike fashion during activation and, similar to the situation in fish, the perivitelline space increases by oocyte shrinkage rather than by membrane elevation. A peculiar observation is that the alveolar contents extrude outside the oocyte surface layers and by hydration form a thick impervious jelly-like structure. Some mammalian oocytes also contain cortical granules which upon activation break open releasing their contents; the zona pellucida hardens and thickens, and this is known as the zona reaction.

In some amphibians, cortical granule exocytosis and elevation of the vitelline coat is remarkably similar to that in the sea urchin. However, the jelly layer apparently plays a different role in these two groups of animal. In the sea urchin, the jelly layer, now on the outside of the fertilization membrane, quickly dissolves. In the frog, the jelly layer swells immensely after fertilization and serves (1) for protection, (2) to allow the oocytes to attach to submerged structures and (3) to keep oocytes spaced and thus allow them enough room for metabolic turnover with the environment. Even in oocytes which lack cortical granules, such as those of the ascidian, there appears to be some sort of exocytosis of cortical material at activation and, in some species at least, the perivitelline space expands. In ascidians, changes in permeability to ions and other molecules provide evidence that the plasma membrane is also reorganized.

The cortical reaction in mammals

The first morphological indication of activation in regulative oocytes is the exocytosis of cortical granules, which are small spherical membrane-bound organelles containing enzymes and mucopolysaccharides, originating as vesicles in the Golgi complex. The cortical reaction in the mammalian oocyte elicits the zona reaction, changing the characteristics of the zona pellucida. A second result of the cortical reaction is that the oocyte plasma membrane now becomes a mosaic of cortical granule membrane and the original plasma membrane. It has long been suggested that the fertilizing spermatozoon, by triggering events such as the cortical reaction, not only activates the oocyte, but at the same time prevents the interaction of supernumerary spermatozoa. Certainly, the alteration to the zona pellucida in the mouse, involving proteinases or glycosidases, causes a zona block with hydrolysis of ZP3 receptors which prevents them from further interaction. The mosaic zygote plasma membrane is also refractory to sperm in many species – this is known as the vitelline block. The appearance of supernumerary spermatozoa in the perivitelline space, for example in the rabbit, has been suggested as an indication of a weak zona reaction and a strong vitelline reaction. In contrast, because perivitelline sperm are rare in rat, mouse, sheep and human oocytes, these species might be considered to have a strong zona reaction.

If we accept the premises that all spermatozoa which reach the oocyte are equally capable of fertilization, and that all areas of the oocyte surface and its extracellular coats are capable of activating spermatozoa, then the cortical reaction is too slow to be considered a block to polyspermy. The cortical reaction may serve to chemically alter the zona pellucida in order to provide a bacterially safe environment for the developing embryo. The fact that only one spermatozoon normally enters the oocyte during in vitro conditions suggests that there is a heterogeneous sperm population, and that there may be restricted areas on the oocyte surface (hot spots) for sperm entry.

The role of cortical reorganization

Cortical reorganization is a common feature of oocyte activation. Although mechanisms differ, the results are often similar. The sea urchin oocyte has been studied in great detail – other oocytes less so. By piecing together all of the information, some general conclusions may be drawn regarding the role of cortical reorganization in embryogenesis. First and foremost, the developing embryo must be protected in some way. In oocytes which lack cortical granules, for example those of ascidians and insects, a protective structure which does not alter much following activation is laid down during oogenesis – i.e. it is preformed. In other animals a different strategy is employed. The oocyte has a relatively thin extracellular coat which hardens after activation, catalyzed by the cortical granule products. In either event, the embryo remains in its protective coat until hatching. A second extracellular structure produced as a result of cortical granule exocytosis is the hyaline layer which serves to keep the dividing blastomeres of the embryo in close contact. The early embryo is a compact mass of continually dividing cells, and the embryo is therefore continually changing shape. Such movement would be hindered if the cells were attached to a rigid structure, so possibly for this reason the embryo is surrounded by the fluid-filled perivitelline space. This gap may also serve as a micro-environment buffering the embryo from changes in the environment.

Reorganization of the plasma membrane appears to be related to the metabolic de-repression of the oocyte and occurs both in oocytes with, and those without, cortical granules. Certainly, this reorganization is dramatic and rapid in granule-containing oocytes and is attained without the participation of the cells' synthetic apparatus. Although we do not know the function of this mosaic plasma membrane, the resulting transient increase in surface area will facilitate the metabolic turnover of the activated oocyte. Finally, the cortical changes will exclude the interaction of supernumerary spermatozoa within a limited range of sperm density, and, in fact, many authors have suggested that such changes have evolved specifically as polyspermy-preventing mechanisms. However, perhaps one should be more objective. Certainly in some animals, i.e. mammals, insects and nematodes, the sperm:oocyte ratio is so low under natural conditions that supernumerary collisions are extremely unlikely and therefore cortical changes may well have other functions, mobilized by the increase in intracellular Ca^{2+}.

Fusion, centrosomes and pronuclei

In marine invertebrates, the tip of the acrosomal tubule makes contact with and then fuses with the oocyte plasma membrane. In mammals, where there is no acrosomal tubule, the spermatozoal plasma membrane in the post-acrosomal region fuses with the oocyte plasma membrane – by fusion we mean that the two membranes become continuous. The process of membrane fusion between gametes (or for that matter between somatic cells) is not understood, but Ca^{2+} and a close approximation of the two membranes is essential. Fusion of gametes seems to be facilitated by the presence of numerous microvilli on the oocyte surface; these have a low radius of curvature which may help to overcome opposing electrostatic charges. In fact, spermatozoa rarely fuse with the microvillus-free areas of the oocyte surface, for example, the area over the second metaphase spindle in mouse oocytes. During fusion, the oocyte cytoplasm rises up in a protuberance around the spermatozoal nucleus to form the fertilization cone. In the sea urchin, microfilaments appear to be involved in the formation and resorption of this structure. It would be interesting to know if some of the enzymes released from the acrosome alter the oocyte plasma membrane, preparing it for the subsequent fusion process. One possibility is that the release of phospholipases and the transient production of lysophospholipids destabilizes the plasma membrane by altering the normal phospholipid components. In mammals and sea urchins, the fertilizing spermatozoon continues flagellar movement for some 20 seconds after attachment to the oocyte surface. There then follows a sudden cessation of flagellar motion, which may occur simultaneously with the process of gamete fusion. In the sea urchin, the spermatozoal tail becomes erect and perpendicular to the oocyte surface. The fertilization membrane elevates around the tail and, during the next 30 seconds, the fertilization cone develops whilst the spermatozoon moves into the oocyte at a rate of 5 µm/s. Once in the cortex, the naked spermatozoal nucleus moves laterally, rotates approximately 180 degrees, and during the next 10 minutes develops into the male pronucleus. The mitochondria and tail of the spermatozoon also enter the cytoplasm but later degenerate.

The process in small mammals is somewhat slower; sperm–oocyte fusion is quite advanced after 3 minutes, the entire incorporation of the sperm head takes 15 minutes, and pronucleus formation takes about 60 minutes. In some mammals (for example the Chinese hamster) the tail is not incorporated, while in others it is incorporated by the progressive fusion of the oocyte and spermatozoal plasma membranes. After incorporation, the middle-piece mitochondria and axial filament of the tail appear to disintegrate. The spermatozoal plasma membrane, however, is integrated into the oocyte plasma membrane and may play a role in development.

Centrosomes

In the previous section, the epigenetic role of soluble sperm factor in oocyte activation was discussed. A second fundamental paternal contribution to embryogenesis is the centrosome. In studies on sea urchins and round worms at the turn of the century, Boveri at the Stazione Zoologica in Naples showed that the male gamete provided the 'division center' for the zygote . He further predicted that the centrosome is a 'cyclical reproducing organ' of the cell. To date, it is generally accepted that the centrosome is of paternal origin. There are notable exceptions: in the mouse and hamster the centrosome is apparently of maternal origin, lending support to the observation that these rodents are poor model systems for human fertilization. In frogs, despite the fact that centrosome inheritance is paternal, the sperm centrosome lacks tubulin, which is essential for the nucleation of microtubules. Tubulin is provided by the oocyte cytoplasm, and therefore in frogs, at least, the functional centrosome is a mosaic of paternal and maternal components.

What then is the centrosome? In somatic cells, the centrosome is composed of two structures called centrioles, placed at right angles to each other and surrounded by dense pericentriolar material. Each centriole is made up of nine triplets of microtubules arranged in a pinwheel array. The centrosome divides during interphase to form the poles of the mitotic spindle, and after division segregates with the chromosomes to each of the daughter cells. In contrast, during oogenesis the centrosomes degenerate after meiosis, leaving the oocyte without a 'division center'. This is then contributed by the sperm during fertilization. The spermatozoon has a functional proximal centriole, close to the nucleus, and a degenerate distal centriole. After the sperm enters the oocyte, a small 'aster' of microtubules grows from the centriole, which directs the migration of the sperm pronucleus to the centre of the oocyte to make contact with the decondensing maternal pronucleus, initiating its migration towards the forming male pronucleus. The zygotic centrosome then duplicates and splits apart during interphase, as microtubules extend from in-between the eccentrically positioned, juxtaposed male and female pronuclei. After duplication, the centrioles migrate to opposite poles during mitotic prophase to set up the first mitotic spindle of the zygote. Although the centrioles are the main organelle associated with cell division, it is now thought that the pericentriolar material may be the principal microtubule organizing centre. In cases of polyspermy, when the oocyte is fertilized by more than one sperm, human oocytes develop multiple sperm asters, each associated with a sperm. During parthenogenesis, where there is no paternal centrosomal contribution, no sperm astral microtubules are nucleated, and cytoplasmic microtubules are instead found throughout the oocyte. In this case, the female centrosome becomes fully functional, duplicating and forming the mitotic spindle poles. Microtubules are present in metaphase-arrested second meiotic spindles in unfertilized oocytes. Although cattle and human oocytes can organize microtubules without sperm entry, this happens later, and less completely, than it does after sperm entry. Defective centrosome function can result in fertilization failure. Six hours post insemination, a small microtubule sperm aster extends from the sperm centrosome, and the activated egg extrudes the second polar body.

Formation of pronuclei

During spermatogenesis, gene expression is completely repressed, DNA replication ceases and sperm chromatin is tightly packed into a nuclear envelope that lacks pores. Transformation of the sperm nucleus into the male pronucleus involves dissassembly of sperm nuclear lamina, chromatin dispersion, enlargement, the disintegration of the nuclear envelope and the formation of a new pronuclear envelope. Once inside the oocyte cytoplasm, the male nucleus

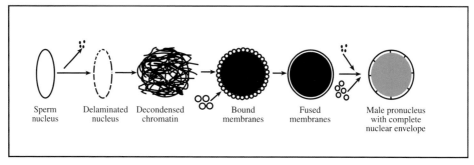

Figure 3.7   Formation of the male sea urchin pronucleus in vitro:
1. Sperm nuclear lamina is solubilized, mediated by PKC
2. Chromatin decondenses inside the delaminated nucleus
3. Membrane vesicles bind to chromatin
4. Chromatin bound membranes fuse
5. Male pronucleus swells, and nuclear lamina assemble with formation of functional nuclear pores. Modified after Collas & Poccia (1992).

undergoes a reverse process of morphological and biochemical transformation that leads to the formation of the male pronucleus. In some species, this process is completed in less than 30 minutes. Most of our information has come from studies of the sea urchin, where the first step is removal of the nuclear envelope. The nuclear lamina is then phosphorylated and disassembled by a cytosolic protein kinase C. Chromatin decondensation follows, and this requires ATP hydrolysis. Membrane vesicles present in the cytosol now bind to the decondensed chromatin in an ATP-dependent fashion, and subsequently fuse together in a GTP-dependent process to form a continous membrane. The nucleus now swells by fusion of additional membrane vesicles and functional nuclear pores found in the cytosol, importing soluble nuclear lamins.

This last process of swelling is dependent on calcium, ATP and GTP. A diagram illustrating pronuclear formation in the sea urchin is shown in Figure 3.7. During this structural modification, specific chromatin proteins are replaced (mammals) or modified (sea urchins) and the chromatin regains its capacity for DNA replication and transcription.

In chapter 1, we saw that oocytes from different animals are blocked at different stages of meiosis (Figure 1.3) Consequently, the sperm nucleus, newly introduced into the oocyte cytoplasm, will find itself in different cytoplasmic environments depending on the species.

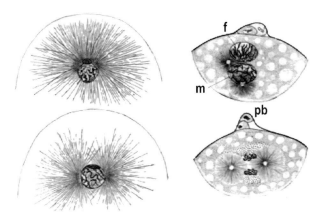

Figure 3.8   A drawing from Wilson (1900) showing (left) the fusion of male and female pronuclei to form the zygote nucleus as in sea urchins. In the majority of animals (and usually in mammals) the pronuclear membranes break down without fusing, allowing the chromosomes to interact in the cytoplasm (frames on the right).

1. In oocytes that are normally fertilized at the germinal vesicle stage, such as some molluscs, germinal vesicle breakdown occurs about 12 minutes after activation. The sperm nucleus decondenses and then swells in conjunction with decondensation of the female pronucleus.
2. Insect oocytes are blocked at the first metaphase, and the sperm forms an aster during the oocyte's 2nd metaphase, but the chromatin does not decondense until the oocyte has completed both meiotic divisions.
3. Vertebrate oocytes are fertilized at second metaphase. In mammals, the first step of nuclear transformation is the reduction of disulphide bonds in nuclear protamines. Dissolution of the sperm nuclear envelope and chromatin decondensation occurs while the oocyte transits from metaphase II to telophase II: during telophase II, the sperm chromatin decondenses as the female pronucleus develops. Sperm protamines are replaced by histones and the male and female pronuclear envelopes develop synchronously.
4. Sea urchin oocytes are fertilized after the completion of meiosis, when the female pronucleus is already formed. Thus, in contrast to the other species, male pronuclear formation occurs in interphase cytoplasm. Within 2 minutes of entry, the sperm nuclear envelope is dissasembled, and within 30 minutes the nucleus swells some 20-fold to form the pronucleus.

Once formed, male and female pronuclei migrate towards each other and subsequently move towards the centre of the oocyte; the sperm aster is involved in this movement. In sea urchins, the envelopes of the two pronuclei fuse to form a zygote nuclear envelope, containing decondensed male and female chromatin. In most other animals (and as originally described for *Ascaris* by E.B. Wilson), the chromosomes in each pronucleus condense and concomitantly the pronuclear envelopes break down without fusing together. The male and female chromosomes then intermix in the cytoplasm and form the metaphase of the first mitotic spindle (Figure 3.8).

Pronucleus formation in mammals

In mammals, during spermatogenesis the sperm nucleus is packed with distinct histones or protamines. The association of nuclear DNA with these highly charged basic amino acids is thought to cause condensation and repression of DNA activity. The rigidity of the mammalian sperm head, necessary for penetration of the zona, is due to extensive disulphide linkage in these protamines. Protamine crosslinking in the human spermatozoon is regulated by Zn^{2+} from the prostrate gland. On entering the oocyte cytoplasm, the sperm nuclear envelope breaks down, the protamines are lost and pronuclear decondensation occurs. A reduced form of glutathione may be responsible for sperm nucleus decondensation. Sperm nucleus decondensing factors seem to be nonspecies specific, since human sperm may decondense when microinjected into amphibian oocytes.

The next step after decondensation is the formation of a new nuclear membrane around the decondensed male and female chromatin to produce the pronuclei. During pronuclear development DNA synthesis and RNA transcription occurs.

Sperm pronucleus development factors are found in limited quantities within the cytoplasm – for example in the hamster a maximum of 5 pronuclei will decondense at any time. Again the factors are not species specific, because human spermatozoa can develop into normal pronuclei in hamster oocytes and form a normal chromosome complement. The migration of the male and female pronuclei to the centre of the oocyte has been studied extensively, particularly in the sea urchin and the mouse. In the mouse, fluorescein conjugated probes for cytoskeletal elements show a thickened area of microfilaments below the cortex of the polar body region. In addition to the spindle microtubules, there are 16 cytoplasmic microtubule organizing centres or foci. Each centrosomal focus organizes an aster. Shortly before the nuclear envelopes disintegrate, the foci condense on the surface of the envelope and the first cleavage ensues.

In the bovine system, sperm incorporation and the conversion of sperm-derived components into the zygote has been explored after tagging sperm with a mitochondrion-specific vital dye. The zygotes were fixed at various times after fertilization for immunochemistry and ultrastructural studies. Results showed that complete incorporation of the sperm depends upon the integrity of oocyte microfilaments, and is inhibited by cytochalasin B, which disrupts microfilaments. After sperm incorporation, the mitochondria were displaced from the sperm midpiece, and the sperm centriole exposed to egg cytoplasm. The microtubule-based sperm aster then formed, initiating union of male and female pronuclei. The dissasembly of the sperm tail occurred as a series of precisely orchestrated events, involving the destruction and transformation of particular sperm structures into zygotic and embryonic components.

Syngamy

'The sun in the egg'

Leopold Auerbach of Breslau, Germany (1828–97) described two protoplasmic vacuoles in a newly fertilized egg, as well as a radiating figure between them. In 1876, Oscar Hertwig identified these vacuoles as the male and female pronuclei, and he observed their fusion. When the two nuclei merged together in syngamy, he described the figure:

> *Es entsteht so vollständig das Bild einer Sonne im Ei.*

> *It arises to completion like a sun within the egg.*

In an analysis of Hertwig's paper, Paul Weindling (1991) proposed, 'This vivid image conveyed the discovery of the moment at which a new life was formed. The metaphor expressed awareness that the force of natural powers was greater than the sum of two cells.'

Further reading

Auerbach, L. (1874) *Organologische Studien.* Breslau.

Boveri, Th. (1902) Über mehrpolige Mitosen als Mittel zur Analyse des Zellkerns. *Verh. d. phys.-med. Ges.* Würzburg N.F. **35**:67–90.

Breitbart (1997) The biochemistry of the acrosome reaction. *Molecular Human Reproduction* **3**(3):195–202.

Cohen-Dayag, A., Tur-Kaspa, I., Dor, J., Mashiach, S. & Eisenbach, M. (1995) Sperm capacitation in humans is transient and correlates with chemotactic responsivness to follicular factors. *Proceedings of the National Academy of Sciences* **92**:11039–43.

Collas, and Poccia, (1992) *Theriogenology* **49**:67–81.

Dale, B. & Monroy, A. (1981) How is polyspermy prevented? *Gamete Research* **4**:151–69.

Dale, B. & DeFelice, L.J. (1990) Soluble sperm factors, electrical events and egg activation. In: (Dale, B. ed.), *Mechanism of Fertilization: Plants to Humans.* Springer, Berlin, Hiedelberg, New York (NATO ASI cell biology ser H 45).

Dale, B., Tosti, E. & Iaccarino, M. (1995) Is the plasma membrane of the human oocyte reorganized following fertilisation and early cleavage? *Zygote* **3(1)**:31–6.

Dale, B., Marino, M. & Wilding, M. (1998) Soluble sperm factor, factors or receptors. *Molecular Human Reproduction* **5**, 1–4.

Davidson (1990) How embryos work: a comparative view of diverse modes of cell fate specification. *Development* **108**:365–89.

Edwards, R.G. (1982) *Conception in the Human Female*. Academic Press, New York.

Eisenbach, M. & Ralt, D. (1992) Precontact mammalian sperm–egg communication and role in fertilization. *American Journal of Physiology* **262**:1095–101.

Fleming, T.A. & Johnson, M.H. (1988) From egg to epithelium. *Annual Review of Cell Biology* **4**:459–85.

Foltz, K.R. & Lennarz, W.J. (1993) The molecular basis of sea urchin gamete interactions at the egg plasma membrane. *Developmental Biology* **158**:46–61.

Gianaroli, L., Tosti, E., Magli, C., Ferrarreti, A. & Dale, B. (1994) The fertilization current in the human oocyte. *Molecular Reproduction Development* **38**:209–14.

Gwatkin, R. (1974) *Fertilization Mechanisms in Man and Mammals*. Plenum Press, New York.

Hertwig, O. (1876) Beiträge zur Kenntniss der Bildung, Befruchtung und Theilung des thierischen Eies. *Morphologische Jahrbuch* **1**:347–434.

Hewitson, L. Simerley, C. & Schatten, G. (1999) ICSI: Unravelling the mysteries. *Alpha Newsletter* vol. 17 (May 1999), and *Nature Medicine*, **5(4)**:431–3.

Holy, J. & Schatten, G. (1991) Spindle pole centrosomes of sea urchin embryos are partially composed of material recruited from maternal stores. *Developmental Biology* **147**:343–53.

Jaffe, L. (1980) Calcium explosions as triggers of development. *Annals of the New York Academy of Science of the USA* **339**:86–101.

Lanzafame, F., Chapman, M., Guglielmino, A., Gearon, C.M. & Forman, R.G. (1994) Pharmacological stimulation of sperm motility. *Human Reproduction* **9(2)**:192–4.

Lauria, A., Gandolfi, E., Enne, G. & Gianaroli, L. (eds.) (1998) *Gametes: Development and Function*. Serono Symposia, Rome.

Lennarz, W.J. (1994) Fertilization in sea urchins: how many different molecules are involved in gamete interaction and fusion? *Zygote* **2(1)**:1–4.

Maro, B., Gueth-Hallonet, C., Aghion, J. & Antony, C. (1991) Cell polarity and microtubule organization during mouse early embryogenesis. *Development Supplement* **10**:17–25.

Myles, D.G. (1992) Molecular mechanism of sperm–egg membrane binding and fusion in mammals. *Developmental Biology* **158**:35–45.

Nuccitelli, R., Cherr, G. & Clark, A. (1989) *Mechanisms of Egg Activation*. Plenum Press, New York.

Ralt et al. (1991) Sperm attraction to follicular factors correlates with human egg fertilizability. *Proceedings of the National Academy of Sciences* **88**:2840–4.

Santella, L., Alikani, M., Talansky, B., Cohen, J. & Dale, B (1992) Is the human oocyte plasma membrane polarized? *Human Reproduction* **7**:999–1003.

Shapiro, S. (1987) The existential decision of a sperm. *Cell* **49**, 293–4.

Sutovsky, P., Navara, C.S. & Schatten, G. (1996) Fate of the sperm mitochondria, and the incorporation, conversion, and disassembly of the sperm tail structures during bovine fertilization. *Biology of Reproduction* **55**:1195–205.

Tesarik, I., Sousa, M. & Testart, J. (1994) Human oocyte activation after intracytoplasmic sperm injection. *Human Reproduction* **9**:511–14.

Tosti, E. (1994) Sperm activation in species with external fertilization. *Zygote* **2(4)**:359–61.

Ward, C.R. & Kopf, G.S. (1993) Molecular events mediating sperm activation. *Developmental Biology* **158**:9–34.

Wassarman, P.M. (1990) Profile of a mammalian sperm receptor. *Development* **108**:1–17.

Wassarman, P.M., Florman, H.M., Greve, I.M. (1985) Receptor-mediated sperm–egg interactions in mammals. In: (Metz C.B. & Monroy, A. eds.), *Fertilization*, vol. 2. Academic Press, New York, pp. 341–60.

Weindling, P.J. (1991) *Darwinism and Social Darwinism in Imperial Germany: The Contribution of the Cell Biologist Oscar Hertwig (1849–1922)*. G. Fischer Verlag, Stuttgart, p. 71.

Wilson, E.B. (1900) *The Cell in Development and Inheritance*. Macmillan, London.

Yanagimachi, R. (1981) Mechanisms of fertilization in mammals. In: (Mastroianni, L. & Biggers, J.D. eds.), *Fertilization and Embryonic Development In Vitro*. Plenum Press, New York, pp. 81–182.

Yanagimachi, R. (1994) Mammalian fertilization. In: (Knobil, E. and Neill, J. eds.) *The Physiology of Reproduction*. Raven Press. New York.

4

First stages of development

After fertilization, the zygote divides by mitosis into a number of smaller cells called blastomeres. This process of division, known as cleavage, is in a sense the opposite to the process of oogenesis: cleavage is a period of intense DNA replication and cell division in the absence of growth, whereas oogenesis is a period of growth without replication or division. Early cleavages are often synchronous, but sooner or later synchrony is lost. The blastomeres become organized in layers or groups, each group having a characteristic rate of cleavage. Although cleavage may be considered a mitotic process as found in adult somatic tissues, there is one important difference: in adult tissue the daughter cells grow following each division and are not able to divide again until they have achieved the original size of the parent cell. The cells in a somatic population thus maintain an average size. During cleavage this is not the case: with each division the resulting blastomeres are approximately half the size of the parent blastomere. As cleavage progresses, the embryo polarizes and differences arise between the blastomeres. Such differences may result from the unequal distribution of cytoplasmic components as already laid down in the oocyte during oogenesis, or from changes occurring in the blastomeres as a result of new embryonic gene transcription during development. Each blastomere nucleus will be subjected to a different cytoplasmic environment, which, in turn, may differentially influence the genome activity. As a result, after the onset of zygote gene activation and subsequent differentiation, eventually the blastomeres set off on their own particular programme of development to give rise to a particular cell line, for example nerve, muscle, etc. Maternal mRNA encoding developmental information is essential in early differentiation, and has been found to persist until gastrulation in some species during specific patterns of gene expression. Localized short- and long-lived maternal mRNAs may regulate initial stages of differentiation.

In mammals, the zygote remains in the oviduct for a few days undergoing

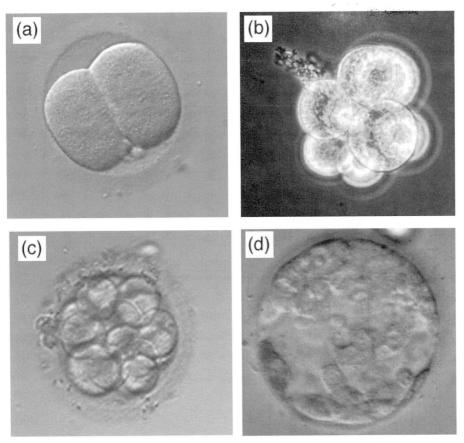

Figure 4.1 The first stages of development in the human: 2-cells (a), 6-cell (b), morula (c), blastocyst (d). By courtesy of Agnese Fiorentino, Naples, Italy.

cleavage divisions, which restore a normal cytoplasmic/nuclear ratio in the cells (Figure 4.1). At about the third cleavage division, the embryo undergoes the process of compaction to form the morula. At this stage, there is a significant increase in RNA and protein synthesis and in the synthetic patterns of phospholipids. At the 32-cell stage, a second morphological change occurs which gives rise to the blastocyst (Figure 4.1d). The form of the blastocyst varies between species, but essentially it is made up of an outer layer of trophectoderm cells and an eccentrically placed inner cell mass layer. The early blastocyst (Day 4/5 in the human) initially shows no increase in size, but it subsequently expands over the next one or two days (Day 5/6) by active accumulation of fluid in the central blastocoelic cavity. Throughout these early stages, the embryo is enclosed in the zona pellucida (ZP), which keeps the cells together prior to compaction and prevents two embryos fusing and forming a

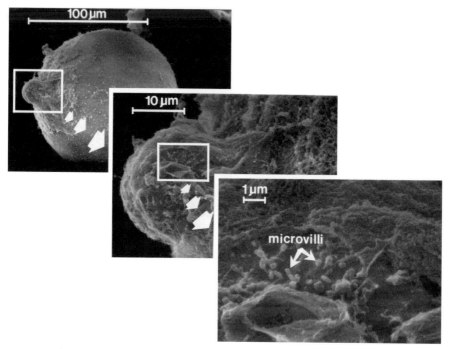

Figure 4.2   Scanning electron micrograph of a hatching human embryo. The microvilli on the surface of the trophectoderm cells are bared owing to internal pressure in the blastocoel and dissolution of the zona pellucida.

chimaera. If the inner cell mass (ICM) divides at this early stage monozygotic (identical) twins may develop.

During the transition from morula to blastocyst, the embryo enters the uterus, where it derives oxygen and metabolic substrates. At the site of implantation, the trophectoderm cells produce proteolytic enzymes which digest a passage through the ZP, as the blastocyst 'hatches' free of the zona. The uterine environment may also contain proteolytic enzymes, but very little is known about the molecular basis for hatching. The exposed cell layers of the hatched blastocyst make firm physical contact and implantation starts. In the human embryo, the first 14–18 days of develement are concerned mainly with the differentiation of various extra-embryonic tissues, and only after this time can separate tissues be identified (Figures 4.2, 4.3 and 4.4).

Activation of the zygote genome

Successful development of a fertilized oocyte beyond the early cleavage stage requires *de novo* initiation and regulation of new embryonic genome

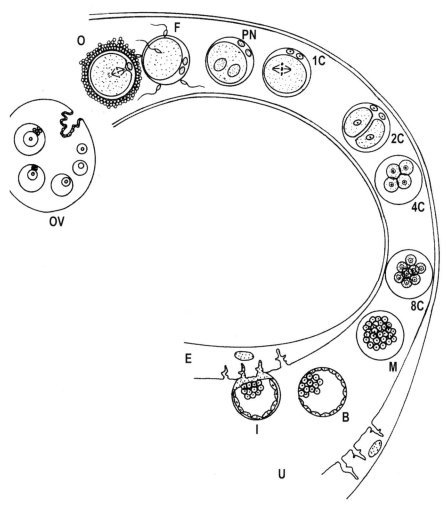

Figure 4.3 Development of the mammalian embryo. The oocytes released from the ovary (OV) enter the ampulla where they are fertilized (F) and then are transported along the fallopian tube, cleaving to generate the morula stage (M). The blastocyst expands, hatches and then implants in the endometrium (E) of the uterus. From Sathananthan et al. (1993).

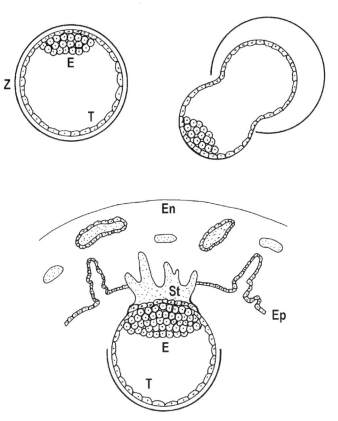

Figure 4.4   Implantation in the mammal. (a) Expanded blastocyst showing the flat layer of trophectoderm cells (T) which will become part of the extra-embryonic tissue and the inner cell mass (E) from which the embryo derives. (b) Shows hatching, probably due in part to the production of a proteolytic-like enzyme by some of the trophectoderm cells. (c) Invasion of the epithelium (Ep) of the endometrium (En).

transcription. The oocyte cytoplasm provides a specialized environment for the newly formed zygotic nucleus, and during the transition from maternal to zygotic gene activation the embryo begins to synthesize its own RNA and protein rather than relying on that inherited from the mother. In the absence of appropriate activation and maintenance of embryonic gene expression, the embryo will simply fail to develop beyond early cleavage stages.

The very early embryo has very little metabolic activity during its first few cleavage divisions; in vitro, it can probably manage excesses and imbalances in culture media because of its low metabolic activity. This situation changes dramatically with the onset of zygote genome activation, when maternal stores are depleted and the genes of the new individual are switched on. Activation of the embryonic genome occurs progressively during preimplantation development:

1. Depletion of maternal RNA transcripts and transcription of new embryonic mRNA
2. Qualitative shift in protein synthesis, and post-translational modification
3. Development of a functional nucleosomal structure, the nuclear organizing region (NOR).

Establishment of the timing of genome activation is likely to depend on the sensitivity of methods available for its detection; new protein synthesis activity has been detected at different stages in different species:

Rabbit	1–2 cell
Mouse	2-cell
Cow	4–8 cell
Human	4-cell
Sheep	8–16 cell
Drosophila	4000 cells
Xenopus	5000 cells

Despite the species-specific differences in onset of embryonic transcription, there is evidence to suggest that a minor degree of transcriptional activity takes place preceding the major activation of the genome. In the mouse, zygote genome activation (ZGA) occurs during the second cell division cycle (2-cell stage) and seems to be regulated by a 'zygotic clock' that measures the time following fertilization rather than the progression through the first cell cycle. ZGA may involve a period of minor gene activation in the 1-cell embryo, followed by a period of major gene activation in the 2-cell embryo. It seems that in mammals ZGA is a time-dependent mechanism rather than a cell cycle-dependent mechanism. Both transcription and translation of nascent transcripts are delayed, and maternal mRNA and zygotic gene transcripts appear to be handled differently (Wiekowski et al., 1991, Schulz & Worrad, 1995, Nothias et al., 1995).

In human preimplantation embryos, reverse transcriptase–polymerase chain reaction (RT–PCR) detected early transcripts for two paternal Y chromosome genes, ZFY and SRY. ZFY transcripts were detected at the pronucleate stage, 20–24 h after in vitro insemination, and at intermediate stages up to the blastocyst stage. SRY transcripts were also detected at 2-cell to blastocyst stages (Ao et al., 1994).

In the mouse and rabbit, a general chromatin-mediated repression of promoter activity appears. Repression factors are inherited by the maternal pronucleus from the oocyte but are absent from the paternal pronucleus; they are not available until sometime during the transition from a late 1-cell to a 2-cell embryo (Wiekowski et al., 1991). This means that paternally inherited genes are exposed to a different environment in fertilized eggs than are maternally inherited genes, a situation that could contribute to genomic imprinting.

Cleavage increases the number of nuclei, which amplifies the number of templates to facilitate the production of specialized proteins needed for the processes of compaction and differentiation to the blastocyst stage. Changes in chromatin structure, rather than changes in the activity of the transcriptional apparatus, may underlie the timing and basis for ZGA. Transcription factors must be available which can bind to the DNA, and a functional physical structure, the Nuclear Organising Region (NOR) develops, producing conformational changes in the DNA structure that will allow the binding of promoters and enhancers of transcription. The formation of the NOR is related to the nuclear:cytoplasmic ratio.

One hypothesis suggests that there is some titratable factor in the cytoplasm that is diluted with increasing nuclear:cytoplasmic ratio, possibly related to cdc25 driving MPF and a kinase cascade which triggers mitosis. The gradual depletion of cdc25 causes a pause in cleavage, which allows time for the nuclear organizing region to develop, and mitosis induces a general repression of promoters prior to initiation of zygotic gene expression. Enhancers then specifically alleviate this repression. Thus, a biological clock delays transcription until both paternal and maternal genomes are replicated; they must then be remodelled from a postmeiotic state to one in which transcription is repressed by chromatin structure. The configuration of this chromatin structure must be such that specific transcription enhancers can then relieve the repression at appropriate times during development. Differential hyperacetylation of histone H4 has also been implicated in the remodelling of maternal and paternal chromatin, and depletion of maternally derived histones has also been suggested as one of the mechanisms involved in ZGA (Adenot et al., 1997).

Chromatin-mediated repression of promoter activity prior to ZGA is similar to what is observed during *Xenopus* embryogenesis; this mechanism ensures that genes are not expressed until the appropriate time in development. When the time is right, positive acting factors such as enhancers can then relieve this repression. The mechanism by which enhancers communicate with promoters seems to change during development, and may depend upon the acquisition of specific co-activators (at the 2-cell stage in mice, perhaps later in other mammals).

Imprinting

A zygotic nucleus has an imprint memory that is retained forever; this controls when genes are expressed. Functional differences between parental chromosomes are heritable, and survive activation of the embryonic genome. Data derived from both pronuclear transplantation experiments and classical genetic experiments indicate that the maternal and paternal genetic contributions to the mammalian zygote nucleus do not function equivalently during subsequent development (Surani et al., 1986). These observations suggest that there is differential 'genome imprinting' during male and female gametogenesis. The molecular mechanism responsible for genome imprinting is unknown, but experimental data gathered to date suggest the following common features:

(1)   The imprint is physically linked to the pronucleus
(2)   The imprint persists through DNA replication and cell division
(3)   The mechanism is capable of affecting gene expression
(4)   The mechanism is capable of switching the identity of the imprint from one sex to the other in successive generations.

One molecular mechanism that could satisfy the first of these criteria is differential DNA methylation during gametogenesis itself, or before formation of the zygote nucleus during embryogenesis (Sapienza et al., 1987). Genomic imprinting must be distinguished from Y-linkage and cytoplasmic and other maternal effects, as processes that influence genetic inheritance. The molecular bases for these critical genetic events require further studies into the initiation and maintenance of imprinting mechanisms.

PCR-based cDNA libraries from single human preimplantation embryos are currently under development, and now provide a new and important resource for the identification and study of novel genes or gene families (Adjaye et al., 1998). Differential display PCR using cDNA libraries as template allows the analysis of stage-specific expression of embryonic genes, and will increase our basic understanding of the molecular control of human development by identifying the time of onset of specific genes. Eventually it may be possible to explore disease-causing mechanisms resulting from mutation of these genes.

The molecular analysis of early gene transcription in human embryogenesis may lead to new avenues of progress in reproductive medicine, in particular assisted reproduction and preimplanation genetic diagnosis.

Compaction

In order to co-ordinate the complex process of cell growth and differentiation during early embryogenesis, the embryonic cells must be in communication. Communicative devices arise early in development and may serve additional roles in the synchronization of early divisions and the determination of the future planes of mitotic spindles. Two types of intercellular junction have been described:

1   Structural tight junctions and desmosomes, which serve to anchor the cells together and also form a permeability seal between cells. Tight junctions are composed of several integral and peripheral proteins, including occludin and cingulin (ZO-1)

2   Low resistance junctions, such as gap junctions, that allow the flow of electrical current and the direct transfer of small molecules, including metabolites and second messengers (cAMP) between blastomeres.

During the first few cleavage divisions to reach the 4–8 cell stage, the individual blastomeres of the developing embryo can be clearly seen. The next stage of embryo development involves compaction, where the blastomeres flatten against each other and begin to form junctions between them, so that the boundaries between blastomeres can no longer be distinguished. The cells of the compacted embryo become highly polarised, and are tightly associated and communicating. This process has been extensively studied in the mouse: surface polarity can be seen by the appearance of dense microvillar and amicrovillar regions, and cytoplasmic polarity can be seen in the distribution of endocytotic vesicles, actin filaments, and the location of the cell nucleus. In the mouse, polarity is maintained in isolated blastomeres following experimental decompaction, and requires neither the prior round of DNA replication, or protein synthesis (Kidder et al., 1985). Therefore, the 4-cell embryo probably contains some of the proteins required for compaction. Although the factors which trigger the timing of its onset are not known, experimental evidence suggests that this may be regulated by post-translational modification of specific proteins such as E-cadherin. The protein E-cadherin (uvomorulin) is expressed in the oocyte, and during all stages of preimplantation development. It is uniformly distributed on the surface of blastomeres, and accumulates in

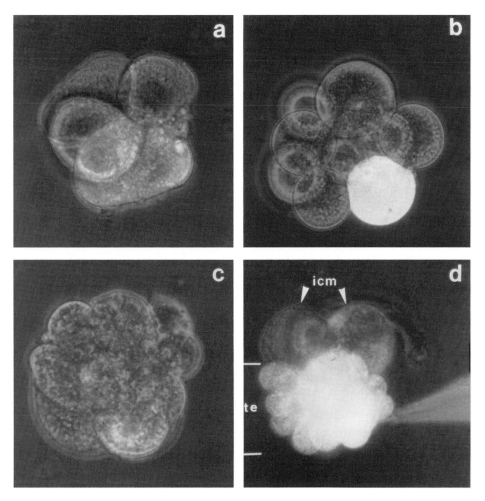

Figure 4.5   Functional expression of gap junctions in the early human embryo shown by microinjection of the low molecular weight tracer lucifer yellow. There is no dye spread in 4 cells (a) 10 cells (b) or morula (c). However, transfer occurs in the blastocyst stage.

the regions of intercellular contact during compaction. E-cadherin phosphorylation can be observed in the mouse 8-cell embryo. Culturing embryos in calcium-free medium prevents compaction, and this also inhibits E-cadherin phosphorylation, but the situation is complex, and precise mechanisms behind the molecular basis for compaction and its timing remain unclear.

In human embryos, tight junctions begin to appear on Day 3, at the 6–10 cell stage, heralding the onset of compaction. Nikas et al. (1996) studied surface morphology of human oocytes and embryos with scanning electron microscopy, and show that unfertilized oocytes one day after insemination were evenly and densely covered with long microvilli. The length and density of microvilli appeared to decrease in fertilized oocytes, and a further decrease was observed in Day 2 and Day 3 embryos with 2–12 cells. There was no evidence of surface polarity of compaction until Day 4, when it was evident in the majority of embryos with 10 or more cells. The microvilli appeared dense again with a polarized distribution over the free surface of the compacted blastomeres. In the mouse, gap junctions are expressed at the 8-cell stage, and their *de novo* assembly during compaction is a time-dependent event. In human embryos, gap junctions are not apparently well developed until the early blastocyst stage, when intercellular communication is clearly seen between ICM cells (Dale et al., 1991; Figure 4.5).

Following compaction, the developing embryo is described as a morula, seen in the human normally four days after fertilization. Whereas cleavage planes up to this stage are apparently random, in the mouse the cleavage planes are no longer random after the 16-cell stage, and subsequent cleavage divisions allocate cells to the interior of the morula. The embryo now shows a significant increase and change of pattern in RNA, protein, and phospholipid synthesis, and this results in a process of differentiation so that cells are allocated to an inner cell mass (ICM), with outer cells forming an epithelial layer of trophectoderm. ICM cells preferentially communicate with each other and not with trophectoderm cells via gap junctions, whereas trophectoderm cells communicate with each other and not with ICM cells.

Between the 16- and 32-cell stage, a second morphological change occurs, known as cavitation. Activation of Na^+, K^+ ATPase systems result in an energy-dependent active transport of sodium pumped into the central area of the embryo, followed by osmotically driven passive movement of water to form a fluid-filled cavity, the blastocoel. The movement of other ions such as chloride and bicarbonate also contributes to blastocoel formation. In vitro, the ionic environment can affect blastocyst formation, and high sodium concentrations can depress the synthesis of mRNAs and proteins. Pumping is only possible because the trophectodermal cells become polarized to form an epithelial layer, but the mechanisms of polarization are unknown. Tight junctions form a continuous belt between trophectoderm cells, and prevent leakage of small ions present in the blastocoel. The cells can be shown by immunohistochemistry to be sitting on a basement membrane, a thin sheet of extracellular matrix material. However, it is not clear whether this basement membrane is a cause or a consequence of trophectodermal cell polarization. The ratio of trophectoderm to ICM cells can be influenced by culture conditions in vitro, and this might have implications for further embryonic/fetal development. Blastocoele formation and expansion is critical for further development, as it is essential for further differentiation of the ICM. This is now bathed in a specific fluid medium, which may contain factors and proteins that will influence cell proliferation and differentiation. The position of cells within the ICM in relation to the fluid cavity might also contribute to the differentiation of the outer cells into primitive endodermal cells. The trophectoderm cells will eventually form the placenta and extra-embryonic tissue. Myxoploidy of trophectoderm cells is a common feature in all animal species, regardless of their implantation mechanisms; i.e., mouse and cow, which differ completely in their mechanism of implantation, show this feature, with chromosome complements of 2n, 4n, 8n in their trophectoderm cells. However, in humans, it could possibly be considered as the initiation of syncitiotrophoblast formation. The regulation of this process, and apparent lack of division in these cells, remains a mystery – but it seems to be related to the appearance of giant cells in the trophectoderm, suggesting that regulation of the nuclear/cytoplasmic ratio is involved. It is interesting to note that there is a counterpart of 'giant cells' in the uterus around the time of implantation. Apoptosis can be seen at the blastocyst stage, localized to the inner cell mass: this may represent a mechanism for the elimination of inappropriate or defective cells.

Causes of embryo arrest

Cleaved embryos do frequently arrest their development in culture, and a great deal of research has been carried out in animal systems to elucidate possible causes and mechanisms. The longest cell division cycle during development is that during which genome activation takes place, when the the final maternal transcripts are degraded and massive synthesis of embryonic transcripts is initiated. Maternal reserves are normally sufficient until transcription begins, but epigenetic effects of defective sperm can lead to accumulation of delays, with resulting arrested development. Antisperm antibodies can have deleterious effects at this stage, by immunoneutralization of proteins that signal division (CS-1) or regulation (Oct-3). After genome activation, the next critical stage is morula/blastocyst transition. Complex remodelling takes place, and poor sperm quality can compromise this transition (see Ménézo & Janny 1997).

Embryonic arrest is frequently a result of events surrounding maturation, but can be a result of any metabolic problem. In bovine and pig oocytes, insufficient glutathione inhibits decondensation of the sperm head and polar body formation, and genetic factors regulate the speed of preimplantation development. Genetic factors implicate enzyme deficiencies or dysfunctional regulation, which may have deleterious effects. In domestic animals, as in humans (Ménézo & Janny, 1997), there is an age-related maternal effect. Maternal age has an effect on embryo quality, especially on blastocyst formation – this may be related to an ATPase dependent Na^+/K^+ pump mechanism, or to a poor stock of mRNA, poor transcriptional and/or post-transcriptional regulation, or accelerated turnover of mRNA. Some maternal mRNAs are present until the blastocyst stage, and may be involved in blastocyst development.

Fluorescent in situ hybridization (FISH) analysis of cleaved human embryos has confirmed that chromosomal aberrations are found in a significant proportion of embryos which develop with regular cleavage and morphology; this undoubtedly contributes to the high wastage of embryos in human IVF.

Paternal factors

Sperm quality may have an influence on embryogenesis and implantation potential. Increasing paternal age is thought to have an influence on fertility, possibly through increased nondisjunction in the sperm. Damage during spermatogenesis may be induced by reactive oxygen species and defective oxidative phosphorylation, or via inherited dysfunctional mitochondrial DNA. Fertilization by a sperm which is diploid, with incomplete decondensation and DNA activation, or inadequate chromatin packaging may cause aneuploidy or lack of genome competence in the embryo. The quality of condensation and packaging of sperm DNA are important factors for the initiation of human embryo development, even after intracytoplasmic sperm injection (ICSI). The centrosome, involved in microtubular organization, is the first epigenetic contribution of the sperm, and correct and harmonious microtubule arrangement is necessary for chromosome segregation and pronuclear migration. An abnormal sperm carrying an imperfect centrosome can disrupt mitosis, provoking problems at the beginning of embryogenesis with the formation of fragments, abnormal chromosome distribution, and early cleavage arrest. Twenty-five per cent of apparently unfertilized eggs have been shown to be fertilized, but with anomalies of cell division. In bulls, there is a positive correlation between spermaster formation at the time of fertilization and the bull's fertility. In the human, paternal Y-linked genes are transcribed as early as the zygote stage, and compromised paternal genetic material could be transcribed at even this early stage, causing fertilization failure or embryonic arrest

Metabolic requirements of the early mammalian embryo in vitro   *Yves Ménézo*

As described earlier, embryo development is initiated from oocyte reserves, accumulated during years prior to and during its growth. When the oocyte is fertilized and starts the process of transcription, the new embryo must maintain an equilibrium between many different parameters:

1. Its endogenous pool of metabolites, largely the result of final stages of oocyte maturation
2. Metabolic turnover of RNA messengers and proteins
3. Active uptake of sugars, aminoacids, and nucleic acid precursors
4. Passive transport, especially of lipids
5. Incorporation of proteins such as albumin which can bind lipids, peptides and catecholamines.

ATP as an energy source is a basic requirement, and mammalian cells can generate ATP either by aerobic oxidation of substrates to CO_2 and H_2O, or by anaerobic glycolysis of glucose to lactic acid. Under in vitro conditions, oocytes and embryos generate ATP by aerobic oxidative metabolism of pyruvate, lactate, amino acids and possibly lipids. As the blastocyst stage is reached, glucose consumption increases. Cumulus cell metabolism undoubtedly influences the concentration of substrates available to the oocyte and embryo in vivo, and in vitro cumulus cells can produce pyruvate for at least 6 days of culture.

The correct balance of electrolytes is always an essential basis for biochemical processes that lead to energy production and cAMP-based regulatory mechanisms. K^+ and HCO_3^- are involved in sperm capacitation, and intracellular pH regulation is a vital aspect of correct homeostasis. HCO_3^- has a particular role in activation, via an increase in cAMP content of sperm. Iron and copper cations appear to arrest embryo development, encouraging free radical formation – therefore EDTA (or penicillamine) in early stage culture media is beneficial as a chelating agent (but not in fertilization medium, as it chelates calcium which is essential for sperm motility, capacitation and acrosome reaction). EDTA appears to be deleterious after genome activation, and should be removed in the second phase of culture.

Prior to genome activation, pyruvate or lactate are primary energy sources;

pyruvate may be the better substrate, as it can remove toxic ammonium ions via transamination to alanine. Glucose has been found to be toxic at this stage, and it has been suggested that glucose and phosphate together may inhibit early embryo development by several different mechanisms, including the induction of glycolyis at the expense of substrate oxidation, through disrupted mitochondrial function. High levels of glucose can lead to excessive free radical formation. However, the biochemistry involved is highly complex, and results vary according to the basic medium used as well as the culture system (see Elliott & Elder, 1997). The toxic effect is dependent upon the overall composition of the media, and in some systems the negative effect of glucose may be counterbalanced b the presence of a correct amino acid balance (see Gardner, 1999). Amino acids and EDTA suppress glycolysis through different combinations, and act in combination to further suppress glycolysis. After genome activation, glucose becomes a key metabolite, required for lipid, amino acid and nucleic acid synthesis. It is also essential for blastocyst hatching, when there is an absolute requirement for C-5 sugars in pentose phosphate pathways. Lipids can be synthesized (through C-2 condensation reactions), accumulated from the surrounding medium or carried with albumin. Cholesterol synthesis is possible, but slow: there is a rate-limiting step at the level of hMG CoA reductase. If synthesis of cholesterol is experimentally inhibited by chetosterol, the embryos arrest and die.

Amino acids are also important regulators of embryo development, with both essential and nonessential amino acids showing specific effects on development and cleavage. However, it is difficult to define exactly which amino acids are in fact essential for the embryo. They are unlikely to be equivalent to the 'essential amino acids' necessary for nutrition of the entire individual. The ratio between different amino acids appears to be more important than their actual concentration in culture media, as they compete with each other for membrane transport systems. Differing affinities for transport mechanisms means that a disequilibirum in the external milieu will be reflected in anomalies of the endogenous pool with potentially deleterious effects on protein synthesis. Active transport mechanisms have been confirmed by the finding that amino acids are found at a higher concentration inside embryos than in the surrounding medium. Reinforcing the complexity of the situation, Lane and Gardner (1997) report that the levels of carbohydrates and amino acids which support excellent development of cleavage stage mouse embryos do not support optimum blastocyst development and differentiation – and the levels of both which do support blastocyst development can actually impair the cleavage stage embryo.

S-amino acids play a particularly important role, in that methionine, via S-adenosyl methionine, is used for transmethylation reactions involving proteins, phospholipids and nucleic acids, and is probably involved in imprinting through this process. Methylation of nucleic acids is known to modulate gene expression and to participate in the mechanism of genomic imprinting. S-amino acids also participate in protecting the embryo from free oxygen radicals. Via cysteine, methionine is used for hypotaurine and taurine synthesis. Cysteine is a precursor of cysteamine and glutathione, and redox coupling between these amino acids helps the embryo to maintain its redox potential and prevent damage from peroxidative reactions. Cysteamine and glutathione play a major role in protecting embryos from the hazards of oxidative stress. Taurine can neutralize toxic aldehyde by-products of peroxidative reactions.

Glycine is an energy source, as it can be deaminated immediately and forms glycollate and glyoxylate (C-2 metabolites), and also acts as a precursor for peptides, proteins and nucleic acids. It is a chelating agent for toxic divalent cations, has an in vitro osmoregulatory role, and is implicated in the regulation of intracellular pH of the embryo.

Deamination reactions are an important part of the biochemical and metabolic processes, and free ammonia is immediately recycled by efficient enzyme systems present in the oviduct. In vitro, in the presence of incubator CO_2, free ammonia forms carbonate and ammonium bicarbonate, both unstable compounds. If the embryo cultures are 'open', without oil, ammonia is liberated and eliminated by the CO_2 atmosphere. However, within microdrops under oil, ammonia can accumulate which is toxic to the embryo – Gardner and Lane (1993) demonstrated severe teratogenic effects in mouse embryos.

At a very early stage, embryos can synthesize purine and pyrimidine bases, precursors of RNA and DNA. These bases can also be actively transported from the surroundings, and there is an exponential increase in the accumulation of these precursors during the transition from morula to blastocyst.

Cleavage patterns

The first cleavage plane in sea urchin embryos is (as in most animals) vertical, extending from the animal to the vegetal pole. The second division is also along the animal–vegetal (A–V) axis, but at right angles to the first. Thus at this stage there are four elongated blastomeres lying side by side (Figure 4.6). The third cleavage plane is equatorial (i.e. perpendicular to the first two planes) and divides the embryo into a tier of four animal blastomeres and a tier of four vegetal blastomeres. From now on the animal blastomeres cleave at one rate,

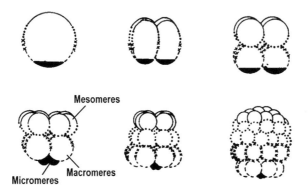

Figure 4.6   Schematic formation of the tier structure of differentiated cells in the regulative sea urchin embryo. Modified after Horstadius (1939).

the vegetal blastomeres at a different rate, and the blastomeres start to differ in size. The 4 animal blastomeres divide meridionally forming a ring of 8 mesomeres, while the 4 vegetal blastomeres cleave horizontally with the cleavage plane shifted towards the vegetal pole. This latter division gives rise to 4 large macromeres and 4 tiny micromeres. Division continues, with the blastomeres becoming smaller and smaller until the embryo assumes a spherical shape, the blastula, consisting of a single layer of cells surrounding a liquid filled cavity, the blastocoel. The segregation of the 4 micromeres is of particular interest: these cells are committed to form the skeleton of the pluteus larva, and they also play an organizing role in embryogenesis.

Spiral cleavage, encountered in the molluscs, annelids and nemerteans, is similar to the above pattern; however, the mitotic spindles are positioned obliquely with respect to the axis and equator of the blastomeres and as a consequence the daughter blastomeres do not lie directly above one another. For example, consider the third cleavage in the mollusc *Trochus*. Each of the four blastomeres divides into a small micromere and a large macromere. Thus, there is an upper tier of 4 micromeres (animal pole) and a lower tier of 4 macromeres (vegetal pole). The quartet of micromeres is however shifted clockwise with respect to the macromeres so that the micromeres lie at the junctions of the lower cells rather than directly over them. Cleavage progresses in this elegant fashion forming spirals of blastomeres until late in development when the pattern becomes modified into one of bilateral symmetry.

Large quantities of yolk tend to slow down the process of cleavage and consequently the pattern of cleavage is extensively modified in yolk-rich oocytes. In amphibian oocytes, the yolk is distributed in a gradient with a maximum at the vegetal pole. Cleavage in these oocytes progresses faster at the animal pole than at the vegetal pole and consequently the animal blastomeres increase in number and decrease in size at a faster rate than the vegetal blastomeres.

In all the previous examples, cleavage is complete or holoblastic, dividing the entire oocyte into a number of small cells. In fish, birds and reptiles, cleavages are incomplete or meroblastic, i.e. they pass through the restricted mass of cytoplasm located at the animal pole and not through the yolk. The embryo develops as a disc of cells perched on top of a yolk mass, the blastodisc. Another type of incomplete cleavage is found in the oocytes of insects. Here the zygote nucleus, lying in the centre of the oocyte, divides several times without the partitioning of the cytoplasm and the resulting nuclei migrate to the cell periphery. The peripheral cytoplasm segments around each nucleus and forms cells which remain in cytoplasmic contact with the central yolk body.

Cytoplasmic segregation and the formation of cell lines

In the previous section, we looked briefly at some of the patterns of cleavage found in the animal kingdom. In some cases, the pattern seems to be related to the constitution of the oocyte as laid down during oogenesis, in particular to the amount and distribution of yolk; in other cases factors controlling the positioning of the mitotic spindles seem to be important. Whichever pattern is employed, cleavage causes a partitioning of cytoplasmic components and this leads to differences in the developmental behaviour of blastomeres and the formation of different cell lines. Consider two classical examples, both marine invertebrate embryos, but quite different in their behaviour.

1. Shortly after fertilization the cytoplasmic components of the ascidian oocyte are redistributed according to a certain pattern and form five distinct territories or plasms (Figure 4.7). During cleavage these plasms become compartmentalized into different blastomeres which in turn give rise to the various cell lines. The first cleavage plane coincides with the A–V axis and divides these plasms equally between the first two blastomeres; in this way the future plane of bilateral symmetry of the larva is established. The left blastomere is committed to become the left half of the larva, the right blastomere to become the right half. Due to the small number of cells in these embryos, it is relatively easy to follow cell lineage from the early cleavage stages. Each plasm gives rise to a particular tissue. For example, the yellow crescent becomes the vegetal posterior part of the embryo and eventually gives rise to the musculature of the tail, while the clear transparent cytoplasm becomes the ectoderm. This

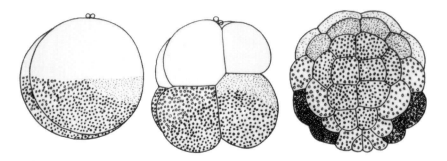

Figure 4.7   In the ascidian embryo segregation of cytoplasmic components generates different plasms that eventually localize to specific groups of cells. The polar bodies mark the animal pole. Modified from Monroy & Moscona (1979).

highly anisotropic structure of the fertilized oocyte prompted embryologists at the turn of the last century to classify such oocytes as mosaic structures.

2. In the sea urchin embryo, the organization of the early embryo is quite different (Figure 4.6). After fertilization there is no obvious segregation of cytoplasmic components and although cleavage results in the compartmentalization of the cytoplasm, the blastomeres retain a certain degree of flexibility. Thus, although each blastomere in situ develops into a certain part of the embryo it retains the capacity to differentiate into other tissue types. This capacity can be demonstrated by simple experimentation. If a blastomere is isolated from a two or four cell embryo, it can reorganize itself and give rise to a whole larva. This phenomenon is called regulation. Amphibian and mammalian blastomeres may also be described as regulative. Blastomeres from mosaic embryos do not have this capacity. For example, if the blastomeres of a two-cell ascidian embryo are physically separated, each blastomere gives rise to what it would have produced if left in situ, i.e. a half larva. There is a limit to the regulative capacity of sea urchin blastomeres, and a gradient of factors essential for normal development lies along the A–V axis of the unfertilized sea urchin oocyte. Blastomeres are only capable of regulation if they possess the vegetal factors. As previously mentioned above, the first two cleavages in the sea urchin are longitudinal and therefore all four blastomeres contain some of the vegetal factors. The third cleavage is equatorial, and if the animal blastomeres are separated from the vegetal blastomeres only the latter cells are capable of forming a whole larva. The elegant implantation experiments of Horstadius in the 1920s and 1930s demonstrated that these vegetal factors are in fact distributed in a gradient. Essentially, in the 64-cell stage embryo there are three tiers of vegetal blastomeres: those nearest the animal blastomeres are nominated Veg 1, the next layer Veg 2, and the micromeres form the distal layer. If an equatorial cut is made through the embryo and the

animal half isolated this will only give rise to a permanent blastula. However, if the micromeres from a second embryo are removed and implanted onto this isolated animal half, a normal embryo will develop. A similar though weaker effect is exerted by implanting the Veg 2 blastomeres, but using the Veg 1 blastomeres results in a defective larva.

The process of embryogenesis is complex, involving cell growth, differentiation and movement.

The mechanism by which nuclear activity may be irreversibly modified by changes in the cytoplasmic environment has been discussed, and indeed this seems to be the key to understanding the phenomenon of cellular differentiation. Such processes are subtle, and to date they have not been clearly elucidated. In the nematode worm *Ascaris*, nuclear differentiation during embryogenesis is more obvious and can be followed by light microscopy. In this worm, the somatic cell line segregates from the germ cell line very early during the course of cleavage. During nuclear division, the cells of the germ line receive the full chromosome complement, whereas in somatic line cells the tips of the chromosomes are structurally modified and eventually cast off. We may conclude that the somatic cells do not require the full genetic complement for development, whereas the germ cells do require a full complement of genes. During later stages of embryogenesis, the somatic cell line differentiates further, forming the various tissues of the adult, but there is no further chromosome elimination.

Further reading

Adenot, P.G., Mercier, Y., Renard, J.P. & Thompson, E.M. (1997) Differential H4 acetylation of paternal and maternal chromatin precedes DNA replication and differential transcriptional activity in pronuclei of 1-cell mouse embryos. *Development* **124(22)**:4615–25.

Adjaye, J., Daniels, R., Monk, M. (1998) The construction of cDNA libraries from human single preimplantation embryos and their use in the study of gene expression during development. *Journal of Assisted Reproduction and Genetics* **15(5)**:344–8.

Ao, A., Erickson, R.P., Winston, R.M.L. and Handyside, A.H. (1994) Transcription of paternal Y-linked genes in the human zygote as early as the pronucleate stage. *Zygote* **2**:281–7.

Asch, R., Simerly, C., Ord, T., Ord, V.A. & Schatten, G. (1995) The stages at which human fertilization arrests: microtubule and chromosome configurations in inseminated oocytes which failed to complete fertilization and development in humans. *Human Reproduction* **10**:1897–1906.

Balinsky, B. (1965) *An Introduction to Embryology*. W.B. Saunders, Philadelphia.

Bavister, B.D. (1995) Culture of preimplantation embryos: facts and artefacts *Human Reproduction Update* **1**:91–148.

Bodmer, C.W. (1968) *Modern Embryology*. Holt, Rinehart and Winston, New York.

Cole, H. & Cupps, P. (1977) *Reproduction in Domestic Animals*. Academic Press, New York.

Cummins, J.M., Jequier, A.M. & Kan, R. (1994) Molecular biology of human male infertility: links with ageing, mitochondrial genetics, and oxidative stress? *Molecular Reproduction and Development* **37**:345–62.

Dale, B. (1983) *Fertilization in Animals*. Edward Arnold, London.

Dale et al. (1991) Gap junctional permeability in early and cleavage arrested ascidian embryos. *Development* **112**:153–60.

Edwards, R.G. & Beard, H.K. (1997) Oocyte polarity and cell determination in early mammalian embryos. *Molecular Human Reproduction* **3**:863–905.

Elliott, T. & Elder, K. (1997) *Blastocyst Culture, Transfer and Freezing*. World Wide Conferences on Reproductive Biology. Ladybrook Publishing, Australia.

Gardner, D. (1998) Changes in requirements and utilization of nutrients during mammalian preimplantation embryo development and their significance in embryo culture. *Theriogenology* **49(1)**:83–102.

Gardner, D.K. (1999) Development of serum-free media for the culture and transfer of human blastocysts. *Human Reproduction* **13, Suppl. 4**:218–25.

Gardner, D.K. & Lane, M. (1993) Amino acids and ammonium regulate mouse embryo development in culture. *Biology of Reproduction* **48**:377–85.

Horstadius, S. (1939) The mechanisms of sea urchin development, studied by operative methods. *Biological Reviews* **14**:132–79.

Janny, L. & Ménézo, Y.J.R. (1994) Evidence for a strong paternal effect on human preimplantation embryo development and blastocyst formation. *Molecular Reproduction and Development* **38**:36–42.

Kidder, G.M. & McLachlin, J.R. (1985) Timing of transcription and protein synthesis underlying morphogenesis in preimplantation of mouse embryos. *Developmental Biology* **112**: 265–75.

Lane, M. & Gardner, D.K. (1997) Differential regulation of mouse embryo development and viability by amino acids. *Journal of Reproductive Fertility* **109**:153.

Majumder, S., DePamphilis, M.L. (1994) Requirements for DNA transcription and replication at the beginning of mouse development. *Journal of Cell Biochemistry* **55(1)**:59–68.

Memili, E. Dominko, T, and First, N. (1998) Onset of transcription in bovine oocytes and embryos. *Molecular Reproduction and Development* **51**:36–41.

Ménézo, Y. & Dale, B. (1995) Paternal contribution to successful embryogenesis. *Human Reproduction* **10**:1326–7.

Ménézo, Y. & Janny, L. (1997) Influence of paternal factors in early embryogenesis. In: (Barrat, C., De Jonge, C., Mortimer, D. & Parinaud, J. eds.), *Genetics of Human Male Infertility*. Editions E.D.K., Paris, 246–57.

Ménézo, Y., Guerin, P. & Janny, L. (1998) Le développment embryonnaire précoce: aspects métaboliques et problemes pathologiques. In: (Hammamah, S. & Ménézo, Y. eds.), *L'ovocyte et l'embryon: de la physiologie à la pathologie*. Ellipses Editions, Paris.

Ménézo, Y., Khatchadourian, C., Gharib, A., Hamidi, J., Greenland, T. & Sarda, N. (1989) Regulation of S-adenosyl methionine synthesis in the mouse embryo. *Life Science* **44(21)**:1601–9.

Monroy, A. & Moscona, A. (1979) *An Introduction to Developmental Biology*. Chicago University Press.

Mortimer, D., Heinman, M., Peters, K. & Catt, J.W. (1998) Inhibitory effects of isoleucine and phenylalanine upon early human development. Abstracts of the 14th Annual meeting of the ESHRE, Göteborg 1998. *Human Reproduction* **13**:218–19.

Nikas, G., Ao, A., Winston, R.M. & Handyside, A.H. (1996) Compaction and surface polarity in the human embryo in vitro. *Biology of Reproduction* **55**:32–7.

Nothias, J.Y., Majumder, S., Kaneko, K.J. & DePamphilis, M.L. (1995) Regulation of gene expression at the beginning of mammalian development. *Journal of Biological Chemistry* **270(38)**:22077–80.

Palermo, G., Munné, S. & Cohen, J. (1994) The human zygote inherits its mitotic potential from the male gamete. *Human Reproduction* **9**:1220–5.

Sapienza, C., Peterson, A.C., Rossant, J., Balling, R. (1987) Degree of methylation of transgenes is dependent on gamete of origin. *Nature* **328(6127)**:251–4.

Sathananthan, H., Ng, S.C., bongo, A., Trounson, A. & Ratnam, S. (1993) *Visual Atlas of Early Human Development of Assisted Reproduction Technology*. Singapore University Press.

Schatten, G. (1994) The centrosome and its mode of inheritance: the reduction of the centrosome during gametogenesis and its restoration during fertilization. *Developmental Biology* **165**:299–335.

Schultz, R.M. (1993) Regulation of zygotic gene activation in the mouse. *Bioessays* **15(8)**:531–8.

Schultz, R.M. (1999) Preimplantation embryo development. In: *Molecular Biology in Reproductive Medicine*. (Fauser, B.C.M. (ed.), Parthenon Publishing, UK, 313–31.

Schultz, R.M. & Worrad, D.M. (1995) Role of chromatin structure in zygotic gene activation in the mammalian embryo. *Seminars in Cell Biology* **6(4)**:201–8.

Shire, J.G. (1989) Unequal parental contributions: genomic imprinting in mammals. *New Biology* **1(2)**:115–20.

Stein, P., Worrad, D., Belyaev, N., Turner, B. & Schultz, R. (1997) Stage-dependent redistributions of acetylated histones in nuclei of the early preimplantation mouse embryo. *Molecular Reproduction and Development* **47**:421–9.

Surani, M.A., Barton, S.C. & Norris, M.L. (1986) Nuclear transplantation in the mouse: heritable differences between parental genomes after activation of the embryonic genome. *Cell* **45(1)**:127–36.

Tucker, M.J., Morton, P.C., Wright, G., Sweitzer, C.L., Ingargiola, P.E. & Chan, S.Y.W. (1996) Paternal influence on embryogenesis and pregnancy in assisted human reproduction. *Journal of the British Fertility Society* **1(2)**, *Human Reproduction* **11**, Natl, Suppl.: 90–5.

Valdimarsson, G. & Kidder, G.M. (1995) Temporal control of gap junction assembly in preimplantation mouse embryos. *Journal of Cell Science* **108** (Pt 4):1715–22.

Van Blerkom, J. & Davis, P. (1995) Evolution of the sperm aster after microinjection of isolated human sperm centrosomes into meiotically mature human oocytes. *Human Reproduction* **10**:2179–82.

Wade, P.A., Pruss, D. & Wolffe, A. (1997) Histone acetylation: Chromatin in action. *Trends in Biochemical Science* **22(4)**:128–32.

Wiekowski, M., Miranda, M. & DePamphilis, M.L. (1991) Regulation of gene expression in preimplantation mouse embryos: effects of the zygotic clock and the first mitosis on promoter and enhancer activities. *Development Biology* **147(2)**:403–14.

Wolffe, A. (1996) Chromatin and gene regulation at the onset of embryonic development. *Reproductive Nutritional Development* **36(6)**:581–607.

5

Endocrine control of reproduction

The previous chapters describe gamete biology at the cellular level. Synchrony is essential for correct embryo development, and to understand synchrony a basic knowledge of reproductive endocrinology is fundamental. Although sexual arousal, erection and ejaculation in the male are obviously under cerebral control, it is less obvious that the ovarian and testicular cycles are also co-ordinated by the brain. For many years after the discovery of the gonado-trophic hormones, follicle stimulating hormone (FSH) and luteinizing hor-mone (LH), the anterior pituitary gland was considered to be an autonomous organ. Animal experiments in which lesions were induced in the hypothalamus clearly demonstrated the mediation of reproductive processes by the nervous system. The hypothalamus, a small inconspicuous part of the brain lying between the midbrain and the forebrain, controls sexual cycles, growth, preg-nancy, lactation and a wide range of other basic and emotional reactions. Despite its small size, the hypothalamus is an extremely complicated structure. Each hypothalamic function is associated with one or more small areas which consist of aggregations of neurons called hypothalamic nuclei. Unlike any other region of the brain, it not only receives sensory inputs from almost every other part of the central nervous system (CNS), but also sends nervous impulses to several endocrine glands and to pathways governing the activity of skeletal muscle, the heart and smooth muscle. In the context of reproduction, several groups of hypothalamic nuclei are connected to the underlying pitu-itary gland by neural and vascular connections.

Gonadotrophin hormone releasing hormone (GnRH) is a neurosecretory product of neurons in the hypothalamus which is transported to the anterior pituitary through the portal vessels. GnRH, a decapeptide with the structure (Pyr)-Glu-His-Trp-Ser-Tyr-Gly-Leu-Arg-Pro-Gly-NH$_2$), is the most import-ant mediator of reproduction by the CNS. Any abnormality in its synthesis, storage, release or action will cause partial or complete failure of gonadal function. GnRH secretion occurs in a pulsatile mode and binds to specific receptors on the plasma membrane of the gonadotroph cells in the pituitary, triggering the inositol triphosphate second messenger system within the cells. This signal induces the movement of secretory granules towards the plasma membrane and eventually the pulsatile secretion of LH and FSH. Continued exposure to GnRH or to a GnRH analogue results in a maintained occupancy of the receptors, uncoupling the receptor from its signal transduction system, and eventually leads to a reduction in LH and FSH secretion (Figure 5.1).

In summary, alterations in the output of GnRH, LH and FSH may be achieved by changing the amplitude or frequency of GnRH, or by modulating the response of the gonadotroph cells. In female primates, gonadotrophin output is regulated by the ovary. Low circulating levels of oestradiol exert a negative feedback control on LH and FSH secretion, and high maintained levels of oestradiol exert a positive feedback effect. High plasma levels of progesterone enhance the negative feedback effects of oestradiol and hold FSH and LH secretion down to a low level. The secretion of FSH, but not LH, is also regulated by non-steroidal high molecular weight (around 30 000) proteins called inhibins found in follicular fluid: inhibin is found at high levels in late follicular phase plasma of fertile women.

The neuroendocrine mechanisms which regulate testicular function are fundamentally similar to those which regulate ovarian activity. The male hypothalamo–pituitary unit is responsible for the secretion of gonadotrophins which regulate the endocrine and spermatogenic activities of the testis, and this gonadotrophin secretion is subject to feedback regulation. A major difference between male and female reproductive endocrinology is the fact that gamete and steroid hormone production in the male is a continuous process after puberty, and not cyclical as in the female. This is reflected in the absence of positive feedback control of gonadotrophin release by testicular products. In the male, LH stimulates the production of testosterone by the Leydig cells and this testosterone in turn regulates LH secretion by reducing the frequency and amplitude of LH peaks. Although less clearly than in the female, inhibin-like molecules in the male have also been found in testicular extracts, which presumably also regulate FSH secretion. In humans, failure of spermatogenesis is correlated with elevated serum FSH levels, perhaps through reduced inhibin secretion by the testis.

LH, FSH, TSH and hCG are heterodimeric glycoprotein molecules that share a common alpha-subunit, and differ by their unique beta-subunit. Only the heterodimers have biological activity. FSH and LH are synthesized in the same cells in the pituitary, the gonadotroph cells, and are secreted in discrete

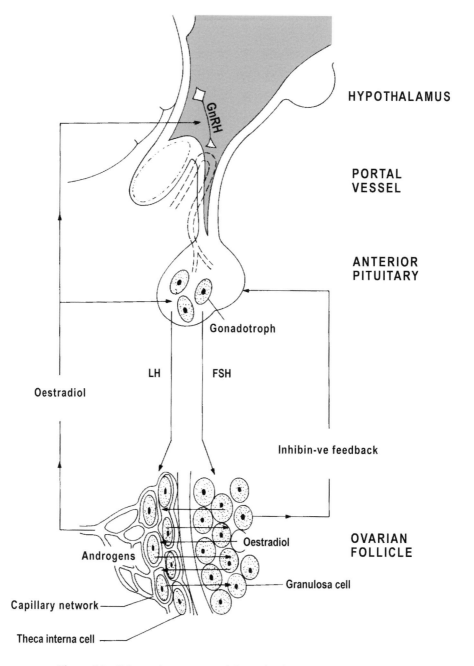

Figure 5.1   Schematic summary of the endocrine control of reproduction in mammals. From Johnson & Everitt (1990).

pulses. In the testis, LH acts on Leydig cells, and FSH on Sertoli cells; males are very sensitive to changes in activity of LH and are relatively resistant to changes in FSH activity. In the ovulatory cycle, FSH stimulates the growth of follicles and increases the rate of granulosa cell production, the aromatization of androgenic precursors, and the appearance of receptors for LH/hCG on granulosa cells. Oestrogens enhance the action of LH on the follicle, and also exert a negative feedback effect on the hypothalamus and pituitary to inhibit further release of gonadotrophins. The levels of oestrogen produced by the granulosa cells increase throughout the follicular phase until a threshold is reached where the negative feedback on gonadotrophin secretion is overridden by a separate positive feedback mechanism which elicits the LH surge – this is the trigger for ovulation. Inhibin is also secreted by the ovary, and reduces pituitary FSH secretion. LH stimulates theca cells to secrete androgens, which are converted to oestrogens by the granulosa cells, and also influences granulosa cell differentiation, i.e. limits their replication and causes luteinization. The 'two cell two gonadotrophin' theory suggests that both FSH and LH are required for oestrogen biosynthesis, and this requires the co-operation of two cell types – theca and granulosa. LH stimulates the formation of progesterone directly from cholesterol in both granulosa and theca cells, and after ovulation the follicle changes rapidly from oestrogen to progesterone dominance within a short period of time.

The specific functions of FSH have been studied with targeted deletions in 'knock-out' mice: FSH-deficient male mice have a decrease in testicular size and epididymal sperm count, but remain fertile. In contrast, homozygous females with the mutation were infertile: their ovaries showed normal primordial and primary follicles, with no abnormalities in oocytes, granulosa, or theca cells, but these failed to develop beyond the preantral stage. The ovaries also lacked corpora lutea, and serum progesterone levels were decreased by 50% compared with normal mice. These studies indicate that, in mice, follicle maturation beyond the preantral stage is FSH-dependent, whereas spermatogenesis can continue in the absence of FSH.

During controlled ovarian hyperstimulation for assisted reproduction, GnRH agonists are used to suppress pituitary release of both LH and FSH. Follicle growth and development can be achieved by the administration of pure FSH alone, in the absence of exogenous LH. However, in women with hypogonadotrophic hypogonadism, who lack both LH and FSH, administration of FSH alone promotes follicular growth, but the oocytes apparently lack developmental competence. The difference between these two patient populations has been attributed to the fact that downregulation with a GnRH agonist leaves sufficient residual LH secretion to support FSH-induced follicular development. The response to FSH in downregulated ART patients is independent of serum LH levels at the time of starting FSH administration. Granulosa cells synthesize oestradiol in response to FSH and LH, and oestradiol levels per retrieved oocyte appear to be correlated to developmental competence of the oocytes. Follicular fluid contains high levels of steroids and enzymes, and aspiration of follicles during ART procedures removes this milieu from its natural environment after follicle rupture in vivo; in addition, follicle flushing removes the cells which would have been incorporated in the new corpus luteum. It is possible that this artificial separation may lead to luteal insufficiency or other subtle consequences on ovarian physiology which are not at present evident.

In vitro experiments using rodent whole follicle culture systems have demonstrated that follicle development to the preantral (Graafian) stage requires FSH, and is unaffected by oestrogens. Oestrogens do however affect the developmental potential of the oocyte. In vitro follicle culture systems in other species are currently under development which will doubtless eventually lead to the elucidation of the precise roles of theses hormones, and the interplay between them necessary to achieve the correct balance for optimum oocyte developmental competence.

Further reading

Austin, C.T. & Short, R.V. (1972) *Reproduction in Mammals.* Cambridge University Press, Cambridge.

Conway, G.S. (1996) Clinical manifestations of genetic defects affecting gonadotrophins and their receptors. *Clinical Endocrinology* **45**:657–63.

Cortvrindt, R., Smitz, J. & Van Steirteghem, A.C. (1997) Assessment of the need for follicle stimulating hormone in early preantral mouse follicle culture in vitro. *Human Reproduction* **12**:759–68.

Johnson, M. & Everitt, B. (1990) *Essential Reproduction.* Blackwell Publications, Oxford.

Kumar, T.R., Wang, Y., Lu, N. & Matzuk, M.M. (1997) Follicle stimulating hormone is required for ovarian follicle maturation but not male fertility. *Nature Genetics* **15**:201–3.

Loumaye, E., Engrand, P., Howles, C.M. & O'Dea, L. (1997) Assessment of the role of serum luteinizing hormone and estradiol response to follicle-stimulating hormone on in vitro fertilization outcome. *Fertility and Sterility* **67**:889–99.

Shenfield, F. (1996) FSH: what is its role in infertility treatments, and particularly in IVF? *Medical Dialogue* **471**:1–4.

Telfer, E.E. (1996) The development of methods for isolation and culture of preantral follicles from bovine and porcine ovaries. *Theriogenology* **45**:101–10.

6

Assisted reproductive technology in farm animals

Artificial insemination

Artificial insemination (AI) has for many years been the predominant method used to increase reproductive potential in agriculture. Although practised in many species, this technique is particularly useful in cattle, where the cost-benefit over natural mating is substantial. In many western countries, the majority of cattle are inseminated artificially. The most common method of semen collection involves the use of an artificial vagina which is designed to simulate natural conditions. This consists of a rigid cylindrical case with a rubber liner, which is lubricated on the inner surface. The space between liner and case is filled with warm water, usually at 40–45 °C, and pressure adjustments may be made by inflating with air. When the male mounts a dummy female the penis is deflected by the operator into the artificial vagina and the ejaculate is collected in a suitably heated receptacle. An alternative method, for use with difficult or young males being taught to mount dummies, is electrojaculation using a rectal probe.

There are significant species differences in the volume of semen and the total number of spermatozoa in an ejaculate. The boar, owing to its large testis and to the short duration of its spermatogenic cycle, produces up to 500 ml of semen containing 45×10^9 of spermatozoa (1×10^8/ml) and can produce even larger volumes of up to 1500 ml. The bull, in contrast, produces an average of 5 ml of semen with a concentration of up to 7×10^9/ml. Whereas a stallion can produce 60 ml with a concentration of 9×10^9/ml, rams produce only 1 ml of semen on average, with a concentration of 3×10^9/ml. The number of spermatozoa that can be exploited from an animal varies greatly and depends on the frequency of semen collection. A mature dairy bull produces about $13\,000 \times 10^6$ spermatozoa per day. In cattle the cervix is held via the rectum so that a pipette can be guided into the uterus to deposit the semen. Normally

1 ml of semen is deposited, with an optimum number of 10 million spermatozoa. In sheep, due to the folding of the cervix, the spermatozoa are deposited within the first fold of the cervix by means of a fine catheter. In this case more spermatozoa are generally required, and 100 million sperm are usually deposited. The pig, however, requires 2000 million spermatozoa diluted to 50–100 ml, delivered via a corkscrew-shaped catheter similar to the shape of the glans penis of the male.

As the fertile lifespan of spermatozoa in the female tract is limited, as is the ovulation period, the timing of insemination is one of the most important factors in AI. The luteinizing hormone (LH) surge controls the induction of ovulation, and oocyte release occurs 36–40 hours after this surge in the cow and human, 24 hours later in the sheep, and 40–42 hours later in the pig. The optimum time for insemination is 10–12 hours before ovulation. Delayed insemination, which may result in the fertilization of aged oocytes, may lead to polyspermy and anomalous development. Accurate diagnosis of oestrous in farm animals is therefore essential for success in AI. The greatest advantages from AI are as a result of developments in semen storage. Storage medium usually contains a cryoprotectant such as egg yolk, glycerol or dimethyl sulphoxide (DMSO), and the semen sample diluted with cryoprotectant is stored at $-196\,^{\circ}\text{C}$ in liquid nitrogen. Not all semen samples freeze–thaw adequately. Cattle and human spermatozoa are easy to freeze–thaw, while ram spermatozoa present more difficulties and boar sperm is very difficult.

The oestrus cycle in cattle and pigs is 21 days, while in sheep it is 16 days. In any group of animals, the cycles are randomly distributed, and pharmacological control of oestrus and ovulation is used for oestrus synchronization to improve the efficiency of AI and for the management of ET cycles. Prostaglandin analogues (Estrumate, Lutalyse, Prosolvin) are used to induce luteolysis when a corpus luteum is present, and this is combined with a progesterone implant (intravaginal or subcutaneously in the ear) to suppress the pituitary. A further dose of prostaglandin analogue is given on removal of the progesterone device.

Today, gonadotrophin releasing hormone (GnRH) analogues such as Buserelin or nafarelin are used to accurately control oestrus in the human. Treatment with exogenous gonadotrophins to induce ovulation is common practice in humans and farm animals alike. This is known as superovulation, and leads to an increased number of ovulated follicles. In all species, however, the limiting factor for productivity is the ability of the uterus to support supernumerary embryos. In many species, excess fetuses will die in the later stages of gestation. However, superovulation in combination with AI is successfully used to produce large numbers of embryos from animals of suitable pedigree. The embryos are then recovered by flushing the uterine cavity for transfer to one or more recipients. A large commercial industry of embryo transfer (ET) on this basis has been well established since the 1950s.

The embryo transfer industry saw little improvement in the technology of donor superovulation for nearly four decades. In vitro fertilization (IVF) of oocytes from the ovaries of valuable donors is now an alternative approach to conventional embryo production, and an effective means of increasing the reproductive efficiency of genetically superior females. In addition, IVF has been used to produce large numbers of embryos for research into the basic developmental and molecular biology of in vitro oocyte maturation and fertilization.

Bovine IVF
(with thanks to R. Brittain)

The first live calves produced as a result of in vitro fertilization of an oocyte were born in the USA, in 1981. This milestone in reproductive biotechnology inspired the development of IVF as the next potential commercial application of assisted reproduction, after AI and conventional transfer of embryos produced in vivo from superovulated donors (ET). Techniques for oocyte retrieval from the ovaries of live cows and heifers were developed from human IVF experience, and, in 1988, Dr Maarten Pieterse at the University of Utrecht in Holland successfully used transvaginal ultrasound recovery techniques in cows. This provided new opportunities for the whole embryo transfer industry, and many organizations now include OPU/IVF as an integral, if not predominant, part of their routine ET activities. A major advantage of the OPU/IVF technique over superovulation and uterine embryo flushing is that it can be performed at almost any stage of the ovarian cycle, usually without the need for superovulation. In routine flushing programmes, the calving interval of the donor is extended by at least two months, further adding to costs. This need not be the case with OPU/IVF. Donors can be rebred to fit a normal calving pattern, and oocyte collection can continue after service and during the first three months of pregnancy.

Donors for OPU are restrained in standing position, sedated, and epidural relaxation is administered. The vulva and perineum are thoroughly cleaned and the ultrasound transducer and needle guide passed into the vagina, lateral to the cervix. An ovary is manipulated rectally and placed against the head of the transducer so that fluid-filled follicles can be visualized on the monitor. Follicular contents are aspirated by passing a needle gently through the vaginal wall and into the ovary. Using constant vacuum pressure, the contents are aspirated through sterile tubing into a vessel containing warmed medium. Temperature of the tubes is controlled, and aspirates scanned under a binocular microscope to identify oocytes for processing in the laboratory. The success of this procedure depends not only on the number of oocytes collected, but also on their quality in terms of further developmental potential.

Post-mortem ovaries can also be used as a source of oocytes for in vitro culture in order to produce large numbers of embryos for research purposes (recent concerns about BSE and viruses make this source generally unsuitable for commercial ET). An average of 12.2 oocytes may recovered from each post-mortem ovary under laboratory conditions, with development of 6.2 blastocysts on average per slaughtered animal. These figures are for ovaries from healthy donors from slaughterhouse origin and are not necessarily comparable to the situation with casualty donors for genetic recovery. The conditions that the ovaries are stored under during transport to the lab, and the time after slaughter that oocytes are aspirated can influence the developmental competence of these oocytes. Optimal results are obtained by aspirating medium-sized follicles, 2.5–8 mm in size, 4 hours after slaughter.

Bovine IVF is carried out at 39 °C, the core temperature of the cow, and involves an initial period of oocyte maturation prior to fertilization and embryo culture. The oocytes and embryos are incubated in groups of 10, in Nunc 4-well dishes or in 50 μl droplets overlaid with oil. An atmosphere of 5% CO_2 in air is used for maturation, and some systems use a reduced oxygen concentration for embryo culture.

Maturation (IVM)

Cows may have two, and occasionally three follicular waves during a single ovarian cycle, each follicular wave lasting 4 to 5 days and usually leading to the ovulation of a single dominant follicle, with degeneration of the rest of the follicular cohort. During this time, the oocyte undergoes the maturation process. Oocytes from the larger follicles at the preovulatory stage may be mature, but the majority of oocytes aspirated at each OPU session are from smaller follicles 2–6 mm in diameter. These require a 24-hour period of maturation in the laboratory, using medium that is supplemented with LH, FSH, oestrogen and fetal calf serum or BSA. When aspirating follicles from slaughterhouse ovaries, oocytes are selected which have visible compact or slightly expanded cumulus layers, and these are similarly matured in vivo.

Fertilization (IVF)

Initial attempts to fertilize oocytes in vitro by direct application of semen were a failure. Successful fertilization was later achieved by using semen retrieved from a cow's uterus 12 hours after service, suggesting that sperm capacitation was a necessary step. After mating or AI, sperm can reach the site of fertilization in the oviduct very rapidly, sometimes within minutes. Ovulation usually takes place 24–30 hours after the onset of oestrus, so that semen is present in the uterus well in advance of the arrival of the egg. This time lag ensures that full capacitation has occurred, and also corresponds to the time required for oocyte maturation. In vitro, it is essential to have a reliable means of artificially capacitating sperm, and heparin is now routinely used. This glycosaminoglycan is present in the reproductive tract of the cow, and is believed to be involved in the natural process of capacitation in the live animal.

There is considerable variation between different bulls in the fertilizing capacity of their semen, not only in terms of fertilization rates, but also in the subsequent yield of embryos. A concentration of between 0.5 and 2 million prepared sperm per millilitre is used for IVF, with an expected fertilization rate in the region of 60–90%. As with maturation, the efficiency of the fertilization process can be markedly influenced by temperature. Spermatozoal penetration in bovine oocytes is less than 1% at 37°C, but can reach up to 90% at 39°C, the core temperature of the cow.

IVF procedures are carried out in media specifically formulated to mimic biochemical constituents of the uterus to promote sperm capacitation, and of the oviduct to simulate the environment needed for oocyte maturation and acquisition of developmental competence for fertilization. Hypotaurine, epinephrine and penicillamine are added in some systems. After a period of 18–24 hours incubation in fertilization medium with the calculated concentration of semen, fertilized oocytes (zygotes), are transferred to the final culture system.

Embryo culture (IVC)

After fertilization, embryos are cultured for a further 7 to 8 days for development to late morula or blastocyst stages, before embryo transfer – unlike the human IVF system, in cows early cleavage stage embryos do not implant.

Early IVF attempts for embryo production were extremely discouraging, as an apparent block in development occurred at the 8–16 cell stage. This developmental arrest was overcome by culturing embryos with the help of intermediate host oviducts, such as rabbits or sheep. Blastocyst stage embryos were then surgically retrieved for embryo transfer. This laborious method was overcome by developing a variety of coculture systems which aimed to mimic the oviductal environment, using cells from the oviduct, granulosa, cumulus or other common cell lines such as Vero or BRL.

Coculture systems have now been replaced with stage-specific, cell-free sequential media supplemented with amino acids, glutamine, lactate and fatty acid-free bovine serum albumin.

In the cattle industry, clinically infertile cows are generally the main candidates for IVF, i.e. cows unable to maintain pregnancy, and not able to produce embryos by superovulation treatment. IVF is also currently used to great advantage in pregnant cows and heifers, and in young maiden heifers prior to service. For research purposes, calves are used as donors, with OPU performed surgically, but to date development to blastocyst remains poor in this system.

There is still a noticeable individual donor variation at each level, in oocyte number and quality, fertilization rate, development to the blastocyst stage, pregnancy rate and fetal survival. None the less, a threefold increase in embryo production can be reached when IVF procedures are used in conjunction with superovulation programmes.

IVF during pregnancy

Pregnancy does not affect follicular wave patterns; for the first three months of gestation, OPU can still be routinely performed. Beyond three months, the weight of the fetus tips the uterus over the inner rim of the pelvis, which then pulls the ovaries forward and makes them difficult to manipulate.

Results

Generally speaking, at least two transferable embryos (blastocysts) should be obtained after each OPU/IVF session, with an expected implantation rate of 50–60% per fresh embryo transferred. Recovery figures for OPU are variable and unpredictable, just as they are for superovulated embryo recoveries. Zero recoveries are not uncommon, and collections of fifty or more oocytes from one OPU session have occasionally been rumoured. IVF with living donors produces approximately 25–40% development of oocytes to the blastocyst stage (higher with large numbers of slaughterhouse oocytes cultured together). In order to produce two transferable embryos per OPU session, at least seven oocytes need to be collected. This figure is frequently attainable with normal, healthy donors, but is unrealistic when dealing with problem or geriatric donors.

It is now generally accepted that more oocytes can be collected and consequently more embryos produced when OPU sessions are performed twice weekly. Aspiration of follicles every 3 or 4 days does not allow sufficient time for the development of a new dominant follicle, so that oestrus is prevented. As the dominant follicle reaches maturity, it suppresses the growth of the smaller, subordinate follicles which are selected for aspiration. OPU performed at, or close to oestrus is therefore usually unsuccessful. If the OPU is carried out once a week, the donors will occasionally come into oestrus, but this is infrequent, especially if they are subfertile. OPU once a fortnight allows a reasonable chance that the donor will be close to ovulation on the day, but this can be prevented with progesterone therapy.

The large calf syndrome

The majority of in vitro produced (IVP) calves are perfectly normal. However, it has become apparent that certain factors in the early in vitro environment of an embryo can sometimes have an adverse influence on fetal development and pre- and postnatal survival. It is not easy to assess the overall incidence of the large calf problem as a result of IVF. An occasional, but significant incidence of fetal oversize and consequent calving difficulty (dystocia) has always been recognized in calves produced from routine ET procedures after transfer of in vivo embryos. Reports accept that about 20% more IVF calves than in vivo produced calves are born above 50 kg and 2% more IVF calves above 60 kg. Recent evidence suggests that peroxidative damage to the trophectoderm cells of blastocyts in vitro may later prejudice the function of the placenta, causing delayed parturition by inadequate transfer of signals from fetus to mother. The major contributor to this artefact is thought to be serum in serum-supplemented or co-culture media.

It is not yet possible to predict safely or realistically how often or under what conditions fetal oversize is likely to occur. Measures can however be taken to minimise the risks:

1. Awareness of extended gestations, with appropriate induction of birth.
2. Selection of sires for IVF that are not known to be high dystocia risks.
3. Use of recipients that are well grown and whose pelvic measurements can be monitored.
4. Adoption of laboratory protocols that are less likely to contain ingredients currently felt to have an adverse influence on the problem, while still maintaining a reliable in vitro system.

Pregnancy results

Fresh IVF embryos produce an approximately 10% lower pregnancy rate compared to in vivo produced embryos, although pregnancy results naturally vary with differing situations, and unexpectedly good and disappointingly bad results can always shatter generalizations. Embryo and recipient quality are fundamental to pregnancy results; transfer of excellent quality IVF blastocysts into perfectly synchronized recipients under optimal conditions should result in a similar pregnancy rate to that expected from in vivo embryos. Morphological assessment of the in vitro embryos can be problematic: the viability of IVF morulae is difficult to appraise by microscopy alone, and some reduction in pregnancy rate may be due to the transfer of Day 7 morulae that have not progressed to the blastocyst stage because they have arrested development.

Results with frozen-thawed in vitro produced embryos were initially discouraging, with rates in the region of 20% lower than with in vivo frozen embryo transfers. However, recent advances in freezing techniques have made it feasible to achieve satisfactory results with thawed IVF embryos approaching those expected from in vivo embryos.

Sex distribution of in vitro produced calves

It has been suggested that more advanced blastocysts from a flush of in vivo produced embryos may result in a predominance of male calves, and a small increase in the birth of male IVF calves has been reported. In the in vitro situation, male and female embryos appear to develop at different speeds and the concept that more rapidly developing blastocysts are likely to be males has been given support. The possibility that Y-chromosome-bearing male sperm may have privileged access to the oocyte in in vitro culture has been suggested. However, some IVF culture conditions produce more rapidly developing embryos than others, and the speed of embryo development is more likely to be due to media constituents, or possibly the time of insemination, than to the sex of the embryo. Preselection of the sex of a calf is now readily available by assessing the Y chromosome of an embryo biopsy, and the sex distribution of IVF embryos should rapidly become apparent. Biopsy results from the sexing process will give an early indication of the male:female ratio; unless one sex has better in utero viability than the other does, this ratio should represent the sex prevalence in calves born. New semen-sorting techniques will soon revolutionize the cattle-breeding industry by providing sexed semen on demand.

On-farm embryo transfer sometimes takes place in adverse conditions, and the fact that it works at all is testimony to the embryo's ability to survive. The amazing power of reproduction is further reinforced by the fact that oocytes can be retrieved from the ovaries of living or recently dead animals, fertilized and cultured in completely foreign environments, and then relocated to grow into new offspring. The in vitro embryo is not quite as tough and resilient, although it is still a remarkable life form. Meticulous attention to detail at all the levels of OPU, IVM, IVF, IVC and transfer of the in vitro embryo is imperative for its survival. There are no short cuts in the IVF process. At each level of interference, the embryo shows a negative response. We now know that there is a slightly lower survival rate of in vivo transferred embryos compared with AI pregnancies. In vitro embryos are at higher risk of not surviving gestation, and frozen, biopsied IVF embryos have their long-term survival further compromised.

As long as progress is cautiously approached, remaining aware of the consequences of embryo intolerance to excessive interference, and with the well-being of donor, calf and recipient as the fundamental priority, in vitro techniques will continue to play a significant role in the genetic improvement of farm animals.

Gender selection

Embryos can be sex-selected either by preimplantation diagnosis after biopsy of an 8- to 10-cell embryo, or by sorting X- from Y-bearing sperm in the ejaculate. The only established difference between X- and Y-chromosome-bearing spermatozoa is the quantity of DNA in the sex chromosome. Many physical, chemical and immunological methods for separating X and Y spermatozoa have been proposed, but as yet there is no conclusive technique for separating sperm. In 1973, it was suggested that human Y spermatozoa are enriched when swimming downwards in albumin columns; since that time, over 100 papers have been published, with both positive and negative reports as to its success in influencing the sex ratio. The only scientifically proven method of separating X- and Y-bearing vital mammalian spermatozoa is the use of a flow cytometry sorter. Spermatozoa are labelled with a fluorescent DNA dye (Bisbenzimide) and exposed to ultraviolet excitation. Spermatozoa are deflected into one or other direction depending on the intensity of the signal, and X- and Y- bearing sperm separately collected. Unfortunately, the technique is slow, allowing only 300 000 spermatozoa to be processed per hour, and therefore it is not suitable for artificial insemination. In addition, it is highly likely that the DNA fluorochrome is teratogenic and, finally, the modified cell sorter is extremely expensive.

Microsurgery in mammalian embryos

Microsurgery was first used to study live mammalian oocytes in the late 1940s, and the 1950s and 1960s saw an increased interest in mammalian experimental embryology. A major influence during this period was T.P. Lin, who performed numerous studies on the technical and experimental nature of oocyte microsurgery. Lin and coworkers also studied the effect of partial microsuction of the egg cytoplasm on the development and transplantation of chromosomes into mammalian oocytes. Microsurgical approaches to the study of early mammalian development progressed with the use of exogenous gonadotrophins to increase the number of oocytes ovulated and consequently the number of preimplantation embryos available for experimental manipulation. A fundamental observation was made in 1968, when a single blastomere taken from an 8-cell rabbit embryo gave rise to a live birth.

During the past 30 years, a fascinating array of manipulations have been carried out on the preimplantation animal embryo. The majority of these experiments have involved the addition or removal of cells, or the transplantation of nuclei. More recently, exogenous DNA has been introduced into the zygote or early embryo to study the function of gene products, the regulation of gene expression and the generation of transgenic animals. Various microsurgical experiments have been devised to study the fate of early differentiating tissues, the contribution of cells from the ICM and the trophectoderm, and the timing of X-chromosome inactivation. In 1961, Andresz Tarkowski first produced a chimera, and in 1968 Richard Gardner generated chimeras by injecting cells into a blastocyst. In addition to intraspecific chimeras, a number of scientists have used interspecific chimeras to study early embryogenesis. This technique enables an embryo from one species to develop within the placenta and uterus of a second species, with subsequent delivery of viable chimeras; this has been achieved using the sheep and the goat.

Another microsurgical approach involves the removal of blastomeres in order to study the fate of partial embryos. In the 1980s, blastomere separation was utilized to produce genetically identical twins, triplets and quadruplets. These techniques have obvious implications in agriculture, where successful sexing of embryos and the production of two or more embryos from one embryo are of enormous cost-benefit to the farmer. Early attempts to transplant whole nuclei in mammalian zygotes to produce clones for animal husbandry were disappointing. On the other hand, the production of transgenic animals by direct microinjection of DNA into one of the zygote pronuclei has been relatively successful.

The term transgene describes novel DNA sequences introduced following laboratory manipulation of the zygote. The majority of transgenic animals have been made by pronuclear injection of naked linear DNA. Approximately 100 linear DNA molecules in a volume of one picolitre are injected into the pronucleus. The DNA is integrated into the recipient DNA during the early cleavage stages and the genetic trait is transmitted to the offspring. A great deal of excitement accompanied a report that foreign DNA mixed with mouse spermatozoa prior to in vitro fertilization, resulted in approximately 30% of pups carrying integrated transgenes. Unfortunately, a concerted international effort to repeat these results has been unsuccessful. The current gene transfer method of choice remains pronuclear injection. Fertilized oocytes are recovered from superovulated donors at the pronuclear stage (i.e. prior to formation of a single diploid nucleus). The injection procedure requires two micromanipulators to support the holding and injection pipettes respectively, and an inverted microscope with Hoffman optics. Embryos are held on a fire-polished glass holding pipette which is connected to a hydraulic control system. A second finely drawn pipette is introduced into the male pronucleus and several hundred copies of the gene construct are injected. Injection is accompanied by pronuclear swelling and probable chromosome damage (mechanical damage may actually be necessary for transgene integration). Injected embryos are incubated briefly to assess survival and then returned to the ampullae of synchronized females. There are developmental and physiological differences between species which reduce the efficiency of gene transfer in farm animals. While mouse pronuclei are readily visible with differential interference contrast (DIC), ungulate embryos contain a large number of lipid granules which tend to obscure internal structure. The pronuclei in the sheep can be seen under DIC in up to 90% of embryos, but in pigs and cattle, centrifugation is required to sequester these granules to one end of the zygote. The efficiency of gene transfer in farm animals is further reduced because small numbers of embryos are obtained per female.

The main disadvantages of pronuclear injection are effects due to the unpredictability of the site of incorporation, and poor reproducibility of experiments due to random incorporation. In addition we can only add, and not remove, sequences. The embryonic stem (ES) cell system is now well documented as an alternative route into the germline of mice which can potentially overcome all of these problems. An additional bonus is the possibility, through ES cells, for the application of site-directed mutagenesis to animals. The ES cell system capitalizes on the capacity of a subpopulation of embryonic cells to proliferate in the undifferentiated state in culture, while maintaining their ability to differentiate fully in vivo (totipotency). When reintroduced into the blastocoele cavity of early embryos, ES cells frequently contribute to the germ line. Hence, pigmented ES cells in albino embryos give rise to chimeric animals whose tissues (including gonads), are a mosaic of host embryo (albino) and ES (pigmented) genotypes. If chimeras are mated to albino females a proportion and, in some cases, all of the offspring will be pigmented, demonstrating the germline transmission of ES-derived DNA.

New technologies such as in vitro maturation, in vitro fertilization, improved culture systems, embryo biopsy and nuclear transfer will dramatically increase the efficiency with which transgenics can be produced. In farm animals, considered effort has been directed towards the introduction of extra copies of growth hormone genes. At the phenotypic level, results have been disappointing and appropriate genes for the improvement of quantitative traits still need to be identified. Engineering of the mammary gland as a source of recombinant protein is promising, although levels of recombinant protein secretion are constrained by our limited understanding of gene expression.

Nuclear transplantation of embryos has brought to the realm of researchers and animal breeders the possibility of producing large quantities of genetically identical animals by cloning. The technology of cloning started in amphibian embryos in the 1950s. Frog eggs were activated by pricking with a glass needle which causes rotation, bringing the animal pole to lie uppermost. The chromosomes are visualized as a black dot that can be extirpated surgically, or can be effectively ablated with laser or ultraviolet irradiation. A proportion of the embryos derived from the transplantation of nuclei from undetermined embryonic cells (blastula and gastrula stage) were able to support development into normal adults indicating that at least some of these cells are totipotent. Studies carried out using nuclei from determined regions of larvae have shown that only around 0.2% will develop to adults and another 4% will arrest at the larval stage (pluripotent nuclei).

As the volume of the mammalian oocyte is one thousand times smaller than that of frog oocytes it is not surprising that more refined methods of microsurgery were required before the development of techniques for nuclear transplantation could be usefully applied to mammals. The successful microinjection of embryonic nuclei into the cytoplasm of rabbit and mouse zygotes suggested that nuclei from later embryonic stages were able to participate with the oocyte genome in supporting preimplantation development. The first report of mice born from nuclear transplantation came from the work of Illmensee and Hoppe in 1981, showing that nuclei derived from the inner cell mass rather than the trophectoderm of mouse blastocysts were able to support development to the morula-blastocyst stage in 34% of the transferred embryos and that 19% of these would develop to term. These reports brought many scientists to speculate that this technique would provide a means of making an infinite number of genetically identical copies from a single embryo. In 1983, McGrath and Solter fused nuclei in a membrane-bound karyoplast to enucleated pronuclear zygotes. Fusion is performed by injecting a small amount of a solution of inactivated Sendai virus which causes the membranes of the karyoplast and the enucleated embryo to fuse within a few minutes of manipulation. Contrary to the poor levels of success obtained using Illmensee and Hoppe's invasive technique, this method proved to be virtually 100% successful.

By using this noninvasive technique, several laboratories have shown that nuclei derived from mouse 2-cell blastomeres are only able to support in vitro development to morula-blastocyst stages. Steen Willadsen in 1986 first reported the development to blastocyst and to term of sheep embryos derived from the transplantation of 8-cell blastomere nuclei to enucleated oocytes. The relevance of these findings was not exclusively related to the ability of a single 8-cell blastomere to support development, as this had already been shown in chimeric studies. The significant feature of this observation was that the resulting fused embryo would develop and differentiate as if commencing from the time of fertilization. This indicates that the oocyte cytoplasm has the capacity to reprogramme the developmental pathway of the donor nucleus.

The success of Ian Wilmut and colleagues (1996, 1997) in cloning adult sheep from a fibroblast derived from the mammary gland (udder) involved starving the adult cell line by nutrient depletion so that they arrested in the G0 resting phase of the cell cycle. This prevents an additional round of DNA replication, and so reduces the incidence of chromosomal abnormalities. Previous attempts used donor cells in S or G2 phases of the cell cycles. When nuclei from S or G2 phase cells are introduced into metaphase II oocytes they tend to

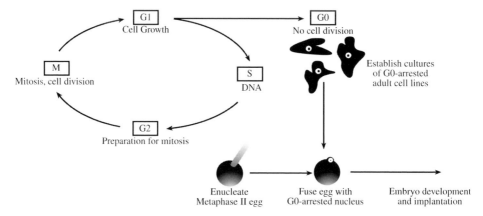

Figure 6.1   Schematic diagram showing the stages involved in nuclear transplantation techniques: cells are first arrested in G0, which prevents a round of DNA replication.

undergo additional DNA replication resulting in aneuploidy (see Figure 6.1). The cloning technique has been repeated in the bovine system, using fibroblast cells from an ear punch.

In general, secondary oocytes are obtained directly from the oviduct either during surgical intervention or at slaughter. One limitation for the use of oocytes as recipient cytoplasm concerns the nucleation procedure. With the exception of the rabbit, metaphase chromosomes cannot be readily visualized in secondary oocytes from farm species due to the presence of large lipid vesicles in the cytoplasm. Consequently, the position of the first polar body is used to indicate the position of the chromosomal plate for aspiration of the chromosomes and surrounding cytoplasm. Noninvasive methods for nuclear transplantation rely on an effective method for fusing the nuclear (karyoplast) and cytoplasmic (cytoplast) portions of two different cells.

Several methods are available for fusion, some of which are either unreliable and toxic, such as polyethylene glycol and lysolecithin, or laborious and dangerous, such as inactivated Sendai virus. Electrofusion has been successfully used to fuse blastomeres and for nuclear transplantation experiments in mammalian embryos derived from species as diverse as mice, rabbit, sheep, cattle and pigs. Fusion seems to be a result of the reversible instability of the plasma membranes in the zone of membrane contact between the cytoplasm and nuclear donor cells. Successful fusion can be attained using a large range of parameters for the direct current fusing pulse. Values of around 1 kV/cm field intensity with durations of 50–100 microseconds are commonly used. Alternating current pulses may be used to align the cells so that their membranes are positioned perpendicular to the electrical field where conditions for fusion are most appropriate. The preceding AC pulse is particularly important when fusing enucleated oocytes to cells with reduced diameters since the polarization caused by the AC field will help to bring their membranes into contact for the DC fusing pulse. Experiments with mouse pronuclear zygotes have indicated that cell cycle stage synchrony between nucleus and cytoplasm is beneficial for further development in vitro. This observation has been further extended to transplantations between 2-cell embryos where asynchronous exchanges were highly deleterious to further development. This effect may be explained either by the disruption of the cell cycle oscillatory mechanisms or by incompatible nucleo-cytoplasmic interactions in controlling critical developmental steps. It is important to note some of the possible disadvantages in the cloning procedure. One aspect concerns the decrease in genetic variability caused by inbreeding. Large foundation populations should be obtained when using cloning in conjunction with multiple ovulation and embryo transfer selection schemes. It is also important to verify the degree to which cytoplasmic inheritance can influence animal production as clones will not only be exposed to different uterine and neonatal environments, but also to a different ooplasm. The possible maternal inheritance of mitochondrial and centriole genomes are examples of differences that may arise between clones derived by nuclear transplantation. Another potential factor for consideration of genetic variation is the random inactivation of X chromosomes in females.

Further reading

Bols, P.E.J. (1997) Transvaginal ovum pick-up in the cow: technical and biological modifications, Ph.D. Thesis University of Gent.

Bousquet, D., Twagiramungu, N., Morin, N., Brisson, C., Carboneay, G. & Durocher, J. (1999) In vitro embryo production in the cow: an effective alternative to the conventional embryo production approach. *Theriogenology* **51**:59–70.

Brackett, R.G., Bousquet, D., Boice, M.L., Donawick, W.J., Evans, J.F. & Dressel, M.A. (1982) Normal development following invitro fertilization in the cow. *Biology of Reproduction* **27**:147–58.

Campbell, K.H., McWhir, J., Ritchie, W.A. & Wilmut, I. (1996) Sheep cloned by nuclear transfer from a cell line. *Nature* **380(6569)**:64–6.

Cibelli, J.B., Stice, S., Golueke, P., Kane, J., Jerry, J., et al. (1998) Cloned transgenic calved produced from nonquiescent fetal fibroblasts. *Science* **280**:1256–8.

Cole, H. & Cupps, P. (1977) *Reproduction in Domestic Animals*. Academic Press, New York.

Farin, P. & Farin, C. (1995) Transfer of bovine embryos produced in vivo or in vitro: survival and fetal development. *Biology of Reproduction* **52(3)**:676–88.

Fulka, J. First, N., Loi, P. & Moor, R. (1998) Cloning by somatic cell nuclear transfer. *Bioessays* **20**:847–51.

Gage, F. (1998) Cell therapy. *Nature* **392**:18–24.

Garry, F., Adams, R., McCann, J. & Odde K. (1996) Postnatal characteristics of calves produced by nuclear transfer cloning. *Theriogen* **45(1)**:141–52.

Goodhand, K.L., Watt, R.G., Staines, M.E., Higgins, L.C., Dolman, D.F., Hutchinson J.S.M. & Broadbent, P.J. (1997) In vivo embryo recovery vs. In vivo oocyte recovery and in vitro embryo production: embryo yields and pregnancy rates in cattle. *Theriogenology* **47**:364.

Gordon, I. & Lu, K. (1990) Production of embryos in vitro and its impact on livestock production. *Theriogenology* **33**:77–87.

Guyader Joly, C., Ponchon, S., Thuard, J.M., Durand, M., Nibart, M., Marquant-le Guienne, B. & Humblot P. (1997) Effects of superovulation on repeated ultrasound guided oocyte collection and in vitro embryo production in pregnant heifers. *Theriogenology* **47**:157.

Hafez, E.S.E. (1974) *Reproduction in Farm Animals.* Lea & Febiger, New York.

Kato, Y., Tani, T., et al. (1998) Eight calves cloned from somatic cells of a single adult. *Science* **282**:2095–8.

King, T. (1966) Nuclear transplantation in amphibia. *Methods in Cell Biology* **2**:1.

Kruip, Th.A.M. & den Daas, J.H.G. (1997 In vitro produced and cloned embryos: effects on pregnancy, parturition and offspring. *Theriogenology* **47**:43–52.

Leibfried, L. & First, N.L. (1979) Characterization of bovine follicular oocytes and their ability to mature in vitro. *Journal of Animal Science* **48**:76–86.

McEvoy, T.G. (1997) Calves: a limiting factor in IVF production. Cook Veterinary Products sponsored IVF Workshop, Cheshire.

McLaren, A. (1984) Methods and success of nuclear transplantation in mammals. *Nature* **309**:671–2.

Meintjes, M., Bellow, M.S., Broussard, J.R., Paul, J.B. & Godke, R.A. (1995) Transvaginal aspiration of bovine oocytes from hormone-treated pregnant beef cattle for IVF. *Journal of Animal Science* 73:967–74.

Palmiter, R. & Brinster, R. (1986) Germline transformation of mice. *Annual Reviews in Genetics* **20**:465–99.

Parrish, J.J., Susko-Parrish, J.L., Wimer, M.A. & First, N.L. (1998) Capacitation of bovine serum by Heparin. *Biological Reproduction* **38**:1171–80.

Pieterse, M.C., Kappen, K.A., Kruip, T.A.M. & Taverne, M.A.M. (1988) Aspiration of bovine oocytes during transvaginal ultrasound scanning of the ovaries. *Theriogenology* **30**:751–62.

Pieterse, M.C., Vos, P.L.A.M., Kruip, Th.A.M., Worth, Y.A., van Beneden, T.H., Willemse, A.H. & Taverne, M.A.M. (1991) Transvaginal ultrasound guided follicular aspiration of bovine oocytes. *Theriogenology* **35**:19–24.

Thompson, J.G., Gardner, D.K., Pugh, A., MacMillan, W. & Teruit, J.J.R. (1995) Lamb birth weight is affected by culture system utilized during in vitgro pre-elongation development of ovine embryos. *Biology of Reproduction* **53**:1385–91.

Thomson, J., Itskovitz-Eldor, J., Shapiro, S., et al. (1998) Embryonic stem cell lines derived from human blastocysts. *Science* **282**:1145–7.

Walker, S.K., Hartwich, K.M. & Seamark, R.F. (1996) The production of unusually large offspring following embryo manipulation: concepts and challenges. *Theriogenology* **45**:111–20.

Willadsen, S.M. (1986) Nuclear transplantation in sheep embryos. *Nature* **320(6057)**:63–5.

Wilmut, I., Schnieke, A.E., McWhir, K., Kind, A.J. & Campbell, K.H. (1997) Viable offspring derived from fetal and adult mammalian cells. *Nature* **385(6619)**:810–13.

7

The clinical in vitro fertilization laboratory

Introduction

In the armoury of medical technology that now exists for the alleviation of disease and improvement in the quality of life, there is nothing to match the unique contribution of assisted reproductive technology. There is no other life experience that matches the birth of a baby in significance and importance. The responsibility of nurturing and watching children grow and develop alters the appreciation of life and health, with a resulting long-term impact upon individuals, families and, ultimately, society. Thus, the combination of oocyte and sperm to create an embryo with the potential to develop into a unique individual cannot be regarded lightly, as merely another form of invasive medical technology, but must be treated with the respect and responsibility due to the most fundamental areas of human life.

Successful assisted reproduction involves the careful co-ordination of both a medical and a scientific approach to each couple who undertake a treatment cycle, with close collaboration between doctors, scientists, nurses and counsellors. Only meticulous attention to detail at every step of each patient's treatment can optimize their chance of delivering a healthy baby. Appropriate patient selection, ovarian stimulation, monitoring and timing of oocyte retrieval should provide the in vitro fertilization (IVF) laboratory with viable gametes capable of producing healthy embryos. It is the responsibility of the IVF laboratory to ensure a stable, nontoxic, pathogen-free environment with optimum parameters for oocyte fertilization and embryo development. The first part of this book reveals the complexity of variables involved in assuring successful fertilization and embryo development in animal systems, together with the fascinating and elegant systems of control which have been elucidated at the molecular level. It goes without saying that human in vitro fertilization must of necessity involve systems of at least equal, if not greater, complexity,

---

The Assisted Conception Treatment Cycle

- Consultation: history, examination, investigation, counselling
- Pituitary downregulation with GnRH agonist
- Baseline assessment
- Gonadotrophin stimulation
- Follicular phase monitoring
- Ultrasound + endocrinology
- HCG administration to induce ovulation
- Oocyte retrieval (OCR)
- In vitro fertilization
- Embryo transfer
- Supernumerary embryo cryopreservation
- Luteal phase support
- Day 15 pregnancy test
- Follow-up pregnancy tests: day 20, 25, 30
- Day 35 ultrasound assessment

---

and it is essential for the clinical biologist to be aware that control mechanisms exist which are exquisitely sensitive to even apparently minor changes in the environment of gametes and embryos, in particular, temperature, pH and any other factors which potentially affect cells at the molecular level. Multiple variables are involved, so the basic science of each step must be carefully controlled, while allowing for individual variation between patients and between treatment cycles. In addition, in this current era of rapidly evolving technology, the success of new innovations in technique and technology can only be gauged by comparison with a standard of efficient and reproducible established procedures. The IVF laboratory therefore has a duty and responsibility not only to ensure that a strict discipline of cleanliness and sterile technique is adhered to throughout all procedures, but also to produce and maintain daily records, with systematic data analysis and reports.

Setting up a laboratory: equipment and facilities

The design of an IVF laboratory should provide a distraction- and accident-free environment in which concentrated attention can be comfortably and safely dedicated to each manipulation, with sensible and logical planning of work stations which are practical and easy to clean. Priority must be given to minimizing the potential for introducing infection or contamination from any source, and therefore the tissue culture area should allow for the highest standards of sterile technique, with all floors, surfaces and components easy to clean on a daily basis. Ideally, the space should be designated as a restricted access area, with facilities for changing into clean operating theatre dress and shoes before entry.

Ambient air quality

The importance of ambient air and the possible consequences of chemical air contamination have been reviewed by Cohen et al. (1997). Whereas most organisms and species are protected to some extent from hazards in their ambient environment through their immune, digestive and epithelial systems, oocytes and embryos in vitro have no such protection, and their active and passive absorption mechanisms are largely indiscriminate. IVF laboratories set up in buildings within polluted areas, or close to industrial manufacturing sites, may be subject to serious chemical air contamination which may be reflected by inadequate pregnancy and live birth rates. Incubators obtain their ambient air directly from the laboratory room; CO_2 is supplied in gas bottles, which may well be contaminated with organic compounds or metallic contaminants. Pressurized rooms using high efficiency particulate air (HEPA) filtration are used by many IVF laboratories, with standards applied to pharmaceutical clean rooms; however, HEPA filtration cannot effectively retain gaseous low molecular weight organic and inorganic molecules.

The four most common air pollutants are:

1. In urban and dense suburban areas, volatile organic compounds (VOC) produced by industry, a variety of cleaning procedures and vehicle and heating exhausts. Instruments such as microscopes, television monitors or furniture (as a result of manufacturing processes) may also produce VOCs.
2. Small inorganic molecules such as N_2O, SO_2, CO.
3. Substances derived from building materials, e.g. aldehydes from flooring adhesives, substituted benzenes, phenol and *n*-decane released from vinyl floor tiles – flooring adhesives have been found to be particularly aggressive in arresting embryo development! Newly painted surfaces frequently present a hazard, as many paints contain substances that are highly toxic in the IVF lab.
4. Other polluting compounds which may be released by pesticides or by aerosols containing butane or iso-butane as a propellant. Liquids such as

floor waxes may contain heavy metals, which have a drastic effect on embryo implantation potential.

Cohen and colleagues conducted a detailed study of chemical air contamination in all areas of their IVF laboratory, which revealed dynamic interactive processes between air-handling systems, spaces, tools, disposable materials and other items unique to their laboratory. Anaesthetic gases, refrigerants, cleaning agents, hydrocarbons and aromatic compounds were found, and some accumulated specifically in incubators. They suggest that there may be an interaction between water-soluble and lipid-soluble solid phases such as those in incubators: whereas some contaminants may be absorbed by culture media, this may be counteracted by providing a larger sink such as a humidification pan in the incubator. Mineral oil may act as a sink for other components. Unfiltered outside air may be cleaner than HEPA filtered laboratory air or air obtained from incubators, due to accumulation of VOCs derived from adjacent spaces or specific laboratory products, including sterile Petri dishes. Manufacturers of compressed air and incubators have no concern for the specific clean air needs of IVF: standards for supplies of compressed gases are based upon criteria which are not designed for cultured and unprotected cells. Testing a new incubator revealed concentrations of VOC > 100-fold higher than those obtained from testing used incubators from the same manufacturer – allowing the emission of gases from new laboratory products is crucial. In view of the fact that it appears impossible to prevent pollution inside the laboratory from the surroundings with current air-conditioning technologies, primary consideration should be given to design of culture spaces and adjacent areas. In order to circumvent this problem of potential hazards in ambient air and culture systems, active filtration units with activated carbon filters and oxidizing material have now been developed specifically for IVF laboratories. These can be placed inside cell-culture incubators (CoDa, GenX, Connecticut, MA, USA) or in the laboratory spaces themselves (Eco-Care, New York, USA).

Laboratory space layout

Careful consideration should be given to the physical manoeuvres involved, ensuring ease and safety of movement between areas, in order to minimize the possibility of accidents. Bench height, adjustable chairs, microscope eye height and efficient use of space and surfaces all contribute to a working environment that minimizes distraction and fatigue. The location of storage areas and equipment such as incubators and centrifuges should be logically planned for efficiency and safety within each working area; the use of mobile laboratory components allows flexibility to meet changing requirements.

Basic essential equipment required for routine IVF includes:

1. Dissecting, inverted, and light microscopes
2. Incubator with accurately regulated temperature and CO_2
3. Centrifuge for sperm preparation
4. Warmed stages or surfaces for culture manipulations
5. Refrigerator/freezer
6. Dry heat oven for drying and sterilizing

A video camera system is also recommended for teaching, assessment and records (patients receive enormous satisfaction and psychological support from observing their oocytes and embryos on a video screen).

When choosing these expensive items of equipment, ensure that not only is each easy to use and maintain, but that servicing and repairs can be quickly and efficiently obtained. Routine schedules of cleaning, maintenance, and servicing must be established for each item of equipment, and checklist records maintained for daily, weekly, monthly and annual schedules of cleaning and maintenance of all items used, together with checks for restocking and expiry dates of supplies.

Incubators

Two types of gas phase have been successfully used: 5% CO_2 in air, and the triple gas mixture of 5% CO_2, 5% O_2, 90% N_2. An atmosphere of 5% CO_2 is required to maintain correct pH in bicarbonate buffered culture media systems in order to maintain a physiological pH of just under 7.5. This equilibrium depends upon the composition of the media used, and is affected by both temperature and atmospheric pressures: some conditions may require a 6% CO_2 in air mixture in order to maintain the correct pH.

Carefully calibrated and accurately controlled CO_2 incubators are critical to successful IVF. The choice of humidified or nonhumidified incubator depends upon the type of tissue culture system used: whereas humidity is required for standard 4-well 'open' culture, the use of an equilibrated humidified overlay of mineral oil allows the use of incubators without humidity. Dry incubators carry less risk of fungal contamination, and are easier to clean. The incubator must be regularly monitored, and readings of the LED display checked and calibrated against independent recordings of temperature and pH monitored by probes placed in a standard 'test' culture system. Temperature stability can be monitored with 24-hour thermocouple readings as part of the standard maintenance schedule.

The inside walls and doors should be washed with sterile water weekly, and a yearly inspection and general servicing by the supplier is recommended. Repeated opening and closing of the incubator affects the stability of the tissue culture environment, and the use of a small benchtop mini-incubator during oocyte retrievals and manipulations helps to minimize disturbance of the storage incubator. Modern mini-incubators specific for IVF culture have recently been introduced designed to overcome problems of pH and temperature consistency and stability encountered with traditional large incubator systems.

Water quality

A reliable source of ultrapure water is a critical factor in the laboratory, particularly if media is prepared 'in house'. Weimer et al. (1998) carried out a complete analysis of impurities that can be found in water: this universal solvent provides a medium for most biological and chemical reactions, and is more susceptible to contamination by other substances than any other common solvent. Both surface and ground water are contaminated with a wide range of substances, including fertilizers, pesticides, herbicides, detergents, industrial waste effluent and waste solvents, with seasonal fluctuations in temperature and precipitation affecting the levels of contamination. Four categories of contaminants are present: inorganics (dissolved cationic and anionic species), organics, particles and microorganisms such as bacteria, algae, mold and fungi. Chlorine, chloramines, polyionic substrates, ozone and fluorine may be added to water during treatment processes, and must be removed from water for cell culture media preparation. In water purification, analysis of the feed water source is crucial to determine the proper filtration steps required, and water-processing protocols should be adapted to meet regional requirements. Processing systems include particulate filtration, activated carbon cartridge filtration, reverse osmosis (RO) and electrodeionization (EDI), an ultraviolet oxidation system, followed by a Milli-Q PF Plus purification before final filtration through a 0.22 μm filter to scavenge any trace particles and prevent reverse bacterial contamination from the environment.

IVF laboratory personnel should be familiar with any subtle variations in their water source, as well as the capabilities of their water purification system, and develop protocols to ensure consistently high-quality ultrapure water supplies. Weimer et al. recommend the following water maintenance schedule for the system that they use in purifying water for media preparation:

Replace carbon and depth filters monthly
Monitor chlorine every 21 days
Chlorine sanitization of RO and EDI system bimonthly
Mock sanitization of RO and EDI system bimonthly
Replace RO pretreatment pack every 3 months
UV recirculation of storage tank
NaOH sanitization storage tank quarterly
NaOH sanitization Milli-Q PF Plus bimonthly
Replace resin purification pack quarterly
Replace 0.22 µm final filter unit monthly
Monitor silica and Total Organic Carbon (TOC) at final product daily.

Supplies

A basic list of supplies is outlined at the end of this chapter; the exact combination required will depend upon the tissue culture system and techniques of manipulation used. Disposable supplies are used whenever possible and must be guaranteed nontoxic tissue culture grade, in particular the culture vessels, needles, collecting system and catheters for oocyte aspiration and embryo transfer.

Disposable high-quality glass pipettes are required for gamete and embryo manipulations; these must be soaked and rinsed with tissue culture grade sterile water and dry heat sterilized before use. In preparing to handle gametes or embryos, examine each pipette and rinse with sterile medium to ensure that it is clean and residue-free.

Daily cleaning routine

During the course of procedures any spillage should be immediately cleaned with dry tissue. No detergent or alcohol should be used whilst oocytes/embryos are being handled. Should it be necessary to use either of the above, allow residual traces to evaporate for a period of at least 20 minutes before removing oocytes/embryos from incubators.

At the end of each day:

1. Heat seal, double bag, and dispose of all waste from procedures.
2. Remove all pipette holders for washing and sterilizing before reuse.
3. Reseal and resterilize pipette canisters.
4. Clean flow hoods, work benches, and all equipment by washing with a solution of distilled water and 7X laboratory detergent (Flow Laboratories), followed by wiping with 70% methylated spirit.
5. Prepare each work station for the following day's work, with clean rubbish bags, pipette holder and Pasteur pipettes.

Washing procedures

If the laboratory has a system for preparation of ultrapure water, particular attention must be paid to instructions for maintenance and chemical cleaning. Water purity is essential for washing procedures, and the system should be periodically checked for organic contamination and endotoxins.

Pipettes

1. Soak new pipettes overnight in fresh Analar or Milli-Q water, ensuring that they are completely covered.
2. Drain the pipettes and rinse with fresh water.
3. Drain again and dry at 100 °C for 1–2 hours.
4. Place in a clean pipette canister (tips forward), and dry heat sterilize for 3 hours at 180 °C.
5. After cooling, record date and use within 1 month of sterilization.

Non-disposable items (handle with non-powered gloves, rinsed in purified water)

1. Soak in distilled water containing 3–5% 7X (flow Laboratories).
2. Sonicate small items for 5–10 minutes in an ultrasonic cleaning bath.
3. Rinse eight times with distilled water, then twice with Analar or Milli-Q water.
4. Dry, seal in aluminium foil or double wrap in autoclave bags as appropriate.
5. Autoclave, or dry heat sterilize at 180 °C for 3 hours.
6. Record date of sterilization, and store in a clean, dust-free area.

Tissue culture media

A great deal of scientific research and analysis has been applied to the development of media which will successfully support the growth and development of human embryos. Many controlled studies have shown fertilization and cleavage to be satisfactory in a variety of simple and complex media (comprehensive reviews are published by Bavister, 1995, and Edwards & Brody, 1995). Metabolic and nutritional requirements of mammalian embryos are complex, stage specific, and, in many cases, species specific: several decades of research in laboratory and livestock animal systems have shown that, although there are some basic similarities, culture requirements of different species must be considered independently. Understanding metabolic pathways of embryos and their substrate and nutrient preferences has led to major advances in the ability to support embryo development in vitro. Rigorous quality control is essential in media preparation, including the source of all ingredients, especially the water, which must be endotoxin-free, low in ion content, and guaranteed free of organic molecules and microorganisms. Each batch of culture media prepared must be checked for osmolality ($285\pm 2\,\mathrm{mOsm/kg}$) and pH (7.35–7.45), and subjected to quality-control procedures with sperm survival or mouse embryo toxicity before use. Furthermore, culture media can rapidly deteriorate during storage, with decrease in its ability to support embryo development, and careful attention must be paid to storage conditions and manufacturers' recommended expiry dates. Commercially prepared, pretested high-quality culture media is now available for purchase from a number of suppliers world-wide, so that media preparation for routine use in the laboratory is not necessary, and may not be a cost-effective exercise when time and quality control are taken into account. A list of available commercial culture media is supplied at the end of this chapter. There is so far no firm scientific evidence that any is superior to another in routine IVF, and choice should depend upon considerations such as quality control and testing procedures applied in its manufacture, cost and, in particular, guaranteed efficient supply delivery in relation to shelf-life. After delivery, the medium may be aliquoted in suitable small volumes, such that one aliquot can be used for a single patient's gamete preparation and culture (including sperm preparation). Media containing HEPES, which maintains a stable pH in the bicarbonate-buffered system, can be used for sperm preparation and oocyte harvesting and washing; however, HEPES is known to alter ion channel activity in the plasma membrane and may well be embryotoxic. The gametes must therefore subsequently be washed in HEPES-free culture medium before insemination and overnight culture.

Media specially designed for 'sperm washing' is also commercially available.

Prior to 1997, single media formulations were used for all stages of IVF. However, during the 1990s, a great deal of research in animal systems led to elucidation of the metabolic biochemistry and molecular mechanisms involved in gamete maturation, activation, fertilization, genomic activation, cleavage, compaction and blastocyst formation. This drew attention to the fact that nutrient and ionic requirements differ during all these different stages. Inappropriate culture conditions expose embryos to cellular stress which could result in retarded cleavage, cleavage arrest, cytoplasmic blebbing, impaired energy production, inadequate genome activation and gene transcription. Blastocyst formation is followed by an exponential increase in protein synthesis, with neosynthesis of glycoproteins, histones and new surface antigens.

Although the specific needs of embryos during their preimplantation development have by no means been completely defined, sequential, stage-specific and chemically defined media are now being developed for use in IVF systems. These endeavour to mimic the natural in vivo situation and take into account the significant changes in embryo physiology and metabolism that occur during the preimplantation period.

Fertilization is invariably successful in very simple media such as Earle's, or a TALP-based formulation, but the situation becomes more complex thereafter (see chapter 4 for details of embryo metabolism).

Serum

Prepared and filtered maternal serum has traditionally been added to IVF culture media, and preparations of human (or bovine) serum albumin were found to be effective replacements during fertilization and cleavage (although blastocyst development was apparently impaired in the absence of maternal serum). Maternal serum is routinely heat-treated to inactivate potentially harmful complement, but this might also destroy beneficial factors and/or create embryotoxic compounds.

Albumin is the major protein constituent of the embryo's environment; it can be incorporated by the embryo, it binds lipids and may help to bind and stabilize growth factors. Theoretically it may not be indispensable, but it does effectively replace serum, and has a major role both in maintaining embryo quality and in preventing gametes and embryos from sticking to glass or plastic surfaces, facilitating their manipulation. Commercial preparations can be highly variable in quality, and recent concerns about blood product transmission of pathogenic agents such as hepatitis and HIV viruses and

Creutzfeld–Jacob disease has made reliable sources of human serum albumin (HSA) increasingly difficult to find. Recombinant technology is now increasingly applied to commercial production of a number of physiological proteins, and recombinant HSA may be available in the future.

In domestic animals, serum has been found to induce a wide range of abnormalities in vitro, and its presence has been associated with the development of abnormally large fetuses (Thompson et al., 1995). Although the mechanisms involved are unresolved, the findings have led to further concerns about the use of serum in human IVF (see chapter 6).

Serum-free media have been introduced, using substitutes such as polyvinyl alcohol (PVA) and hyaluronate to replace albumin. PVA is a synthetic polymer, and, although it has been shown to support human IVF culture (Rinehart et al., 1998), it is a nonphysiological compound, and any long-term effects or consequences may remain undetected for some time. Hyaluronate is a glycosaminoglycan found at increased levels in the uterus around the time of implantation (Zorn et al., 1995), and the human embryo expresses its receptor throughout preimplantation development (Campbell et al., 1995). It is also known to form an antiviral and anti-immunogenic layer around the embryo, to increase angiogenesis, and to facilitate the rapid diffusion of transfer medium into the viscous uterine fluid environment. It may also be involved in the initial phases of attachment of the blastocyst to the endometrium. Hyaluronate has no protein moieties, and can therefore be synthesized and isolated in a pure form. Preliminary trials indicated that its presence not only replaced albumin in culture, but also significantly increased the implantation rate of resultant mouse blastocysts (Gardner, 1999).

Growth factors

Growth factors play a key role in growth and differentiation from the time of morula/blastocyst transition. However, defining their precise role and potential for improving in vitro preimplantation development is complicated by factors such as gene expression both of the factors and their receptors. There is also the potential of ascribing positive effects to specific factors when the result may in fact be due to a combination of a myriad of other causes. The mammalian blastocyst expresses ligands and receptors for several growth factors, many of which can cross-react, making it difficult to interpret the effects of single factors added to a medium. Insulin, LIF, EGF/TGFα, TGFβ, PDGG, HB-EGF have all been studied in IVF culture, and, although it is clear that these and other growth factors can show an influence on in vitro blastocyst development and hatching, further assessment remains an area of research – a comprehensive review was published by Kane et al. in 1997. It has been suggested that the mechanism whereby serum induces abnormalities in domestic animal systems may involve the overexpression of certain growth factors – there is no doubt that complex and delicate regulatory systems are involved.

Culture of embryos in 'groups' rather than singly has been found to improve viability and implantation in some systems: it is possible that autocrine/paracrine effects or 'trophic' factors exist between embryos. However, observed effects of 'group' culture will inevitably be related to the composition of the culture medium and the precise physical conditions used for embryo culture, especially the ratio of embryo: medium volume.

Follicular flushing

Ideally, if a patient has responded well to follicular phase stimulation with appropriate monitoring and timing of ovulation induction by human chorionic gonadotrophin (hCG) injection, the oocyte retrieval may proceed smoothly with efficient recovery of oocytes without flushing the follicles. If the number of follicles is low or the procedure is difficult for technical reasons, follicles may be flushed with a physiological solution to assist recovery of all the oocytes present. Balanced salt solutions such as Earle's (EBSS) may be used for follicular flushing, and heparin may be added at a concentration of 2 units/ml. HEPES buffered media can also be used for flushing. Temperature and pH of flushing media must be carefully controlled, and the oocytes recovered from flushing media subsequently washed in culture media before transfer to their final culture droplet or well.

Quality control procedures

IVF laboratories should have an effective Total Quality Management (TQM) system that can monitor all procedures and components of the laboratory. This must include not only pregnancy and implantation rates, but also a systematic check and survey of all laboratory material, supplies, equipment and instruments. Standard Operating Procedures should be available to all laboratory personnel, which describe not only the detailed method to be applied to each procedure, but also products, equipment and relevant quality control measures, with quality standards or specifications for each aspect of the testing procedure. All equipment must have a clear and readily accessible manual, together with a log-book of maintenance, servicing, and routine checks. A system that monitors individual performance of members of the team, with regular appraisal, is also helpful in maintaining an optimal standard of results.

The ultimate test of quality control must rest with pregnancy and live birth rates per IVF treatment cycle. An ongoing record of the results of fertilization, cleavage, and embryo development provide the best short-term evidence of good quality control (QC). Daily records in the form of a laboratory log-book are essential, summarizing details of patients and outcome of laboratory procedures: age, cause of infertility, stimulation protocol, number of oocytes retrieved, semen analysis, sperm preparation details, insemination time, fertilization, cleavage, embryo transfer and cryopreservation. It is also essential to record details of media and oil batches for reference, along with the introduction of any new methods or materials used. A range of bioassays to detect toxicity and suboptimal culture conditions have been tried, such as human sperm survival, hamster sperm survival, somatic cell lines, and the culture of mouse embryos from either the 1-cell or 2-cell stage. The validity of a mouse embryo bioassay has been questioned as a reliable assay for extrapolation to clinical IVF: it assumes that the requirements of human and mouse embryos are the same, and we know that this is a false assumption. The mouse embryo cannot regulate its endogenous metabolic pool before the late 2-cell stage; this is not the case for human or bovine embryos. Mouse embryos will develop from the 2-cell stage onwards in a very wide variety of cell culture media, without discrimination. Whilst none of the systems currently available can guarantee the detection of subtle levels of toxicity, they can be helpful in identifying specific problems. Any bioassay done routinely and frequently with baseline data for comparing deviations from the norm will be helpful in minimizing the random introduction of contaminants into the system, and is a useful investment of time and resources in an IVF lab.

New batches of media, oil, material or supplies used in the culture system, if not pretested, should be tested before use, and in routine IVF culture a normal fertilization rate in the order of >70% and cleavage rate of >95% is expected. The cleavage rate is important, as a block at the 2PN stage indicates a serious problem. At least 65% of inseminated oocytes should result in cleaved embryos on Day 2. The physico-chemical limits of culture media testing are also crucial: osmolarity must be within the limits of 275 and 305 mOsm, with a total variation of no more than 30 mOsm. pH must be within the limits of 7.2–7.5, with a maximal variation of 0.4 units of pH. Larger variations in either parameter indicate poor technique/technology and inadequate controls during manufacture, leading to poor reproducibility.

Tissue culture plastics have on occasion been found to be subject to vari-ation in quality: even within a single 4-well plate, well to well variations have been observed, and rinsing plates with media before use may be a useful precaution. Studies have shown that oil can interact with different plastic supports, and this can affect embryo development. Manufacturers of plastic-ware used for tissue culture may change the chemical formulation of their products without notification, and such changes in manufacture of syringes, filters and culture dishes may sometimes be embryotoxic. Embryos are very sensitive quality control indicators: firstly, in any block at the 2PN stage, and, secondly, in the appearance of the blastomeres and the presence of fragmenta-tion. The early human embryo should be bright and clear, without granules in the cytoplasm. During cell division, the nucleocytoplasmic ratio is important. If osmolarity of the culture medium is low, the size of the embryo increases relative to the volume of the cytoplasm, and cytoplasmic blebs are formed in order to compensate and reach the adequate N/C ratio for entering mitosis. However, in doing so, the embryo loses not only cytoplasm but also mRNA and proteins, which are necessary for further development.

Suggested useful routine QC procedures include the following:

1. Sperm survival test

Select a normal sample of washed prepared spermatozoa and assess for count, motility and progression. Divide the selected sample into 4 aliquots: add test material to 2 aliquots, and equivalent control material (in current use) to 2 aliquots. Incubate one control and one test sample at 37 °C, and one of each at room temperature. Assess each sample for count, motility and progression after 24 and 48 hours (a computer-aided system can be used if available). Test and control samples should show equivalent survival. If there is any doubt, repeat the test.

2. Culture of surplus oocytes

Surplus oocytes from patients who have large numbers of oocytes retrieved may be used to test new culture material. Culture at least 6 oocytes in the control media, and a maximum of 4 in test media.

3. Multipronucleate embryo culture

Oocytes which show abnormal fertilization on day 1 after insemination can be used for testing new batches of material. Observe, score and assess each embryo daily until Day 6 after insemination.

4. *Culture of 'spare' embryos*

Surplus embryos after embryo transfer which are not suitable for freezing can also be used for testing new culture material. Observe, score, and assess each embryo daily as above. Embryo development to the blastocyst stage is regarded as evidence of adequate culture conditions, and blastocysts assessed to be of good quality may be cryopreserved.

Tissue culture systems

Vessels successfully used for in vitro fertilization include test tubes, 4-well culture dishes, organ culture dishes and Petri dishes containing microdroplets of culture medium under a layer of paraffin or mineral oil. Whatever the system employed, it must be capable of rigidly maintaining fixed stable parameters of temperature, pH and osmolarity. Human oocytes are extremely sensitive to transient cooling in vitro, and modest reductions in temperature can cause irreversible disruption of the meiotic spindle, with possible chromosome dispersal. Analyses of embryos produced by IVF have shown that a high proportion are chromosomally abnormal, and it is possible that temperature-induced chromosome disruption may contribute to the high rates of preclinical and spontaneous abortion that follow IVF and gamete intrafallopian transfer (GIFT). Therefore, it is essential to control temperature fluctuation from the moment of follicle aspiration, and during all oocyte and embryo manipulations, by using heated microscope stages and heating blocks or platforms.

An overlay of equilibrated oil as part of the tissue culture system confers specific advantages:

1. The oil acts as a physical barrier, separating droplets of medium from the atmosphere and airborne particles or pathogens.
2. Oil prevents evaporation and delays gas diffusion, thereby keeping pH, temperature and osmolality of the medium stable during gamete manipulations, protecting the embryos from significant fluctuations in their microenvironment.
3. Oil prevents evaporation: humidified and pre-equilibrated oil allows the use of nonhumidified incubators, which are easier to clean and maintain.

It has been suggested that oil could enhance embryo development by removing lipid-soluble toxins from the medium; on the other hand, an oil overlay prevents free diffusion of metabolic by-products such as ammonia, and accumulation of ammonia in culture media is toxic to the embryo. The use of an oil overlay also influences oxygen concentration in the medium, with resulting effects on the delicate balance of embryo metabolism; as mentioned previously, it can absorb and concentrate harmful volatile organic compounds.

Oil preparation

Mineral, paraffin or silicone oil should be sterile as supplied, and does not require sterilization or filtration. High temperature for sterilization may be detrimental to the oil itself, and the procedure may also 'leach' potential toxins from the container. Provo and Herr (1998) reported that exposure of mineral oil to direct sunlight for a period of 4 hours resulted in a highly embryotoxic overlay, and they recommend that washed oil should be shielded from light and treated as a photoreactive compound. Contaminants have been reported in certain types of oil. Washing procedures remove water-soluble toxins, but non water-soluble toxins may also be present which will not be removed by washing. Therefore it is prudent not only to wash, but to test every batch of oil before use with, at the very least, a sperm survival test as a quality control procedure. In 1995, Erbach et al. suggested that zinc might be a contaminant in silicone oil, and found that washing the oil with EDTA removed a toxicity factor that may have been due to the presence of zinc. Some mineral oil products may also contain preservatives such as alpha-tocopherol. Oil can be carefully washed in sterile disposable tissue culture flasks (without vigorous shaking) with either Milli-Q water, sterile saline solution or a simple culture medium without protein or lipid-soluble components, in a ratio of 5:1 oil:aq. The oil can be further 'equilibrated' by bubbling 5% CO_2 through the mixture before allowing the phases to separate and settle. Washed oil can be stored either at room temperature or at 4 °C in equilibrium with the aqueous layer, or separated before storage, but should be prepared at least 2 days prior to its use. Oil overlays must be further equilibrated in the CO_2 incubator for several hours (or overnight) before introducing media/gametes/embryos.

Serum supplements

Commercially prepared media are supplied complete, and do not require the addition of any supplements; most contain a serum substitute such as 'albuminar', human serum albumin. If maternal serum is used in the culture system, it must be homologous; pooled or donor sera are not recommended, even after thorough viral screening.

Preparation of maternal serum

Collect 20 ml of the patient's blood by venepuncture, maintain in an ice bucket, and spin immediately, before the sample clots. Remove the supernatant serum, and leave it to clot for approximately 30–60 minutes. Remove the clot by compressing it around a Pasteur pipette, and heat inactivate the serum at 56 °C for 45 minutes. Cool, and then filter through two millipore filters of 0.45 μm and 0.22 μm in sequence. Store at 4 °C. Maternal serum must not be used in cases of immunological or idiopathic infertility, or in cases with a previous history of unexplained failed fertilization.

Basic equipment required for the IVF laboratory

Embryology

CO_2 incubator
Dissecting microscope
Inverted microscope
Heated surfaces for microscope and manipulation areas
Heating block for test tubes
Laminar flow cabinet
Oven for heat-sterilizing
Small autoclave
Water bath
Pipette 10–100 μl Eppendorf
Pipette 20–1000 μl Eppendorf
Refrigerator
Supply of medical grade CO_2

Supply of 5% CO_2 in air
Wash bottle + Millex filter for gas
Rubber tubing
Pipette canisters
Mineral or paraffin oil
Culture media

Glassware for media preparation
Osmometer (for media preparation)
Weighing balance
Millipore Bell filter unit for filtering media

Tissue culture plastics: (Nunc, Corning, Sterilin)
Flasks for media and oil: 50 ml, 175 ml
Culture dishes: 60, 35 mm
OCR (oocyte retrieval) needles
Test-tubes for OCR: 17 ml disposable
Transfer catheters: embryo, GIFT, IUI
Syringes
Needles
Disposable pipettes: 1, 5, 10, 25 ml
'Pipetus' pipetting device
Eppendorf tips, small and large
Millipore filters: 0.22, 0.8 μm
Glass Pasteur pipettes (Volac)
Pipette bulbs
Test-tube racks
Spirit burners + methanol or gas Bunsen burner
Rubbish bags
Tissues
Tape for labelling
7X detergent (Flow)
70% ethanol
Sterile gloves

Oil: Boots, Squibb, Sigma, Medicult
Supply of purified water: Milli-Q system or Analar
Glassware for making culture media: beakers, flasks, measuring cylinder

Details of IVF media can be obtained from the following manufacturing companies:

Medicult: Møllehaven 12, DK-4040 Jyllinge, Denmark
Scandinavian IVF Science AB, Mölndalsvägen 30A, PO Box 14105, Göthenburg, Sweden
Ham's F-10, EBSS: Flow Laboratories, UK
HTF: Irvine Scientific, USA

Cook IVF: 12 Electronics Street, Brisbane Technology Park, Eight Mile Plains, Queensland 4113, Australia

Sage BioPharma, Inc. 944 Calle Amanecer, Suite L., San Clemente, CA 92673, USA

Further reading

Almeida, P.A. & Bolton, V.N. (1996) The effect of temperature fluctuations on the cytoskeletal organisation and chromosomal constitution of the human oocyte. *Zygote* **3**:357–65.

Angell, R.R., Templeton, A.A. & Aitken, R.J. (1986) Chromosome studies in human in vitro fertilisation *Human Genetics* **72**:333–9.

Ashwood-Smith, M.J., Hollands, P. & Edwards, R.G. (1989) The use of Albuminar (TM) as a medium supplement in clinical IVF. *Human Reproduction* **4**:702–5.

Augustus, D. (1996) Cell culture incubators: tips for successful routine maintenance. *Alpha Newsletter* vol. 4, April 1996.

Bavister, B.D. (1995) Culture of preimplantation embryos: facts and artifacts. *Human Reproduction update* **1(2)**: 91–148.

Bavister, B.D. & Andrews, J.C. (1988) A rapid sperm motility bioassay procedure for quality control testing of water and culture media. *Journal of In Vitro Fertilization and Embryo Transfer* **5**:67–8.

Boone, W.R., Johnson, J.E., Locke, A.J., Crane, M.M. & Price, T.M. (1999) Control of air quality in an assisted reproductive technology laboratory. *Fertility and Sterility* **71**:150–4.

Campbell, S., Swann, H.R., Aplin, J.D., Seif, M.W., Kimber, S.J. & Elstein, M. (1995) CD44 is expressed throughout pre-implantation human embryo development. *Human Reproduction* **10**:425–30.

Cohen, J., Gilligan, A., Esposito, W., Schimmel, T. & Dale, B. (1997) Ambient air and its potential effects on conception *in vitro*. *Human Reproduction* **12(8)**:1742–9.

Danforth, R.A., Piana, S.D. & Smith, M. (1987) HIgh purity water: an important component for success in in vitro fertilization. *American Biotechnology Laboratory* **5**:58–60.

Davidson, A., Vermesh, M., Lobo, R.A. & Paulsen, R.J. (1988) Mouse embryo culture as quality control for human in vitro fertilisation: the one-cell versus two-cell model. *Fertility and Sterility* **49**:516–21.

Dumolin, J.S., Menheere, P.P., Evers, J.L., Kleukers, A.P., Oueters, M.H., Bras, M. & Geraedts, J.P. (1991) The effects of endotoxins on gametes and preimplantation embryos cultured in vitro. *Human Reproduction* **6**:730–4.

Edwards, R.G. & Brody, S.A. (1995) Human fertilization in the labortory. In: *Principles and Practice of Assisted Human Reproduction*. W.B. Saunders & Co., Philadelphia, Pennsylvania, 351–413.

Elder, K. & Elliott, T., (1998) Troubleshooting and Problem Solving in IVF. *Worldwide Conferences on Reproductive Biology*. Ladybrook Publishing, Australia.

Elliott, T. & Elder, K. (eds.) (1997) Blastocyst culture, transfer, and freezing. *Worldwide Conferences on Reproductive Biology*. Ladybrook Publishing, Australia.

Erbach, G.T., Bhatnagar.,P., Baltz, J.,M. & Biggers, J.D. (1995) Zinc is a possible toxic contaminant of silicone oil in microdrop cultures of preimplantation mouse embryos. *Human Reproduction* **10**:3248–54.

Fleetham, J. & Mahadevan, M.M. (1988) Purification of water for in vitro fertilization and embryo transfer. *Journal of In Vitro Fertilization and Embryo Transfer* **5**:171–4.

Fleming, T.P., Pratt, H.P.M. & Braude, P.R. (1987) The use of mouse preimplantation embryos for quality control of culture reagents in human in vitro fertilisation programs: a cautionary note. *Fertility and Sterility* **47**:858–60.

Gardner, D. (1999) Development of new serum-free media for the culture and transfer of human blastocysts. *Human Reproduction* **13, Suppl. 4**:218–25.

George, M.A., Braude, P.R., Johnson, M.H. & Sweetnam, D.G. (1989) Quality control in the IVF laboratory: in vitro and in vivo development of mouse embryos is unaffected by the quality of water used in culture media. *Human Reproduction* **4**:826–31.

Johnson, C., Hofmann, G. & Scott, R. (1994) The use of oil overlay for in vitro fertilisation and culture. *Assisted Reproduction Review* **4**:198–201.

Kane, M.T., Morgan, P.M. & Coonan, C. (1997) Peptide growth factors and preimplantation development. *Human Reproduction Update* **3(2)**: 137–57.

Ma, S., Kalousek, D.K., Zouves, C., Yuen, B.H., Gomel, V. & Moon, Y.S. (1990) The chromosomal complements of cleaved human embryos resulting from in vitro fertilisation. *Journal of In Vitro Fertilization and Embryo Transfer* **7**:16–21.

Marrs, R.P., Saito, H., Yee, B., Sato, F. & Brown, J. (1984) Effect of variation of in vitro culture techniques upon oocyte fertilization and embryo development in human in vitro fertilization procedures. *Fertility and Sterility* **41**:519–23.

Matson, P.L. (1998) Internal and external quality assurance in the IVF laboratory. *Human Reproduction Supplement* **13**, Suppl. 4:156–65.

Ménézo, Y. (1998) Why culture media should mimic nature. *Alpha Newsletter* **13**:8.

Mortimer, D. & Quinn, P. (1996) Bicarbonate-buffered media and CO_2. *Alpha Newsletter* vol. 4, April 1996.

Naaktgeboren, N. (1987) Quality control of culture media for in vitro fertilisation. *In Vitro Fertilisation Program*, Academic Hospital, Vrije Universiteit, Brussels, Belgium. Annal Biologie Clinique (Paris) **45**:368–72.

Pearson, F.C. (1985) *Pyrogens: Endotoxins, LAL Testing, and Depyrogenation*. Marcel Dekker, Inc., pp. 98–100, 206–11.

Pellestor, F., Girardet, A., Andreo, B., Anal, F. & Humeau, C. (1994) Relationship between morphology and chromosomal constitution in human preimplantation embryos. *Molecular and Reproductive Development* **39**:141–6.

Pickering, S.J., Braude, P.R., Johnson, M.H., Cant, A. & Currie, J. (1990) Transient cooling to room temperature can cause irreversible disruption of the meiotic spindle in the human oocyte. *Fertility and Sterility* **54**:102–8.

Plachot, M., De Grouchy, J., Montagut, J., Lepetre, S., Carle, E., Veiga, A., Calderon, G., Santalo, J. (1987) Multicentric study of chromosome analysis in human oocytes and embryos in an IVF programme *Human Reproduction* **2**:29.

Provo, M.C. & Herr, C. (1998) Washed paraffin oil becomes toxic to mouse embryos upon exposure to sunlight. *Theriogenology* **49(1)**:214.

Purdy, J. (1982) Methods for fertilization and embryo culture in vitro. In: (Edwards, R.G. & Purdy, J.M. eds.) *Human Conception In Vitro*. Academic Press, London, p. 135.

Quinn, P., Warner, G.M., Klein, J.F. & Kirby, C. (1985) Culture factors affecting the success rate of in vitro fertilization and embryo transfer. *Annals of the New York Academy of Sciences* **412**:195.

Rinehart, J.S., Bavister, B.D. & Gerrity, M. (1988) Quality control in the in vitro fertilization laboratory: comparison of bioassay systems for water quality. *Journal of In Vitro Fertilization and Embryo Transfer* **5**:335–42.

Rinehart, J., Chapman, C., McKiernan, S. & Bavister, B. (1998) A protein-free chemically defined embryo culture medium produces pregnancy rates similar to human tubal fluid (HTF) supplemented with 10% synthetic serum substitute (SSS). Abstracts of the 14th Annual meeting of the ESHRE, Göteborg 1998. *Human Reproduction* **13**:59.

Staessen, C., Van den Abbeel, E., Carle, M., Khan, I., Devroey, P. & Van Steirteghen, A.C. (1990) Comparison between human serum and Albuminar-20(TM) supplement for in vitro fertilization. *Human Reproduction* **5**:336–41.

Thompson, J.G., Gardner, D.K., Pugh, A., MacMillan, W. & Teruit, J.J.R. (1995) Lamb birth weight is affected by culture system utilized during in vitro pre-elongation development of ovine embryos. *Biology of Reproduction* **53**:1385–91.

Wales, R.G. (1970) Effect of ions on the development of preimplantation mouse embryos in vitro. *Australian Journal of Biological Sciences* **23**:421–9.

Weimer, K.E., Anderson, A. & Stewart, B. (1998) The importance of water quality for media preparation. *Human Reproduction Supplement* **13, Suppl. 4**:166–72.

Yovich, J.L., Edirisinghe, W., Yovich, J.M., Stanger, J. & Matson, P. (1988) Methods of water purification for the preparation of culture media in an IVF-ET programme. *Human Reproduction* **3**:245–8.

Zorn, T.M.T., Pinhal, M.A.S., Nader, H.B., Carvalho, J.J., Abrahamsohn, P.A. & Diedrich, C.P. (1995) Biosynthesis of glucosaminoglycans in the endometrium during the initial stages of pregnancy of the mouse. *Cell Molecular Biology* **41**:97–106.

Semen analysis and preparation for assisted reproductive techniques

At least 50% of couples referred for infertility investigation and treatment are found to have a contributing male factor. Male factor infertility can represent a variety of defects, which result in abnormal sperm number, morphology or function. Detailed analysis of sperm assessment and function are important for accurate diagnosis, and are described in detail in numerous textbooks of practical andrology and semen analysis. A comprehensive review of semen analysis is beyong the scope of this book, and only details relevant to assisted conception treatment will be described here.

The World Health Organization (WHO) laboratory manual describes standard conditions for the collection of semen samples, their delivery and the standardization of laboratory assessment procedures. The WHO standards indicate that a 'normal' semen sample contains at least 20×10^6 spermatozoa/ml, with at least 50% exhibiting good to excellent forward progressive movement within 60 minutes after ejaculation. The introduction of external quality control and quality assurance schemes in semen assessment have highlighted the fact that accurate analysis of seminal fluid is notoriously difficult to standardize, with many technical variables, and the quality of semen analysis in different laboratories can be highly variable (Matson, 1995). This implies that diagnosis and treatment modality chosen for a patient could differ according to the laboratory carrying out the assessment. Without good semen analysis data, patients may be offered inappropriate treatments or no treatment at all: it is essential that an assisted reproductive service should ensure that staff are adequately and correctly trained in basic semen assessment techniques according to WHO guidelines. Even the most confident of labs should have a discipline of monitored standards. The recent introduction of intracytoplasmic sperm injection (ICSI) now provides effective in vitro fertilization (IVF) treatment for even the most severe cases of male infertility which were previously felt to be beyond hope, and the fact that fertilization can be achieved from semen with 'hopeless' sperm parameters has forced a review of standard semen analysis and sperm function testing. This chapter will address only the basic principles required in the practical features of sperm preparation procedures for assisted conception techniques.

Semen assessment

Collection of semen samples

The male partner must be provided with a clearly labelled standard sterile disposable plastic pot. Reusable glass containers must NOT be used (certain types of glass are toxic, and residues of detergent used for washing are also toxic). The time of sample collection should be clearly recorded on the label. An accompanying form may be completed, describing details of length of abstinence, recent illness, medication taken, smoking and alcohol consumption.

Samples previously assessed as having high viscosity benefit from collection into pots containing 1 ml of medium. In cases of immunological infertility, when the mixed antiglobulin reaction (MAR), immunobead or tray agglutination (TAT) tests indicate the presence of antisperm antibodies in the semen, the sample should be collected into medium containing 50% serum albumin. Immediate processing of these samples on a buoyant density gradient helps to minimize antibody binding to sperm.

Liquefaction

Allow the specimen to liquefy naturally on the bench; liquefaction should be complete within 30 minutes. Before proceeding with the analysis, mix the specimen thoroughly; note and record the colour, and whether the sample runs freely on pipetting. Viscous samples are difficult to pipette, leaving sticky strands. High viscosity will interfere with accurate assessment of motility and density, and repeated aspiration through a pipette or needle can help to break down the viscosity.

Measure the volume using a graduated pipette or syringe

Assessment of density and motility

Accurate assessments of sperm density can be calculated using a haemocytometer to count a sample of immobilized sperm, and this method (as described in the WHO manual) should be employed for diagnostic purposes. However, when the purpose of assessment is the selection of an appropriate method of preparing the sample for assisted conception procedures, it may be practical to use a method which allows simultaneous judgment of motile and immotile concentrations, as well as type of sperm motility. Fixed-depth counting chambers (Makler, Horwell or disposable chambers) allow simultaneous assessment of density and motility in order to choose the most appropriate method of sperm preparation. Place the required sample volume on the chamber, according to the manufacturer's instructions, and examine microscopically using a ×20 objective. It has been demonstrated that the results of assessment using fixed-depth counting chambers will vary according to the volume of sample applied, and to the time delay between applying the sample and the coverslip; standardization of precise technical detail is therefore essential.

Before performing the count, note the following features of the specimen:

(a)   The presence of debris and cells other than spermatozoa, such as red or white blood cells;

(b)   agglutination of spermatoza and type if present (H-H, T-T, H-T).

Examine the counting grid and count the number of *motile* sperm in 20 squares. If the count appears on initial observation to be less than 10 million/ml, all 100 squares should be counted. Count the *total* number of sperm in the same group of squares, and calculate motility:

> *Sperm density in millions/ml* = *the number of sperm in 10 squares of the grid.*
> *Motility*   = *No. of motile sperm in $\underline{n}$ number of squares*
> $\times$ *100 divided by total number of sperm in $\underline{n}$*
> *squares*

Progression

Progression is assessed on a scale of 0–4 (The Macleod Scale)

0   immotile sperm
1   motile sperm with no progressive forward movement
2   slow forward progressive movement
3   moderate forward progressive movement
4   rapid, regular forward progression

Morphology

A normal, fertile semen sample contains a very high proportion of morphologically abnormal forms, and the significance of abnormal sperm morphology is not entirely understood. Although sperm of abnormal morphology evidently have reduced fertilizing potential, the true anomalies present in abnormal sperm cells have only partially been characterized; a correlation has been found with specific deficiencies such as poor zona pellucida binding and penetration, poor response to agonists that modulate intracellular calcium concentrations, and with biochemical markers such as reactive oxygen species production and enhanced creatine phosphokinase activity. Sperm condensation quality and sperm morphology studies suggest that the quality of chromatin packaging in human sperm, as assessed by its binding capacity for specific dyes and fluorochromes, can be used as an adjunct to the assessment of morphology. Sperm of poor morphology may possess loosely packaged chromatin, and this may contribute to a failure in sperm decondensation during fertilization.

Detailed morphology assessment is carried out by counting a stained slide preparation using bright-field optics at 1000 magnification as described in the WHO manual. Figure 8.1 shows examples of sperm morphology. The normal head has an oval shape with a length:width ratio of 1.50:1.75. A well-defined acrosomal region should cover 40–70% of the head area. No neck, midpiece or tail defects should be evident, and cytoplasmic droplets should constitute no mor than one-third the size of a normal sperm head. All borderline forms are classified as abnormal.

Mix a drop of semen on a slide with a drop of 1% formaldehyde in 0.01 mol/L phosphate buffer, and stain with 1% eosin in distilled water followed by 10% nigrosin in distilled water. Cover with a cover slip, and count 200 sperm with a scoring system according to strict Kruger criteria:
(Prestained slides are also available: Blustain, Irvine Scientific)

- (1) Abnormal heads
- (2) Tail abnormality
- (3) Midpiece abnormalities
- (4) Immature forms.

Calculate the percentage of each abnormal form, and add together the percentages to yield the total percentage of abnormal forms in the sample.

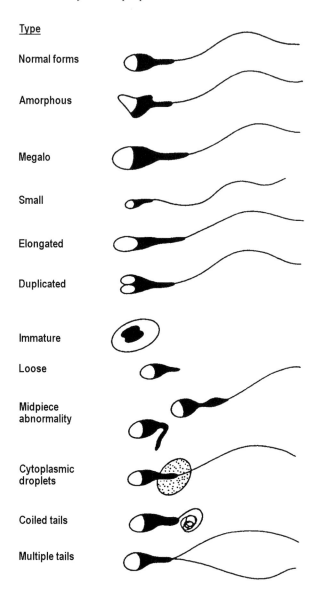

Figure 8.1   Common abnormalities found in human sperm morphology.

Chromatin staining

Damaged chromatin will take up the following dyes:

1. Chromomycin (CMA3) staining

Fix prepared semen samples or semen smears in 3:1 v/v of methanol/glacial
    acetic acid, at 4°C for 5 minutes
Treat each slide for 20 minutes with 100 μl CMA3 solution: 0.25 mg/ml in
    McIlvane's buffer, pH 7.0 containing 10 mM $MgCl_2$
Evaluate the slides using fluorescent microscopy

2. Aniline Blue Staining (AAB)

Fix the samples in 3% buffered glutaraldehyde for 30 min.
Stain the slides with 5% aqueous Aniline Blue and mix with 4% acetic acid
    (pH 3.5) for 7 minutes. Three classes of head staining can be noted:
    unstained (grey/white)
    partially stained
    entire sperm head dark blue intensity.

Antisperm antibodies

Kits (SpermMar, FertiPro N.V, Belgium, Micron, UK) are available for antisperm antibody screening in semen samples; the Mixed Antiglobulin Reaction
(MAR) test will nonspecifically detect IgG, IgA or IgM antibodies, and specific
latex particle Immunobeads (BioRad) can be used to distinguish between the
different categories of antibody. The MAR test offers a rapid and simple
screening test for antisperm antibodies, which can be performed as part of the
routine semen analysis. Advance knowledge of the presence of antisperm
antibodies can significantly improve the outcome of fertilization by allowing
appropriate steps to be taken in sample collection and preparation which will
decrease the binding of antibodies to the sperm and thus facilitate fertilization.

Preparation of sperm for in vitro fertilization/GIFT/intrauterine insemination

At the time of oocyte retrieval or intrauterine insemination (IUI), the laboratory should already be familiar with the male partner's semen profile, and can
refer to features which might influence the choice of sperm preparation method

used. The choice of sperm preparation method or combination of methods depends upon the assessment of:

- the motile count
- ratio between motile : immotile count
- volume
- presence of antibodies, agglutination, pus cells or debris

Sterile technique must be used throughout

Ejaculated semen is a viscous liquid composed of a mixture of testicular and epididymal secretions containing spermatozoa, mixed with prostatic secretions produced at the time of ejaculation. This seminal plasma contains substances which inhibit capacitation and prevent fertilization. The purpose of sperm preparation is to concentrate the motile spermatozoa in a fraction which is free of seminal plasma and its debris. Although sperm can be prepared by simple washing and centrifugation, the method applied to early IVF practice, this method also concentrates cells, debris and immotile sperm, the presence of which jeopardizes fertilization. Aitken et al. (1987) have demonstrated that white cells and dead sperm in semen are a source of reactive oxygen species which can initiate lipid peroxidation in human sperm membranes. Peroxidation of sperm membrane unsaturated fatty acids leads to a loss of membrane fluidity, which inhibits sperm fusion events during the process of fertilization. When preparing sperm for assisted conception it is advantageous to separate motile sperm from leucocytes and dead sperm as effectively and efficiently as possible. However, if intracytoplasmic sperm injection is the treatment of choice, sperm fusion events are of course bypassed, and direct high-speed centrifugation of these suboptimal sperm samples does not appear to jeopardize fertilization by ICSI.

Sperm samples which show moderate to high counts ($>35 \times 10^6$ motile sperm/ml) with good forward progression and motility can be prepared using a basic overlay and swim-up technique. Discontinuous buoyant density gradient centrifugation is the method of choice for samples which show:

1. Low motility;
2. Poor forward progression;
3. Large amounts of debris and/or high numbers of cells;
4. Antisperm antibodies.

At the end of each preparation procedure, the pH of the resulting samples is adjusted by gassing gently with 5% CO_2, and samples are stored at room temperature until final preparation for insemination.

Standard swim-up or layering

Pipette 2 ml of culture medium into a round-bottomed disposable test tube. Gently pipette approximately 1.5 ml neat semen underneath the medium (being very careful not to disturb the interface formed between the semen and the medium). Tightly cap the tube and allow it to stand at room temperature for up to 2 hours. The ejaculate can also be divided into several tubes for layering if necessary. Harvest the resulting top and middle clouded layers into a conical test-tube and spin at 200 g for 5 minutes. Remove the supernatant and resuspend the pellet in 2 ml medium. Centrifuge again, discard the supernatant, and resuspend the pellet in 1 ml medium. Assess this sample for count and motility, gas the surface gently with 5% CO_2 in air, and store at room temperature prior to dilution for the insemination procedure.

Alternatively, 2 ml of medium can be gently layered over the semen sample in its pot, which provides a larger interface surface area. After 10–45 minutes, suspend an aliquot of this layer in 1 ml of medium, and process as above.

The time allowed for swim-up should be adjusted according to the quality of the initial sample: the percentage of abnormal sperm which will appear in the medium increases with time, and continues to do so after normal motile density has reached its optimum level.

Pellet and swim-up

This method is used when the semen has been collected into medium or medium + serum. It is also useful for viscous samples (once the viscosity has been decreased, by vigorous pipetting or syringing) and when the total volume of semen is very low. This method is not recommended when motility is very poor or when there is a large degree of cellular contamination and debris (the sperm will be concentrated with this prior to the swim-up).

1. Mix semen and medium and centrifuge once. *N.B.* In some cases (i.e. oligo/asthenospermia) much more semen will need to be prepared, and the volume of medium used should be increased accordingly. As a general rule be careful not to take far more of the semen than is required.
2. Carefully remove all the supernatant and then very gently pipette about 0.75 ml of medium over the pellet, taking care not to disturb it.
3. Allow the sperm to swim-up into the medium. If the sample has poor motility it sometimes helps to lay the centrifuge tube on its side.

　　　　– 10 minutes is sufficient for very motile sperm (activity 3–4)
　　　　– 1 hour plus may be required for poorly motile sperm.
　　　　In general do not leave for too long, as some cells and debris will become resuspended.
　　4.　Carefully remove supernatant from pellet and place in a clean centrifuge tube.
　　5.　Centrifuge again, resuspend in medium, assess count and motility, and gas with CO_2 before storing at room temperature.

This method has the disadvantage of exposing motile sperm to peroxidative damage during centrifugation with defective sperm and white cells. Aitken (1990) has shown that unselected sperm exhibit higher levels of reactive oxygen species production in response to centrifugation than the functionally competent sperm selected prior to centrifugation by the layering method. Sperm that are selected prior to centrifugation produce much lower levels of reactive oxygen species and their functional capacity is not impaired.

Discontinuous buoyant density gradient centrifugation

Following the withdrawal of Percoll (Pharmacia) for use in human ART programmes in 1996, buoyant density gradient 'kits' for sperm preparation are now commercially available. These are based upon either coated silica particles, a mixture of Ficoll and Iodixanol, or highly purified arabinogalactan. Individual experiences comparing the use of these products have reported no significant differences between them. Buoyant density gradients apparently protect the sperm from the trauma of centrifugation, and a high proportion of functional sperm can be recovered from the gradients. Discontinuous two- or three-step gradients are simple to prepare and highly effective in preparing motile sperm fractions from suboptimal semen samples. A single layer of 90–100% density can also be used for simple filtration by layering the sample on top of the column and allowing the sperm to migrate through the density medium, where they can be harvested from the bottom of the test tube.

Methods

Manufacturers' instructions should be followed for the different commercial preparations, but 'recipes' can be adapted according to each individual semen sample, in particular with respect to volumes, speed of centrifugation, and length of centrifugation. In general, a longer centrifugation *time* increases the recovery of both motile and immotile sperm; normal immotile sperm are only decelerated by the particles, and after long spinning they will reach the bottom of the gradient. Higher centrifugation *speeds* increase the recovery of motile sperm, and also of lower density particles; therefore, if the gradients are spun at a higher speed, a shorter time should be used. Debris, round cells, and abnormal forms with amorphous heads and cytoplasmic droplets never reach the bottom of the tube because of their low density. Gradients with larger volumes result in improved filtration, but decreased yield. The three layers of a mini-gradient improve filtration, and the smaller volumes improve recovery of sperm from severely oligospermic samples. Large amounts of debris can disrupt gradients and prevent adequate filtration. Samples with a large amount of debris should be distributed in smaller volumes over several gradients. Severely asthenozoospermic samples, with a normal sperm density but poor motility can also be distributed over a series of mini-gradients.

Isotonic gradient so·lution

10 × concentrated EBS (or other media concentrate)	10 ml
5% human serum albumin	9 ml
Sodium pyruvate	3 mg
Sodium lactate @ 60%	0.37 ml
1 M HEPES	2 ml
Gentamicin sulphate, 5 mg/ml	2 ml

Mix, and filter this solution through a 0.22 μm Millipore filter,

Add 90 ml density gradient preparation
Store at + 4°C for up to 1 week.

Two-step gradient, 80/40
Can be used for all samples which contain more than four million motile sperm/ml. Should be used for all specimens with known or suspected anti-sperm antibodies

80%: 8 ml isotonic + 2 ml culture medium
40%: 4 ml isotonic + 6 ml culture medium

1. Gradients: pipette 2.0–2.5 ml of 80% into the bottom of a conical centrifuge tube.
    Gently overlay with an equal volume of 40%.
    Layer up to 2 ml of sample on top of the 40% layer.
2. Centrifuge at 600 *g* for 20 minutes.
    Cells, debris, and immotile/abnormal sperm accumulate at the interfaces, and the pellet should contain functionally normal sperm. Recovery of a good

pellet is influenced by the amount of debris and immotile sperm which impede the travel of the good sperm.

3. Carefully recover the pellet at the bottom of the 80% layer, resuspend in 1 ml of medium, and assess (even if there is no visible pellet, a sufficient number of sperm can usually be recovered by aspirating the bottom 20–50 µl of the 80% layer).
4. If the sample looks sufficiently clean, centrifuge for 5 minutes at 200 g, resuspend the pellet in fresh medium, and assess the final preparation.
5. If there is a high percentage of immotile sperm, centrifuge at 200 g for 5 minutes, remove the supernatant, carefully layer 1 ml fresh medium over the pellet, and allow the motile sperm to swim up for 15–30 minutes. Collect the supernatant and assess the final preparation.

If at least 10^6 motile sperm/ml have been recovered, spin at 200 g for 5 minutes and resuspend in fresh medium. This will be the final preparation to be diluted before insemination, therefore the volume of medium added will depend upon the calculated assessment.

Mini-gradient (95/70/50)

95%	9.5 ml Percoll + 0.5 ml culture medium	
70%	7.0 ml	3.0 ml
50%	5.0 ml	5.0 ml

1. Gradients: make layers with 0.3 ml of each solution: 95, then 70, then 50.
2. Dilute the semen 1:1 with culture medium, and centrifuge at 200 g for 10 minutes.
3. Resuspend the pellet in 0.3 ml culture mediumn, and layer over mini-gradient (resuspend in a larger volume if it is to be distributed over several gradients).
4. Centrifuge at 600 g, for 20–30 minutes.
5. Recover the pellet(s), resuspend in 0.5 ml culture medium, and assess count and motility. Proceed exactly as for two-step gradient preparation: either centrifuge at 200 g for 5 minutes and resuspend the pellet, or layer over the pellet for a further preparation by swim up. The concentration of the final prepration should be adjusted to a sperm density of approximately one million motile sperm per ml if possible (Figure 8.2).

NB: if a sample is being prepared for ICSI, note that residual PVP-coated particles in the preparation will interact with polyvinylpyrrolidone (PVP), resulting in a gelatinous mass from which the sperm cannot be aspirated!! Careful washing of the preparation to remove all traces of gradient preparation is essential when handling samples for ICSI.

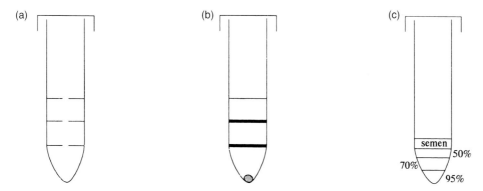

Figure 8.2   Buoyant density gradients. (a,b) Two-step gradients before and after centrifugation: (c) Mini-gradient.

Sedimentation method or layering under paraffin oil

This method is useful for samples with very low counts and poor motility. It is very effective in removing debris, but requires several hours of preparation time.

1. Mix the semen with a large volume of medium, pipetting thoroughly to break down viscosity etc. and wash the sample by dilution and centrifugation twice.
2. Alternatively: process the entire sample (undiluted) on an appropriate discontinuous buoyant density gradient.
3. Resuspend the pellet in a reduced volume of medium so that the final motile sperm concentration is not too dilute.
4. Layer this final suspension under paraffin oil (making one large droplet) in a small Petri dish. Place in a desiccator and gas with 5% CO_2.
5. Leave at room temperature for 3–24 hours. The duration of sedimentation depends upon the amount of cells, debris and motile spermatozoa; a longer period is usually more effective in reducing cells and debris, but may also reduce the number of freely motile sperm in the upper part of the droplet.
6. Carefully aspirate motile sperm by pipetting the upper part of the droplet. Aspiration can be made more efficient by using a fine drawn pipette and also by positioning the droplet under the stereomicroscope, to ensure that as little debris as possible is collected.

High-speed centrifugation and washing

Cryptozoospermic (or nearly cryptozoospermic) samples which must be prepared for ICSI can be either centrifuged directly (without dilution) at $1800\,g$ for

5 minutes, or diluted with medium and then centrifuged at 1800 g for 5 minutes.

Wash the pellet with a small volume of medium (0.5 ml approximately) and centrifuge at 200 g for 5 minutes. Recover this pellet in a minimal volume of medium (20–50 μl), and overlay with mineral oil. Single sperm for microinjection can then be retrieved from this droplet using the micromanipulator.

It is important to bear in mind that every semen specimen has different characteristics and parameters, and it is illogical to treat each specimen identically. All preparation methods are adaptable in some way: layering can be carried out in test-tubes, but a wider vessel increases the area exposed to culture medium and decreases the depth of the specimen, increasing the potential return of motile sperm from oligoasthenospermic samples. Centrifugation times for buoyant density gradients may be adjusted according to the quality of the specimen to give optimum results. It is important to tailor preparation techniques to fit the parameters of the semen specimen, rather than to have fixed recipes. A trial preparation prior to oocyte retrieval may be advisable in choosing the suitable technique for particular patients.

Chemical enhancement of sperm motility prior to insemination

Pentoxifylline is a methyl-xanthine derived phosphodiesterase inhibitor which is known to elevate spermatozoal intracellular levels of cyclic adenosine 3′5′ monophosphate in vitro. It has been postulated that the resulting increase in intracellular adenosine triphosphate (ATP) enhances sperm motility in samples which on assessment show poor progressive motility, with an increase in fertilization and pregnancy rates for suboptimal semen samples. 2-Deoxyadenosine has also been used to achieve a similar effect.

The protocol involves a 30 minute preincubation of prepared sperm with the stimulant; the resulting sperm suspension is then washed to remove the stimulant, and the preparation is used immediately for insemination.

Stock solutions:

1 mM PF: dissolve 22 mg Pentoxifylline (Hoechst) in 10 ml medium
3 mM 2-DA: dissolve 8 mg 2-deoxyadenosine in 10 ml medium
Gas with 5% CO_2 to adjust pH
Store at 4 °C for a maximum period of one month

> **Methods of sperm preparation**
>
> - Overlay and swim-up, multiple overlay
> - Discontinuous buoyant density gradients
>   mini: 95/70/50%
>   two-step: 40/80, 45/90, 47.95%
>   one-step: 95%
> - High-speed centrifugation and washing
>   sedimentation under oil
>   'fishing' with micromanipulator
>   swim-out under oil
>   *Be flexible: use and adapt a combination of methods*

Procedure:

1. Gas and warm PF or 2-DA solutions, and also an additional 10 ml medium.
2. 35–40 minutes prior to insemination time, add an equal volume of PF or 2-DA solutions to the sperm preparation suspension.
3. Incubate at 37 °C for 30 minutes.
4. Centrifuge, 5 minutes 200 g, and resuspend pellet in warm medium.
5. Analyse the sperm suspension for count and motility, dilute to appropriate concentration for insemination, and inseminate oocytes immediately.

Sperm preparation for ICSI

A combination of sperm preparation methods can be used:

Extremely oligospermic/asthenozoospermic samples cannot be prepared by buoyant density centifugation or swim-up techniques.

1. Centrifuge the whole sample, 1800 g, 5 minutes, wash with medium, and resuspend the pellet in a small volume of medium.
2. Apply this sample directly to the injection dish, without PVP, or add an aliquot of the suspension to a drop of HEPES buffered medium without PVP.
3. If possible, use the injection pipette to select a moving sperm with apparently normal morphology from this drop and transfer it into the PVP drop. If PVP is not to be used for the injection procedure transfer the sperm into another drop of HEPES buffered medium without PVP.
4. If there is debris attached to the sperm, clean it by pipetting the sperm back and forth with the injection pipette.

5. If the sperm still has some movement in the PVP drop, immobilize it and proceed with the injection as previously described.
6. It may sometimes be helpful to connect the sperm droplet to another small medium droplet by means of a bridge of medium, and allow motile sperm to swim out into the clean droplet.

No motile sperm

Even if the results of semen analysis have shown no motile sperm to be present, it may be possible to see occasional slight tail movement in a medium drop without PVP. If absolutely no motile sperm are found, immotile sperm may be used. The fertilization rate with immotile sperm is generally lower than that with motile sperm, and oocytes with a single pronucleus are seen more often in these cases. Previous assessment with a vital stain may be helpful before deciding upon ICSI treatment.

The hypo-osmotic swelling test (HOS)

The HOS test assesses the osmoregulatory ability of the sperm, and therefore the functional integrity of its membranes. It can be used to discriminate viable from non-viable sperm cells in a sample which has zero or little apparent motility. The test is based upon the ability of live spermatozoa to withstand the moderate stress of a hypo-osmotic environment – they react to this stress by swelling of the tail. Dead spermatozoa whose plasma membranes are no longer intact do not show tail swelling. HOS test diluent is a solution of 150 mOsm/kg osmolarity, and can be made by dissolving 7.35 g sodium citrate and 13.51 g fructose in 1000 ml of reagent-grade water. Mix an aliquot of the sample with approximately $10 \times$ the volume of diluent, incubate at $37\,^{\circ}$C for 30 minutes, remix and transfer one drop of the mixture to a clean microscope slide. Cover with a coverslip, and examine using phase-contrast microscopy at a magnification of $\times 400$–500 for the presence of swollen (coiled) tails. Osmotically incompetent and dead spermatozoa swell so much that the plasma membrane bursts, allowing the tail to straighten out again.

100% abnormal heads

If the semen analysis shows 100% head anomalies, it may still be possible to find the occasional normal form in the sample. In cases where no normal forms are found, the fertilization and implantation rates may be lower; however, debate continues about this subject, and individual judgment should be applied to each case, with careful assessment of several different semen samples.

Fertilization and pregnancy have now been demonstrated using samples from men with globozoospermia, a 100% head anomaly where all sperm lack an acrosomal cap; however, recent evidence suggests that such defects which are genetically determined have a high probability of being transmitted to the offspring, and debate continues as to whether it is ethically advisable to offer treatment to these men.

Sticky sperm

Sperm which have a tendency to stick to the injection pipette make the injection procedure more difficult. If the sperm is caught in the pipette, try to release it by repeatedly aspirating and blowing with the injection system.

Excessive amounts of debris

Large amounts of debris in the sperm preparation may block the injection pipette, or become attached to the outside of the pipette. A blocked pipette may be cleared by blowing a small amount of the air already in the pipette through it (or by using 'Sonic Sword' from Research Instruments). Debris attached to the outside of the injection pipette can be cleaned by rubbing the pipette against the holding pipette, against the oocyte, or against the oil at the edge of the medium drop. It may be necessary (and preferable) to change the pipette if it cannot be quickly cleared.

Retrograde ejaculation and electroejaculation: sperm preparation

When treating patients with ejaculatory dysfunction, with or without the aid of electroejaculation, both antegrade and retrograde ejaculation (into the bladder) are commonly found. When retrograde ejaculation is anticipated, the bladder should first be emptied via a catheter, and approximately 20 ml of culture medium then instilled. After ejaculation, the bladder is again emptied, and the entire sample centrifuged. The resulting pellet(s) can then be resuspended in medium and processed on appropriate density gradients. As with all abnormal semen samples, a flexible approach is required in order to obtain a suitable sample for insemination.

Obstructive and nonobstructive azoospermia: epididymal and testicular sperm

1. Epididymal sperm can be obtained by open microscopic surgery or by percutaneous puncture, using a 21 g 'butterfly' or equivalent needle to aspirate fluid. If large numbers of sperm are found, they can be processed by buoyant density gradient centrifugation or even by swim-up techniques. Samples with fewer sperm can be washed and centrifuged with IVF medium a number of times, and the concentrated sample is then added to microdroplets in the injection dish. Motile spermatozoa 'swim out' to the periphery of the droplets, where they can be collected and transferred to clean drops of medium or PVP for injection later.

2. Testicular sperm is obtained by open biopsy or by percutaneous needle biopsy, and there are a variety of approaches to sample processing:

   i. Crush the biopsy sample between two microscope slides, and expose sperm by shredding the tissue either with glass slides, by needle dissection, by dissection using microscissors, or by maceration using a microgrinder. Concentrate the debris by centrifugation and examine under high-power microscopy to look for spermatozoa. Large quantities of debris are invariably present, and it may be difficult to find sperm (especially with cases of focal spermatogenesis). Further processing steps will depend upon the quality of the sample: it may be loaded onto a small single-step buoyant density gradient, or sperm simply harvested 'by hand' under the microscope. Use a large needle, assisted hatching pipette or biopsy pipette to collect and pool live sperm in a clean drop of medium.

   ii. Tubules in the biopsy sample can be carefully unravelled under the dissecting microscope, using fine watchmakers' forceps. Cut the tubules into small lengths of 1–2 cm, and 'milk' the contents by squeezing from the middle to an open end. The cells can be picked out of the dish and placed onto the ICSI microscope for examination, or into a centrifuge tube of clean medium for further preparation. An alternative approach is to slit the segments of tubule rather than 'milking' to release the cells. Fresh testicular sperm are often immotile and combined with Sertoli cells, but free-swimming sperm are usually seen after further incubation. Pregnancies have been achieved from testicular sperm incubated up to three days after the biopsy procedure, but the proportion of motile sperm in a testicular biopsy sample is usually highest after 24 hours' incubation. Incubation at 32 °C instead of 37 °C may also be of benefit (Van den Berg, 1998). If fresh sperm is to be used, the biopsy procedure should be carried out the day before the planned oocyte retrieval. If the sperm are to be cryopreserved, a higher proportion of frozen testicular sperm have been found to retain their motility on thawing if they have been incubated for 24–48 hours before freezing.

Spermatid identification

In some cases of severe testicular dysfunction, no spermatozoa can be found either in the ejaculate or in testicular tissue, but precursor cells (round, elongating, or elongated spermatids) may be identified. Although pregnancies and live births have been achieved following injection of these cells, fertilization and pregnancy rates are dramatically lower than following the use of mature spermatozoa, and the value, as well as the ethics, of offering this therapy is still open to question.

Although staining techniques under light or electron microscopy allow identification and classification of the different stages of spermiogenesis, from a practical standpoint, it can be difficult to confidently identify and isolate immature sperm cells in a wet preparation. Under Hoffman Modulation Contrast systems, four categories of spermatids can be observed and identified according to their shape, amount of cytoplasm, and size of tail: round, elongating, elongated and mature spermatids just prior to their release from Sertoli cells.

Round spermatids must be distinguished from other round cells such as spermatogonia, spermatocytes, polymorphonuclear leukocytes, lymphocytes and erythrocytes. Their diameter (6.5 μm to 8 μm) is similar to that of erythrocytes (7.2 μm) and small lymphocytes. Round spermatids may be observed at three different phases: golgi, cap and acrosome phase (where the nucleus moves towards a peripheral position). When the cell is rotated, a centrally located smooth (uncondensed) nucleus can be seen, and a developing acrosomal structure may be observed as a bright spot or small protrusion on one side of the cell, adjacent to the spermatid nucleus.

Sertoli cell nuclei are very flat and transparent, with a prominent central or adjacent nucleus, whereas the ROS is a three-dimensional round cell. (Figures 8.3, 8.4).

When attempting to isolate ROS from a biopsy sample, the first search criteria is size – look for cells which are approximately the same size as an erythrocyte, and which contain a smooth, regular, centrally located nucleus surrounded by a thin, smooth rim of cytoplasm. Sometimes you can see the acrosomal vesicle as a bright round spot next to the nucleus in Phase I spermatids, or as a darker thin region spread over one of the poles of the nucleus in phase 2 spermatids. Phase 3 is a transition between round and elongated forms – elongated spermatids have an elongated nucleus at one side of the cell, and a larger cytoplasmic region on the other side, surrounding the developing tail. Cells suspected to be round spermatids are transferred to a clean droplet of medium for further examination under × 400 magnification, together with a few RBCs for comparison. Roll the cells gently with the injection pipette until the surface 'button' (developing acrosomal structure) can be clearly seen.

The methodology for ROS isolation is a major factor affecting the outcome of spermatid injection, and the morphological criteria used are highly susceptible to intra and extra observer variations. An embryologist should feel confident with the technique and criteria before working with spermatid cells.

Sperm preparation: equipment and materials

Semen sterile collection pot 60 ml
Microscope (phase is useful)
Counting chamber (Makler, Sefi Medical Instruments, POB 7295, Haifa
    31070 Israel, or Horwell Haemocytometer)
Centrifuge with swing-out rotor (Mistral 1000, MSE)
Centrifuge tubes (15 ml, Corning)
Microscope slides
Coverslips
Disposable test-tubes: 4 ml, 10 ml
Culture media
Buoyant Density Media:
    Pure Sperm (Scandinavian IVF AB)
    IxtaPrep (MediCult)
    Sil-Select (MICROM)
    Isolate (Irvine Scientific)
Glass Pasteur pipettes
Disposable pipettes: 1, 5, 10 ml
Spirit burner + methanol or gas Bunsen burner
Plastic ampoules or straws for sperm freezing
Sperm cryopreservation media (chapter 11)
Supply of liquid nitrogen and storage Dewars

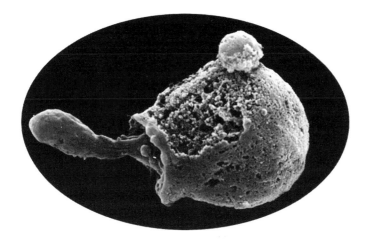

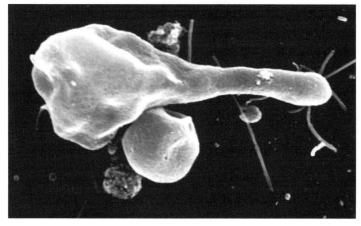

Figure 8.3   Scanning electron micrographs of early spermatid detected in azoospermic ejaculate. Courtesy of Professor B. Bartov, Israel.

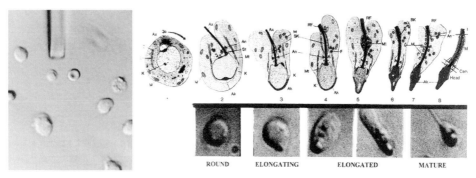

Figure 8.4   Developing sperm. Courtesy of M. Nijs and P. Vanderzwalmen, Belgium.

Further reading

Aitken, R.J. (1988) Assessment of sperm function for IVF. *Human Reproduction* **3**:89–95.

Aitken, R.J. (1989) The role of free oxygen radicals and sperm function. *International Journal of Andrology* **12**:95–7.

Aitken, R.J. (1990) Evaluation of human sperm function. *British Medical Bulletin* **46**:654–74.

Aitken, R.J. & Clarkson, J.S. (1987) Cellular basis of defective sperm function and its association with the genesis of reactive oxygen species by human spermatozoa. *Journal of Reproductive Fertility* **81**:459–69.

Aitken, R.J., Comhaire, F.H., Eliasson, R., Jager, S., Kremer, J., Jones, W.R., de Kretser, D.M., Nieschlag, G., Paulse, C.A., Wang, C. & Waites, G.M.H. (1987) *WHO Manual for the Examination of Human Semen and Semen–Cervical Mucus Interaction.* 2nd edn, Cambridge University Press, Cambridge, England.

Avery, S.M. & Elder, K.T. (1992) Semen assessment and preparation. In: (Brinsden, P.R. & Rainsbury, P.A. eds.), *In Vitro Fertilization and Assisted Reproduction.* The Parthenon Publishing Group, UK, pp. 171–85.

Avery, S.M., Marriott, V., Mason, B., Riddle, A. & Sharma, V. (1987) An assessment of the efficiency of various sperm preparation techniques. Presented at Vth World Congress on IVF and ET, *Programme Supplement* **85**:p. 58.

Braude, P.R. & Bolton, V.N. (1984) The preparation of spermatozoa for in vitro fertilization by buoyant density centrifugation. In: (Feichtinger, W. & Kemeter, P. eds.), *Recent Progress in Human In Vitro Fertilisation.* Cofese, Palermo, pp. 125–34.

Cohen, J., Edwards, R.G., Fehilly, C., Fishel, S., Hewitt, J., Purdy, J., Rowland, G., Steptoe, P.C. & Webster, J. (1985) In vitro fertilization: a treatment for male infertility. *Fertility and Sterility* **43**: 422–32.

Comhaire, F., Depoorter, B., Vermeulen, L. & Schoonjans, F. (1995) Assessment of sperm concentration. In: (Hedon, B., Bringer, J. & Mares, P. eds.) *Fertility & Sterility: A Current Overview (IFFS-95).* The Parthenon Publishing Group, New York, London, pp. 297–302.

Dravland, J.E. & Mortimer, D. (1985) A simple discontinuous Percoll gradient for washing human spermatozoa. *IRCS Medical Science* **13**:16–18.

Elder, K. & Elliott, T. (1998) The use of testicular and epididymal sperm in IVF. *Worldwide Conferences on Reproductive Biology*, Ladybrook Publishing, Australia.

Elder, K.T., Wick, K.L. & Edwards, R.G. (1990) Seminal plasma anti-sperm antibodies and IVF: the effect of semen sample collection into 50% serum. *Human Reproduction* **5**:179–84.

Edwards, R.G., Fishel, S.G., Cohen, J., Fehilly, C.B., Purdy, J.M., Steptoe, P.C. & Webster, J.M. (1984) Factors influencing the success of in vitro fertilization for alleviating human infertility. *Journal of In Vitro Fertilization and Embryo Transfer* **1**:3–23.

Franken, D. (1998) Sperm morphology: a closer look – is sperm morphology related to chromatin packaging? *Alpha Newsletter* **14**:1–3.

Glover, T.D., Barratt, C.L.R., Tyler, J.P.A. & Hennessey, J.F. (1990) *Human Male Fertility and Semen Analysis.* Academic Press, London.

Hall, J., Fishel, S., Green, S., Fleming, S., Hunter, A., Stoddart, N., Dowell, K. & Thornton, S. (1995) Intracytoplasmic sperm injection versus high insemination concentration in-vitro fertilization in cases of very severe teratozoospermia. *Human Reproduction* **10**:493–6.

Hamamah, S. & Gatti, J-L. (1998) Role of the ionic environment and internal pH on sperm activity. *Human Reproduction* **13 Suppl. 4**:20–30.

Jager, S., Kremer, J. & Van-Schlochteren-Draaisma, T. (1978) A simple method of screening for antisperm antibodies in the human male: detection of spermatozoa surface IgG with the direct mixed antiglobulin reaction carried out on untreated fresh human semen. *International*

Journal of Fertility **23**:12.

Makler, A. (1978) A new chamber for rapid sperm count and motility evaluation. *Fertility and Sterility* **30**:414.

Matson, P.L. (1995) External quality assessment for semen analysis and sperm antibody detection: results of a pilot scheme. *Human Reproduction* **10**:620–5.

Menkveld, R., Oettler, E.E., Kruger, T.F., Swanson, R.J., Acosta, A.A. & Oeninger, S. (1991) *Atlas of Human Sperm Morphology*. Williams & Wilkins, Baltimore, MD.

Mortimer, D. (1991) Sperm preparation techniques and iatrogenic failures of in-vitro fertilization. *Human Reproduction* **6(2)**:173–6.

Mortimer, D. (1994) *Practical Laboratory Andrology*. Oxford University Press, New York.

Rainsbury, P.A. (1992) The treatment of male factor infertility due to sexual dysfunction. In: (Brinsden, P.R. & Rainsbury, P.A.) *In Vitro Fertilization and Assisted Reproduction*. The Parthenon Publishing Group, UK.

Sakkas, D., Urmer, F., Bizzaro, D., Minicardi, G., Bianchi, P.G., Shoukir, Y. & Campana, A. (1998) Sperm nuclear DNA damage and altered chromatin structure: effect on fertilization and embryo development. *Human Reproduction* **13, Suppl. 4**:11–19.

Sousa, M., Barros, A. & Tesarik, J. (1998) Current problems with spermatid conception. *Human Reproduction* **13**:255–8.

Stewart, B. (1998) New horizons in male infertility: the use of testicular and epididymal sperm in IVF. *Alpha Newsletter* **13**:1–3.

Van den Berg, M. (1998) In: (Elder, K. & Elliott, T. eds.), *The Use of Epidemiological and Testicular Sperm in IUF*. World Wide Conferences on Reproductive Biology, Ladybrook Publishing, Australia.

Van der Ven, H., Bhattacharya, A.K., Binor, Z., Leto, S. & Zaneveld, L.J.D. (1982) Inhibition of human sperm capacitation by a high molecular weight factor from human seminal plasma. *Fertility and Sterility* **38**:753–5.

Vanderzwalmen, P., Zech, H., Birkenfeld, A., Yemini, M., Betini, G., Lejeune, B., Nijs, M., Segal, L., Stecher, A., Vandamme, B., van Rosendaal, E. & Schoysman, R. (1997) Intracytoplasmic injection of spermatids retrieved from testicular tissue: influence of testicular pathology, type of selected spermatids and oocyte activation. *Human Reproduction* **12**:1203–13.

World Health Organization (1999) *WHO Laboratory Manual for the Examination of Human Semen and Semen–Cervical Mucus Interaction*. Cambridge University Press, Cambridge.

Yovich, J.L. (1992) Assisted reproduction for male factor infertility. In: (Brinsden, P.R. & Rainsbury, P.A. eds.), *In Vitro Fertilization and Assisted Reproduction*. The Parthenon Publishing Group, UK.

Yovich, J.M., Edirisinghe, W.R., Cummins, J.M. & Yovich, J.L. (1990) Influence of pentoxifylline in severe male factor infertility. *Fertility and Sterility* **53**:715–22.

9

Oocyte retrieval and embryo culture

Programmed superovulation protocols

Programmed superovulation protocols now provide a convenient and effective means of scheduling and organizing a clinical IVF programme, allowing oocyte retrievals to be performed on specific days of the week, or in 'batches'. A standard protocol that can be used to maximize the number of oocytes recovered uses downregulation with gonadotrophin releasing hormone (GnRH) agonist, commencing in the luteal phase of the previous cycle, and ovarian stimulation with purified follicular stimulating hormone (FSH) by subcutaneous injection.

There are many variations of this standard protocol, and individual ART programmes apply the same strategy with a variety of different drugs and schedules. Downregulation with a GnRH agonist may begin either in the luteal or the follicular phase ('long protocol') of the previous menstrual cycle, and can be administered with a depot preparation such as decapeptyl, goserelin or leuprolide, by daily subcutaneous injections, or daily intranasal sniffs. It may also be administered from Day 1 of the treatment cycle and continued until ovulation induction with hCG ('short protocol', sometimes also known as 'flare protocol'). The 'Ultrashort protocol' uses only three doses of the agonist, on days 2, 3 and 4 of the treatment cycle. Treatment cycles may also be scheduled by programming menstruation using an oral contraceptive preparation such as Norethisterone 5 mg TDS. The 'standard' protocols are not always suitable for every patient, and every treatment regime should be tailored according to the patient's medical history and response to any previous ovarian stimulation. Patients with suspected polycystic ovarian disease (PCO) and those with limited ovarian reserve ('poor responders') require careful management and individualized treatment regimes. Simplified treatment schedules using GnRH antagonists in combination with recombinant gonadotrophins are currently under development and clinical trial, and may lead to a 'revolution' in ovarian stimulation therapy in the near future. One example of a 'standard' protocol, using luteal phase downregulation, is described below:

Protocol

1. Commence downregulation on Day 19–21 of the cycle, depending upon menstrual history and cycle length. Rx: Nafarelin (Synarel, Searle) two sniffs (400 mg twice daily), or Buserelin (Suprefact, Hoechst) 500 µg subcutaneously daily.
2. Programmed cycles allow for 6–12 days of stimulation, varied according to the individual patient's age, cause of infertility and previous history.
3. Before starting follicular stimulation: confirm downregulation with baseline assessments
   – ultrasound pelvic scan
   – plasma assays for oestrogen, luteinizing hormone (LH) and progesterone. If any of the endocrine parameters are elevated (oestradiol (E2) > 50 ng/ml, LH >5.0 IU/ml, P4 >2.0 ng/ml), stimulation is postponed and the assays repeated after 2–4 further days of downregulation.
4. Standard starting dose of gonadotropin for stimulation = two or three ampoules daily, (150–225 IU) varied according to age of patient and previous history, etc. Polycystic ovary (PCO) patients start with one ampoule, (75 IU) and are carefully monitored.
5. Ovulation is induced by subcutaneous administration of human chorionic gonadotrophin hormone (hCG) 5000–10 000 units (Profasi, Serono UK) when at least one leading follicle ≥ 18 mm diameter.
6. Oocyte retrieval is scheduled 34–36 hours after hCG injection. Luteal support per vaginum (PV) Utrogestan capsules, 100 mg three times daily (Besins-Iscovesco), Cyclogest pessaries 200 mg PV twice daily (Hoechst), or Gestone 50 mg daily by intramuscular injection (Ferring) is commenced on the day after hCG administration.
7. Oocyte retrieval procedures are performed by vacuum aspirating follicles under vaginal ultrasound guidance. Disposable needles are used, which may have a double- or single-lumen, according to the team's preference for aspiration of follicles with or without further rinsing or 'flushing' (the COOK IVF K-MAR Complete System provides an efficient vacuum aspiration and infusion system). Aspirates are collected into heated 15 ml Falcon tubes.

   Oocyte retrieval can be safely carried out as an out-patient procedure, using either local anaesthesia, intravenous sedation or light general anaesthesia. An experienced operator can collect an average number of oocytes (i.e. 8–12) in a

Drug treatment for scheduled cycles

- Pituitary downregulation with GnRH agonist: Synarel (Syntex) by intranasal administration, twice daily or Suprefact (Hoechst) by daily subcutaneous injection
- Baseline endocrinology and ultrasound assessment to confirm down-regulation
- Ovarian stimulation with Metrodin HP or Gonal F(Serono)
- Follicular phase monitoring after one week of stimulation

> cycle day 19–21 start   baseline   monitoring
>
> downregulation for 10–14 days   stimulation..8–12 days   36 hours......OCR......ET
> Synarel
>
>   or...FSH.........................hCG
> Suprefact   Utrogestan
>   or Cyclogest..........

Baseline assessment: ultrasound

- Ovaries: Size, position
             Shape, texture
             Cysts
             Evidence of PCO
- Uterus: Endometrial size, shape, texture & thickness
             Fibroids
             Congenital or other anomalies/abnormalities
- Hydrosalpinges, loculated fluid

Baseline assessment: endocrinology

- Oestradiol: less than 50 pg/ml
- LH: less than 5 IU/l.
- Progesterone: less than 2 ng/ml
    If any values are elevated:
        continue GnRH agonist treatment
        withhold stimulation
        reassess 3–7 days later
- If LH remains elevated:
        withhold stimulation
        increase dose of GnRH agonist
- (FSH: less than 10 IU/l without downregulation)

Ovarian stimulation
- Pure FSH by subcutaneous self-injection
- Starting dose:
    According to age and/or history
    - age 35 or younger: 150 IU/day
    - age over 35:   225 IU/day
      depending on previous response,
    - up to 300–450 IU daily
- Begin monitoring after 7 days of stimulation
  (*adjusted according to history and baseline assessment*)

Cycle monitoring

Stimulation Day 8 assessment
- Ultrasound assessment
    Follicle size 14 mm or less: review in 2 or 3 days
    Follicle size 16 mm or greater: review daily
- Plasma oestradiol
- Plasma LH
    review as necessary

Induction of ovulation

- hCG 10 000 IU by subcutaneous injection when:
    Leading follicle is at least 17–18 mm in diameter
    2 or more follicles > 14 mm in diameter
    Endometrium:
        at least 8 mm in thickness with
        trilaminar 'halo' appearance
    Oestradiol levels approx.
        100–150 pg/ml per large follicle
- Oocyte retrieval scheduled for 34–36 hours post-hCG

---

10 to 20 minute time period, and the patient can usually be discharged within 2 to 3 hours of a routine oocyte collection.

Preparation for each case

The embryologist is involved in the management of each in vitro fertilization (IVF) case from the time that the treatment cycle is initiated, and there should be a system which ensures that all members of the laboratory staff can be familiar with the treatment plan for each patient. The laboratory staff should also ensure that all appropriate consent forms have been signed by both

partners, including consent for special procedures and storage of cryopreserved embryos. Study all details of any previous assisted conception treatment,
including response to stimulation, number and quality of oocytes, timing of
insemination, fertilization rate, embryo quality and embryo transfer procedure, and judge whether any parameters at any stage could be altered or
improved in the present cycle. A repeat semen assessment may be required at
the beginning of the treatment cycle, especially if the male partner has suffered
recent illness, stress or trauma which could affect spermatogenesis. If necessary, a back-up semen sample may also be cryopreserved after this assessment.

The risk of introducing any infection into the laboratory via gametes and
samples must be absolutely minimized: note details of screening tests such as
human immunodeficiency virus (HIV) and hepatitis B and C at the beginning
of the treatment cycle, and repeat if necessary.

After administration of hCG to induce ovulation, the embryologist should
again examine the case notes and prepare the laboratory records for the
following day's oocyte retrievals, with attention to the following details:

1. Previous history, with attention to laboratory procedures: any modifications
   required?
2. Semen assessment: any special preparations or precautions required for
   sample collection or preparation?
3. Current cycle history: number of follicles, endocrine parameters, any sugges-
   tion of ovarian hyperstimulation syndrome?

Laboratory case notes, media, culture vessels and tubes for sperm preparation
are prepared during the afternoon prior to each case, with clear and adequate
labelling throughout. Tissue culture dishes or plates are equilibrated in the
CO_2 incubator overnight.

The choice of culture system used is a matter of individual preference and
previous experience; two systems which are both widely and successfully used
by different IVF groups are described here:

Microdroplets under oil

Pour previously equilibrated mineral oil into 60 mm Petri dishes which have
been clearly marked with each patient's surname.

Using either a Pasteur pipette or adjustable pipettor and sterile tips, carefully place 8 or 9 droplets of medium around the edge of the dish. One or two
drops may be placed centrally, to be used as wash drops.

Examination of the follicular growth records will indicate approximately how many drops/dishes should be prepared; each drop may contain one or two oocytes. Droplet size can range from 50 to 250 μl per drop.

Four-well plates

Prepare labelled and numbered plates containing 0.5–1 ml of tissue culture medium and equilibrate overnight in a humidified incubator. Each well is normally used to incubate three oocytes. Small Petri dishes with approximately 2 ml of HEPES-containing medium may also be prepared, to be used for washing oocytes immediately after identification in the follicular aspirates. This system may also be used in combination with an overlay of equilibrated mineral oil.

Oocyte retrieval (OCR) and identification

Before beginning each OCR procedure.

1. Ensure that heating blocks, stages, and trays are warmed to 37 °C.
2. Prewarm collection test-tubes and 60 mm Petri dishes for scanning aspirates.
3. Prepare a fire-polished Pasteur pipette + holder, a fine-drawn blunt Pasteur pipette as a probe for manipulations, and 1 ml syringes with attached needles for dissection.
4. Check names on dishes and laboratory case notes with medical notes.

Examine follicular aspirates under a stereo dissecting microscope with transmitted illumination base and heated stage. Aliquot the contents of each test tube into two or three Petri dishes, forming a thin layer of fluid which can be quickly, carefully and easily scanned for the presence of an oocyte in the follicular tissue. Low-power magnification ($\times 6$–12) can be used for scanning the fluid, and oocyte identification verified using higher magnification ($\times 25$–50).

The oocyte usually appears within varying quantities of cumulus cells and, if very mature, may be pale and difficult to see (immature oocytes are dark and also difficult to see). Granulosa cells are clearer and more 'fluffy', present in amorphous, often iridescent clumps. Blood clots, especially from the collection needle, should be carefully dissected with 23-gauge needles to check for the presence of cumulus cells.

When an oocyte/cumulus complex (OCC) is found, assess its stage of maturity by noting the volume, density and condition of the surrounding coronal and cumulus cells. If the egg can be seen, the presence of a single polar body indicates that it has reached the stage of metaphase II.

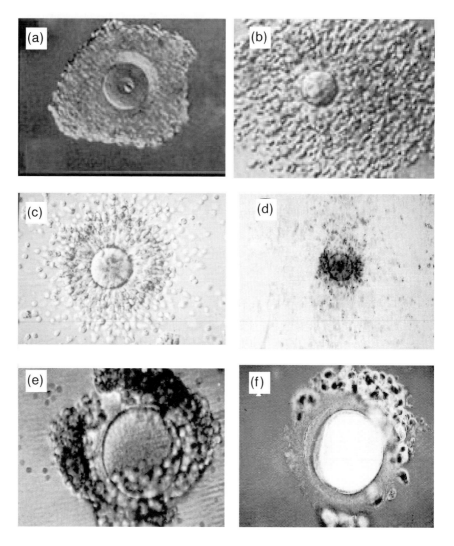

Figure 9.1   Stages of human oocyte maturation normally encountered in ART.
(a) Germinal vesicle; (b) immature, metaphase I; (c) preovulatory metaphase II;
(d) postmature; (e) luteinized; (f) atretic.

There are reports relating the OCC appearance with maturity and fertilizing
capacity of the oocyte, and the following scheme can be used for assessment:

1. *Germinal vesicle*: the oocyte is very immature. There is no expansion of the
    surrounding cells, which are tightly packed around the egg. A large nucleus
    (the germinal vesicle) is still present and may occasionally be seen with the
    help of an inverted microscope. Maturation occasionally takes place in vitro

from this stage, and germinal vesicles are preincubated for 24 hours before insemination (Figure 9.1a).

2. *Metaphase I*: the oocyte is surrounded by a tightly apposed layer of corona cells, and tightly packed cumulus may surround this with a maximum size of approximately five egg diameters. If the oocyte can be seen, it no longer shows a germinal vesicle. The absence of a polar body indicates that the oocyte is in metaphase I, and these immature eggs can be preincubated for 12–24 hours before insemination (Figure 9.1b).

3. *Metaphase II*

   (a) *Preovulatory* (harvested from Graafian follicles): this is the optimal level of maturity, appropriate for successful fertilization. Coronal cells are still apposed to the egg, but are fully radiating; one polar body has been extruded. The cumulus has expanded into a fluffy mass (although beware the possibility that some may have been lost in aspiration) and can be easily stretched (Figure 9.1c).

   (b) *Very mature*: the egg can often be seen clearly as a pale orb; little coronal material is present and is dissociated from the egg. The cumulus is very profuse but it still cellular. The latest events of this stage involve a condensation of cumulus into small black (refractile) drops, as if a tight corona is reforming around the egg (Figure 9.1d).

   (c) *Luteinised*: the egg is very pale and often is difficult to find. The cumulus has broken down and becomes a gelatinous mass around the egg. These eggs have a low probability of fertilization, and are usually inseminated with little delay (Figure 9.1e).

   (d) *Atretic*: granulosa cells are fragmented, and have a lace-like appearance. The oocyte is very dark, and can be difficult to identify (Figure 9.1f).

Gross morphological assessment of oocyte maturity is highly subjective, and subject to inaccuracies. Since 1990, micromanipulation procedures have been widely introduced into routine IVF; because the procedure involves completely denuding oocytes from surrounding cells using hyaluronidase, nuclear maturity and cytoplasm can be accurately assessed. It is now apparent that gross OCC morphology does not necessarily correlate with nuclear maturity. Alikani et al. (1995) used intracytoplasmic sperm injection (ICSI) to analyse its developmental consequences in dysmorphic human oocytes. Of 2968 injected oocytes, 806 (27.2%) were classified as dysmorphic on the basis of cytoplasmic granularity, areas of necrosis, organelle clustering, vacuolation or accumulating saccules of smooth endoplasmic reticulum. Anomalies of the zona pellucida and nonspherical oocytes were also noted.

No single abnormality was found to be associated with a reduction in fertilization rate, and fertilization was not compromised in oocytes with multiple abnormalities. Overall pregnancy and implantation rates were not altered in patients in whom at least one oocyte was dysmorphic; however, exclusive replacement of embryos which originated from dysmorphic oocytes led to a lower implantation rate, and a higher incidence of biochemical pregnancies. They suggest that aberrations in the morphology of oocytes, possibly a result of ovarian hyperstimulation, are of no consequence to fertilization or early cleavage after ICSI. It is possible that embryos generated from dysmorphic oocytes have a reduced potential for implantation and further development.

Van Blerkom and Henry (1992) reported aneuploidy in 50% of oocytes with cytoplasmic dysmorphism; it is not clear whether oocyte aneuploidy is a fundamental developmental phenomenon, or a patient-specific response to induced ovarian stimulation. In 1996, the same group related the oxygen content of human follicular fluid to oocyte quality and subsequent implantation potential. They propose that low oxygen tension associated with poor blood flow to follicles lowers the pH and produces anomalies in chromosomal organization and microtubule assembly, which might cause segregation disorders. Schmutzler et al. (1998) suggest that oocyte morphology is related to serum oestradiol concentration, and that this can be correlated to implantation potential.

Evidence has further accumulated to suggest that the status of the ovary plays a significant role in determining implantation potential of individual oocytes. Heterogeneity of follicles may have a significant impact on oocyte competence and embryo viability, and factors that contribute to the heterogeneity of follicles may provide markers of implantation. Gregory and Leese (1996) and Gregory (1998) studied cell proliferation and biochemical activity of cumulus and granulosa cells isolated from individual follicles in vitro, and were able to relate specific features with implantation potential. They suggest that extent and quality of cumulus cell proliferation, together with their in vitro oestradiol production, provide a marker of implantation potential. Oestradiol production by cumulus cells 24 hours after oocyte collection was significantly higher in pregnant cycles than in cycles where there was a failure of implantation, and oestradiol production by cumulus in vitro may provide a further marker of implantation potential. This information is available to the embryologist prior to embryo transfer, and could act as an objective marker of embryo viability.

Expression of 11βhydroxysteroid dehydrogenase (11βHSD) by granulosa cells in vitro showed a direct negative correlation with implantation; they suggest that this may be related to regulation of intrafollicular cortisol. In-

Oocyte collection

1 Scan follicular aspirates immediately, on a heated microscope stage
2 Wash oocytes, if necessary dissect free of blood clots or granulosa cells
3 Transfer immediately to culture system
4 At the end of the procedure, assess oocytes for quality and maturity, and record optimum time for insemination
5 For microdroplet/oil system, prepare oil dish(es) for insemination, and equilibrate in the incubator
6 Maintain stable pH and temperature throughout

trafollicular cortisol increases significantly after the LH surge, and it is possible that cortisol, and its regulation by 11βHSD, is involved in oocyte maturation and ovulation.

In a further study, they measured blood flow to individual follicles by power colour doppler ultrasound, and confirmed the observations of Van Blerkom et al. (1997) in correlating follicular blood flow with implantation; the incidence of triploid zygotes was also found to be significantly higher when oocytes were derived from follicles with poor vascularity. Follicular vascularity may also influence free cortisol levels in follicular fluid by promoting its diffusion across the follicle boundary.

R. Homburg and M Shelef (1995) reviewed the factors affecting oocyte quality, including morphology, chromosome anomalies, age, follicular micro-environment (in relation to ovulation induction protocol) and endocrine factors. They concluded that nuclear maturity is an important factor in the assessment of oocyte quality, and that the environment of the oocyte has a significant effect upon its quality. LH plays a central role in the maturation process of the oocyte, and an imbalance in the secretion of LH may upset the mechanisms involved. LH is required for completion of the first meiotic division, and inappropriate secretion of LH impairs oocyte quality. A working hypothesis has been proposed which suggests that inappropriately high levels of LH cause a premature maturation of the oocyte, causing it to become physiologically aged, less readily fertilized and, if embryo implantation occurs, it may be more prone to early abortion.

High follicular phase LH levels are a poor prognosis for IVF and pregnancy, and patients with a poor previous history of IVF, including poor oocyte and embryo quality, may benefit from management with long-term GnRH down-regulation and LH monitoring during the follicular phase.

In view of the complexity of all the elegant biochemistry and physiology involved in the development of a competent oocyte, and the delicate balance that must be required within each contributing component and compartment, it seems miraculous indeed that the application of essentially ill-defined strategies has led to the successful birth of so many children. The UK database for 1994 (H.F.E.A., 1996) revealed that from nearly 50 000 embryos transferred, only 11.4% implanted. This enormous wastage of embryos reinforces the fact that a great deal more research is required to identify and define factors involved in the development of competent oocytes and viable embryos.

Insemination

Oocytes are routinely inseminated with a concentration of 100 000 normal motile sperm per ml. If the prepared sperm show suboptimal parameters of motility or morphology, the insemination concentration may be accordingly increased. Some reports have suggested that the use of a high insemination concentration (HIC) may be a useful prelude before deciding upon ICSI treatment for male factor patients.

Microdroplets under oil

At the end of the oocyte retrieval procedure, prepare insemination dishes by pouring mineral oil into the appropriate number of 60 mm Petri dishes, and equilibrate these in the incubator along with the collected oocytes in their collection dishes.

Preovulatory oocytes are inseminated after 3–4 hours preincubation in vitro. Each oocyte is transferred into a drop containing motile sperm at a concentration of approximately 100 000 per ml.

1. Assess the volume of sperm suspension required according to the number of oocytes, and make an appropriate dilution of prepared sperm in a test-tube. Check the dilution by examining a drop of suspension on a plain glass slide under the microscope: it should contain 20 normal motile sperm per high power field ($\times 10$). Adjust the dilution accordingly until the number of progressively motile normal sperm appears adequate.
2. Adjust the pH of the suspension by gently blowing 5% CO_2 over the surface, and incubate at $37\,^{\circ}C$ for 30 minutes.
3. Place droplets of the sperm suspension under previously prepared and equilibrated oil overlays.
4. Examine each oocyte before transfer to the insemination drop; it may be necessary to dissect the cumulus in order to remove bubbles, large clumps of granulosa cells or blood clots.

5. Prepare labelled 35 mm Petri dishes containing equilibrated oil at this time. These will be used for culture of the zygotes after scoring for fertilization the following day.

If the oocyte culture droplets have been created to a measured (e.g. 240 µl) volume, the oocytes can be inseminated by adding 10 µl of prepared sperm suspension that has been adjusted to 2.5 million per ml (final concentration approximately 100 000 sperm per ml, or 25 000 per oocyte).

Four-well dishes

Add a measured volume of prepared sperm suspension to each well, to a total concentration of approximately 100 000 progressively motile sperm per well.

Traditionally inseminated oocytes are incubated overnight in the presence of the prepared sperm sample; however, sperm binding to the zona normally takes place within one to three hours of insemination, and the oocytes can be washed free of excess sperm after three hours' incubation.

Scoring of fertilization on Day 1

Embryo dissection

Inseminated oocytes are dissected 17–20 hours following insemination in order to assess fertilization. Oocytes at this time are normally covered with a layer of dispersed coronal and cumulus cells, which must be carefully removed so that the cell cytoplasm can be examined for the presence of two pronuclei and two polar bodies, indicating normal fertilization.

Scoring for pronuclei should be carried out within the appropriate time span, before pronuclei merge during syngamy – cleaved embryos with abnormal fertilization are indistinguishable from those with 2PN. Abnormal fertilization is observed in human IVF at a rate of approximately 5% of fertilized oocytes, and is generally attributed to polyspermy or nonextrusion of the second polar body. FISH analysis of 3PN embryos has revealed that 80-89% are mosaic.

The choice of dissection procedure is a matter of individual preference, and sometimes a combination of methods may be necessary for particular cases. Whatever the method used, it must be carried out carefully, delicately and speedily, taking care not to expose the fertilized eggs to changes in temperature and pH.

Dissection techniques

1. *Needle dissection:* use two 26-gauge needles attached to 1 ml syringes, microscope at × 25 magnification. Use one needle as a guide, anchoring a piece of cellular debris if possible; slide the other needle down the first one, 'shaving' cells from around the zona pellucida, with a scissors-like action.
2. *'Rolling':* use one 23-gauge needle attached to a syringe, and a fine glass probe. With the microscope at × 12 magnification, use the needle to score lines in each droplet on the base of the plastic dish. Adjust the magnification to × 25, and push the egg gently over the scratches with a fire polished glass probe until the adhering cells are teased away.

   Great care must be taken with either technique to avoid damaging the zona pellucida or the egg either by puncture or overdistortion. Breaks or cracks in the zona can sometimes be seen, and a small portion of the egg may extrude through the crack (this may have occurred during dissection or during the aspiration process). Occasionally, the zona is very fragile, fracturing or distorting at the slightest touch. In cases such as this, it is probably best not to continue the dissection. If no pronuclei have been seen, immediate reinsemination may be considered as a precaution.
3. *Narrow-gauge pipetting:* usee the microscope at × 25 magnification, and choose a drawn-out pipette with a diameter slightly larger than the egg. Attach a bulb or holder to the pipette, and aspirate 2 cm of clean culture medium into it, providing a protective buffer. This allows easy flushing of the egg, and prevents it from sticking to the inside surface of the pipette.

   Place the pipette over the egg and gently aspirate it into the shaft.

   If the oocyte does not easily enter, change to a larger diameter pipette (however, if the diameter is too large, it will be ineffective for cumulus removal).

   Gently aspirate and expel the egg through the pipette, retaining the initial buffer volume, until sufficient cumulus and corona is removed, allowing clear visualization of the cell cytoplasm and pronuclei.

Making narrow-gauge pipettes

The preparation of finely drawn pipettes with an inner diameter slightly larger than the circumference of an egg is an acquired skill which requires practice and patience. Hold both ends of the pipette, and roll an area approximately 2.5 cm below the tapered section of the pipette over a gentle flame (Bunsen or spirit burner). As the glass begins to melt, quickly pull the pipette in both directions to separate, and carefully and quickly (before the glass has a chance to cool) break the pipette at an appropriate position. It is important that the tip should have a clean break, without rough or uneven edges; these will damage the egg during dissection. Always examine the tip of each pipette to ensure that it is of accurate diameter, with smooth clean edges.

Systems are now available which offer an alternative to hand-pulled pipettes, and better control than is possible with 'old-fashioned' rubber bulbs (mouth pipetting is now actively discouraged by some regulatory authorities). COOK IVF provide a 'Flexipet' pipetting device with sterile disposable polycarbonate capillaries supplied with inner diameters of 140, 160 and 600 μm. A similar device known as 'The Stripper' is a 3 μl gel sequencing pipette supplied by Drummond Scientific. Tips (known as sequencing bores), can be purchased in different sizes, and must be sterilized before use.

Scoring of pronuclei

An inverted microscope is recommended for accurate scoring of fertilization; although the pronuclei can be seen with dissecting microscopes, it can often be difficult to distinguish normal pronuclei from vacuoles or other irregularities in the cytoplasm. Normally fertilized eggs should have two pronuclei, two polar bodies, regular shape with intact zona pellucida, and a clear healthy cytoplasm. A variety of different features may be observed: the cytoplasm of normally fertilized eggs is usually slightly granular, whereas the cytoplasm of unfertilized eggs tends to be completely clear and featureless. The cytoplasm can vary from slightly granular and healthy-looking, to brown or dark and degenerate. The shape of the egg may also vary, from perfectly spherical to irregular (Figure 9.2). A clear halo of peripheral cytoplasm 5–10 μm thick is an indication of good activation and reinitiation of meiosis.

Single pronucleate zygotes obtained after conventional IVF have been analysed by fluorescent in situ hybridization (FISH) to determine their ploidy: of 16 zygotes, 10 were haploid and 6 were diploid (4 XY and 2 XX). It seems that during the course of their interaction, it is possible for human gamete nuclei to associate together and form diploid, single pronucleate zygotes. These findings confirm a newly recognized variation of human pronuclear interaction during syngamy, and the authors suggest that single pronucleate zygotes which develop with normal cleavage may be safely replaced (Levron et al., 1995).

Details of morphology and fertilization should be recorded for each zygote, for reference when choosing embryos for transfer on Day 2.

Remove zygotes with normal fertilization at the time of scoring from the insemination drops or wells, transfer into new dishes or plates containing

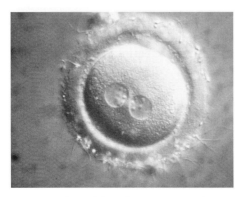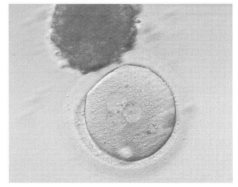

Figure 9.2   Phase contrast micrographs of fertilized human eggs. (a) Normal fertilization: two pronuclei, one polar body (courtesy of Dr P. Matson, Australia). (b) Abnormal fertilization: three pronuclei.

pre-equilibrated culture medium, and return them to the incubator for a further 24 hours of culture. Those with abnormal fertilization such as multi-pronucleate zygotes, must be cultured separately, so that there is no possibility of their being selected for embryo transfer; after cleavage these are indistinguishable from normally fertilized oocytes.

Although the presence of two pronuclei confirms fertilization, their absence does not necessarily indicate fertilization failure, and may instead represent either parthenogenetic activation, or a delay in timing of one or more of the events involved in fertilization. A study has shown that in 40% of oocytes with no sign of fertilization 17–27 hours after insemination, 41% had the appearance of morphologically normal embryos on the following day, with morphology and cleavage rate similar to that of eggs with obvious pronuclei on Day 1. However, 30% of these zygotes arrested on Day 2, compared with only 7% of 'normally' fertilized oocytes (Plachot et al., 1993), and they showed a reduced implantation rate of 6% compared with 11.1%. Cytogenetic analysis of these embryos revealed a higher incidence of chromosomal anomalies (55% versus 29%), and a high rate of haploidy (20%), confirming parthenogenetic activation. Nine per cent were triploid, and 26% mosaic (Plachot et al., 1988).

Delayed fertilization with the appearance of pronuclei on Day 2 may also be observed, and these embryos tend to have an impaired developmental potential. Oehninger et al. (1989) suggest that delayed fertilization can be attributed to morphological or endocrine oocyte defects in 37% of their cases, and sperm defects in 14.8%. Thirty-three per cent of the cases studied had no obvious association with either oocyte or sperm defects.

Reinsemination

Although oocytes which fail to demonstrate clear pronuclei at the time of scoring for fertilization can be reinseminated, this practice has been widely questioned scientifically. Fertilization or cleavage may then be seen on Day 2, but this may be as a consequence of the initial insemination, and the delay in fertilization may be attributed either to functional disorders of the sperm, or maturation delay of the oocyte. These embryos generally have a poor prognosis for implantation; however, complete failure of fertilization on Day 1 is a devastating crisis for the couple, and extremely difficult for them to accept without further attempted action. As everyone who has experience of IVF will testify, even the most unlikely and improbable circumstances can sometimes result in the birth of a healthy baby.

The reinsemination procedure should be carried out as early as possible. If the husband is not available to produce a second sample within 26–28 hours of the oocyte retrieval, the original insemination sample should be re-examined for motility and used at least as an interim measure.

Selection of surplus pronucleate embryos for cryopreservation

If a large number of oocytes have two clearly visible pronuclei on Day 1, a selected number can be kept in culture for transfer on Day 2, and the remainder considered for pronucleate stage cryopreservation. The decision as to the number of embryos to be frozen at the pronucleate stage should take into consideration the patient's previous history regarding cleavage and quality of embryos. Embryos to be frozen should have a regular outline, distinct zona and clearly visible pronuclei. The cryopreservation procedure must be initiated while the pronuclei are still visible, before the onset of syngamy.

Embryo quality and selection for transfer

Historically, embryo transfer was carried out two days (approximately 48–54 hours) after oocyte retrieval. Recent evidence suggests that it is possible to select zygotes at the pronuclear stage based upon PN alignment, and trials of zygote transfer on Day 1 have achieved acceptable pregnancy rates. Scott & Smith 1998 suggest a scoring system to define the criteria that can be observed in zygotes at the pronucleate stage to indicate optimal implantation potential: close alignment of nucleoli in a row, adequate separation of pronuclei, heterogeneous cytoplasm with a clear 'halo', and cleavage within 24–26 hours.

Activated oocytes may also be transferred to the uterus within one hour of performing ICSI (AOT, activated oocyte transfer), and satisfactory pregnancy rates make this also a valid alternative to selected patient groups (Dale et al., 1999).

On Day 2, cleaved embryos may contain from 2 to 8 blastomeres. Embryo transfer one day later, on Day 3, does not jeopardize pregnancy rates, and is advocated as a means of selecting better quality embryos, by the elimination of those who show early cleavage arrest in vitro. 'Faster cleaving' embryos, i.e. those with the highest cell number at the time of assessment, are felt to have better implantation potential.

Blastocyst transfer

The transfer of blastocysts on Day 5 or 6 may have the advantage of allowing better synchrony between the embryo and endometrium, as well as eliminating those embryos which are unable to develop after activation of the zygote genome due to genetic or metabolic defects. Until recently, in vitro culture systems could not support blastocyst development adequately, without the use of a supporting feeder cell layer (co-culture). Sequential, stage-specific media have now been introduced which greatly enhance the rate of blastocyst formation in vitro without the need for co-culture, and it has been suggested that Day 5 transfer of blastocysts rather than earlier transfer of cleavage stage embryos will significantly enhance implantation potential. The aim of extended culture is to produce blastocysts with better implantation potential than cleavage stage embryos, so that transfer of only one or two blastocysts may result in successful pregnancy, thus reducing the number of multiple gestations and increasing the overall efficiency of IVF. Extended culture helps to identify those embryos with little developmental competence, as well as facilitating the synchronization of embryonic stage with uterine endometrial development.

Blastocyst culture also allows trophectoderm biopsy and assessment of embryo metabolism as further tests of embryo viability. Current data suggest that blastocyst transfer has a place in the treatment of selected groups of patients, in particular those with a high risk of multiple gestation or in whom a multiple pregnancy represents an obstetric disaster. An important prerequisite for blastocyst culture is an optimal IVF laboratory culture environment; there is no advantage in extended culture unless satisfactory implantation rates are already obtained after culture to Day 2 or 3. In patients who develop three or more good-quality 8-cell embryos on Day 3, extended culture to blastocyst stage has achieved implantation rates in the order of 40% per embryo, with pregnancy rates of at least 65% per transfer (Gardner Schoolcraft, 1999; Elder

& Elliott, 1999). This strategy has also been used in the treatment of patients who carry chromosomal translocations; chromosome translocations cause a delay in the cell cycle, and abnormal or slowly developing embryos are eliminated during in vitro culture. Several normal pregnancies have been successfully established after transfer of healthy blastocysts in a group of patients carrying translocations (Ménézo et al., 1999, personal communication).

The ability to identify healthy viable blastocysts is an important factor in the success of blastocyst transfer, and a grading system has been devised which takes into consideration the degree of expansion, hatching status, the development of the inner cell mass and the development of the trophectoderm (Gardner & Schoolcraft, 1999). Satisfactory implantation rates after blastocyst transfer are only achieved with selection after careful assessment of all morphological parameters available.

If embryos are to be cultured beyond Day 2 for potential blastocyst development, the culture medium should be changed on Day 2 or Day 3 to a stage-specific formulation, with careful rinsing of the embryos in the new medium before placing in culture.

Selection of embryos for transfer

In selecting embryos for transfer, the limitations of evaluating embryos based on morphological criteria alone are well recognized: correlations between gross morphology and implantation are weak and inaccurate, unless the embryos are clearly fragmenting. Objective criteria for evaluating embryos are possible, but these methods are available only in specialized laboratories with research facilities, and are not practical for a routine clinical IVF laboratory without access to specialized equipment and facilities. Culture media can be assayed to measure individual embryos' metabolic activity and secretions, and fluorescent in situ hybridization (FISH) techniques are used to determine aneuploidy and examine specific chromosomes after polar body or blastomere biopsy. These techniques have provided an increasing body of knowledge about embryo viability and implantation potential, and there is no doubt that this will have an increasing impact upon embryo selection for transfer in routine IVF.

In an attempt to more clearly define morphological criteria that might be used for embryo assessment, Cohen et al. carried out a detailed analysis using videocinematography (1989). Immediately before embryo transfer, embryos were recorded on VHS for 30–90 seconds, at several focal points, using Nomarski optics and an overall magnification of × 1400. The recordings were subsequently analysed by observers who were unaware of the outcome of the IVF procedure, and they objectively assessed a total of 11 different parameters:

Cell organelles visible	Cellular extrusions
Blastomeres all intact	Cytoplasmic vacuoles
Identical blastomere size	Blastomeres contracted
Smooth membranes	
Dark blastomeres	% variation in zona thickness
Cell–cell adherence	% extracellular fragments

Nine parameters were judged (+) or (−), and variation in zona thickness and percentage of extracellular fragments were given a numerical value. Analysis of these criteria showed that the most important predictor of fresh embryo implantation was the percentage of variation in thickness of the zona pellucida. Embryos with a thick, even zona had a poor prognosis for implantation; those whose zona had thin patches also had 'swollen', more refractile blastomeres, and had few or no fragments.

In analysing frozen-thawed embryos, the best predictor of implantation was cell–cell adherence. The proportion of thawed embryos with more than one abnormality (77%) was higher than that of fresh embryos (38%) despite similar implantation rates (18% versus 15%).

Fragments

Most IVF embryologists would agree that fragmentation is the norm in routine IVF, but it is not clear whether this is an effect of culture conditions and follicular stimulation, or a characteristic of human development. The degree of fragmentation varies from 5 or 10% to 100%, and the fragments may be either localized or scattered. Alikani and Cohen (1995) used an analysis of patterns of cell fragmentation in the human embryo as a means of determining the relationship between cell fragmentation and implantation potential, with the conclusion that not only the degree, but also the pattern of embryo fragmentation determine its implantation potential.

Five distinct patterns of fragmentation which can be seen by Day 3 were identified:

1. <5% of the volume of the perivitelline space occupied by fragments.
2. All or most fragments localized, concentrated in one area of the perivitelline space, with five or more normal cells visible.

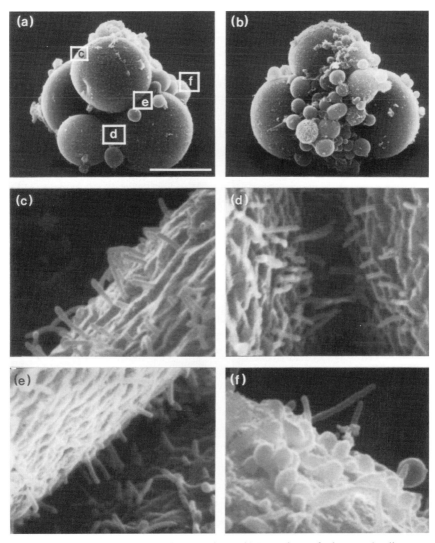

Figure 9.3   Scanning electron micrographs. (a, b) Two views of a human 4-cell embryo showing 20% fragmentation (c–e) magnification of corresponding areas showing regular short microvilli of vital blastomeres and intercellular areas; (f) magnification of the surface of a cytoplasmic fragment showing irregular blebs and protrusions (Dale et al., 1995).

3. Fragments scattered throughout, and similar in size.
4. Large fragments, indistinguishable from blastomeres, and scattered through-out the perivitelline space (PVS); usually associated with very few cells.
5. Fragments throughout the PVS, appearing degenerate such that cell bound-aries are invisible, associated with contracted and granular cytoplasm.

Implantation potential was greatest in types 1 and 2, and diminished in types 3 and 4. In 15 years of clinical embryology, there are no definitive reports on the causes of fragmentation, although speculations include high spermatozoal numbers and consequently high levels of free radicals, temperature or pH shock, and stimulation protocols. Observed through the scanning electron microscope, the surface of fragments is made up of irregularly shaped blebs and protrusions, very different to the regular surface of blastomeres, which is organized into short, regular microvilli (Figure 9.3). Interestingly, pro-grammed cell death in somatic cells also starts with surface blebbing, and is caused, in part, by a calcium-induced disorganization of the cytoskeleton. We can speculate that similar mechanisms operate within human embryos, but we have so far no scientific evidence that this is the case. Brenner et al. (1997) first reported a study of human embryonic transcription of specific genes that regulate apoptosis during the preimplantation period. Two genes are involved in apoptosis: *bax* and *bcl-2*; bax is a regulatory gene which promotes cell death, and *bcl-2* functions to enhance cell survival in various cell types. *Bax* mRNA is expressed at all stages of preimplantation human embryonic development – transcripts are both maternal and embryonic, and varying levels are expressed at different stages of oocyte maturation. *Bcl-2* mRNA can be found in 2c, 8c, 16c embryos and morulae – but in fewer embryos. The ratio of bcl-2 to bax expression may be the critical determinant of cell fate, such that increased *bcl-2* leads to extended survival, and increased levels of *bax* accelerate cell death in an incremental fashion. It is unusual to have active gene transcription in zygotes, because the human embryonic genome is normally first activated at the 4c–8c stage. Activation of *bcl-2* transcription upon fertilization may play a unique role in protection of the preimplantation embryo from apoptosis, and elucidation of a genetic mechanism of preimplantation death and survival may have implications relevant for successful IVF and preimplantation genetic diagnosis.

There does appear to be an element of programming in this partial embry-onic autodestruction, as embryos from certain patients, irrespective of the types of procedure applied in successive IVF attempts, are always prone to fragmentation. Fragments may be removed during micromanipulation for assisted hatching, and there is growing evidence that fragment removal may improve implantation. Surprisingly, fragmented embryos, repaired or not, do implant and often come to term. Sophisticated time-lapse photography tech-nology has enabled in situ imaging of cleaving embryos, with imaging amplifi-cation to minimize light exposure which might be potentially harmful to them. This technique has clearly demonstrated that an individual embryo can radically change its morphological appearance in a short period of time: fragments which are apparent at a particular moment in time can be subsequently absorbed with no evidence of their prior existence (Hamberger et al., 1998).

This demonstrates the highly regulative nature of the human embryo, as it can apparently lose over half of its cellular mass and still recover, and also confirms the general consensus that the mature oocyte contains much more material than it needs for development. The reasons why part, and only part, of an early embryo should become disorganized and degenerate are a mystery. Different degrees of fragmentation argue against the idea that the embryo is purposely casting off excess cytoplasm, somewhat analogous to the situation in annelids and marsupials that shed cytoplasmic lobes rich in yolk, and favours the idea of partial degeneration. Perhaps it involves cell polarization, where organelles gather to one side of the cell. It is certain that pH, calcium and transcellular currents trigger cell polarization, which may in certain cases lead to an abnormal polarization, and therefore to fragmentation. These areas are for the moment wide open to speculation, and studies are in progress.

Attempts have been made to improve the implantation potential of human embryos by intrusive methods such as assisted hatching, zona removal, excising cytoplasmic fragments, and ooplasmic donation (Cohen et al., 1998). Although reported results following assisted hatching are variable, it has raised implantation rates in some centres when applied to selected embryos (see chapter 12).

Removal of all fragments from highly fragmented spare embryos carefully matched with other embryos with similar morphology and development rate that were only zona drilled, resulted more frequently in the formation of single cavity blastocysts in the fragment-free embryos, indicating that some intercellular fragments may inhibit cell–cell contact.

Cytoplasmic donation

In a few cases of multiple implantation failure, cytoplasm was removed from a donor egg, and injected into the patients' oocyte. This method is highly experimental, and the correct indications and appropriate methodology are yet to be elucidated. Areas of investigation include the effect of maturation promoting factor (MPF), the consequences of polarity in the egg, whether specific sites are better than others, the role of mitochondria, etc. During 1996–98, the extraction and injection technique was attempted in 16 patients with multiple implantation failures and poor embryo development: 9 became pregnant, 1 miscarried and 5 have delivered apparently normal single infants.

Three failed procedures occurred in couples with male factor infertility. (J. Cohen, personal communication, 1999). At least 10 other pregnancies have been obtained with this method in 3 other IVF centres.

Embryo transfer

Current standard morphological criteria used in evaluating embryo quality prior to transfer include: rate of division judged by the number of blastomeres, size, shape, symmetry and cytoplasmic appearance of the blastomeres, the presence of anucleate cytoplasmic fragments, and the appearance of the zona pellucida. Although this assessment is recognized to be arbitrary and unsatisfactory, it is quick, noninvasive, easy to carry out in routine practice, and does help to eliminate those embryos with the poorest prognosis.

Embryos have been arbitrarily classified based upon these criteria:

Grade 1
Embryos have even, regular spherical blastomeres with moderate refractility (i.e. not very dark) and with intact zona. Allowance must be made for the appearance of blastomeres that are in division or that have divided asynchronously with their sisters, e.g. 3-, 5-, 6- or 7-cell embryos. These may be uneven but are perfectly normal. As always, individual judgement is important, and this is a highly subjective assessment. Grade 1 embryos have no, or very few, fragments (less than 10%) (Figure 9.4a).

Grade 2
Embryos have uneven or irregular shaped blastomeres, with mild variation in refractility and no more than 10% fragmentation of blastomeres (Figue 9.4b).

Grade 3
Embryos show fragmentation of no more than 50% of blastomeres. The remaining blastomeres must be at least in reasonable (Grade 2) condition and with refractility associated with cell viability; the zona pellucida must be intact (Figure 9.4c).

Grade 4
More than 50% of the blastomeres are fragmented, and there may be gross variation in refractility. Remaining blastomeres should appear viable (Figure 9.4d).

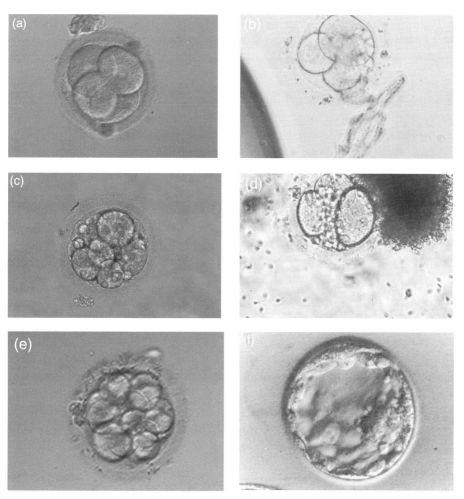

Figure 9.4   Photographs of morphological variations in human embryos 2 days after fertilization in vitro. (a) Four regular blastomeres, no fragments; (b) uneven blastomeres, approximately 10% fragmentation; (c) four blastomeres, approximately 20% fragmentation; (d) three blastomeres, approximately 50% fragmentation; (e) human embryo at morula stage, initiating compaction; (f) human expanded blastocyst showing inner cell mass, trophectoderm and blastocoelic cavity. By courtesy of Agnese Fiorentino, Naples, Italy.

Grade 5
Zygotes with two pronuclei on Day 2, either as a result of delayed fertilization or reinsemination on Day 1.

Grade 6
Embryos are nonviable, with lysed, contracted or dark blastomeres.

It is important to bear in mind that the time during which the assessment and judgment is made represents only a tiny instant of a rapidly evolving process of development. Embryos can be judged quite differently at two different periods in time, as may be seen if a comparison is made between assessments made in the morning, and later in the day immediately before transfer. Individual judgment should be exercised in determining which embryos are selected. In general, those embryos at later stages and of higher grades are preferred, but the choice is often not clear cut. The Grade 2 category covers a wide range of morphological states but, provided the blastomeres are not grossly abnormal, a later stage Grade 2 embryo may be selected in preference to an earlier stage Grade 1 embryo. Attention should also be paid to the appearance of the zona pellucida and to the pattern of fragmentation. Embryos of Grade 3 or 4 are transferred only where no better embryos are available. If only pronucleate embryos are available on Day 2, they should be cultured further and transferred only if cleavage occurs.

The recent application of preimplantation genetic diagnosis by FISH analysis of biopsied blastomeres has shown a surprising discrepancy between gross morphology and genetic normality of embryos. Even the most 'beautiful' Grade 1 embryos may have numerical chromosomal anomalies, whilst those judged to be of 'poorer' quality, with uneven blastomeres and fragments, may have a normal chromosome complement. In a FISH analysis of a large number of embryos using DNA probes that bind to specific regions of the target chromosomes, Harper et al. (1995) identified several different patterns of chromosome arrangement:

1. Uniformly diploid for the probes examined
2. Uniformly abnormal, such as Down's or Turner's syndrome
3. Mosaic, where both diploid cells and aneuploid, haploid or polyploid nuclei are present
4. Chaotic embryos, where every nucleus shows a different chromosome complement – the incidence of these embryos is related to individual patients.

Multinucleated blastomeres have been reported, from karyotyping and FISH analysis; the presence of such blastomeres may be more common in arrested embryos, and may occur more readily in some patients. Nonmosaic aneuploidy in normally developing embryos increases with maternal age (Munné et al., 1995a,b), and some groups have used FISH analysis of biopsied polar bodies to eliminate aneuploid oocytes in these patients (Verlinsky et al., 1995, 1996, Munné et al., 1995b).

With respect to the data accumulated from preimplantation genetic diagnosis, an interesting fact to bear in mind is that few cells (possibly only a single cell from an 8-cell embryo) differentiate to the embryo itself: the majority contribute to the cytotrophoblast and fetal membranes. In the mouse, experimental production of tetraploid/diploid conceptuses suggests that a mechanism exists to exclude chromosomally abnormal cells from the primitive ectoderm lineage, or they are selectively lost later (James & West, 1994).

Another surprising feature found as a result of PGD studies is the regular occurrence of mosaicism in preimplantation embryos. Fluorescent in situ hybridization studies have been applied to blastomeres from abnormally fertilized, developmentally arrested and normally developing embryos from IVF patients (see chapter 12). Mosaic aneuploidy results from loss or gain of a chromosome from some cells during postzygotic development, and there is evidence to suggest that one of the mechanisms involved is mitotic nondisjunction, which causes a reciprocal loss and gain. Both aneuploid and ploidy mosaicism seem to be generated after the first cleavage division, typically at the second division (Delhanty et al., 1997).

Remaining embryos

After embryo transfer, remaining embryos of Grades 1 or 2 which show less than 20% fragmentation at the time of assessment may be cryopreserved on Day 2 or Day 3. Embryos of suboptimal morphology at this time can be transferred into stage-specific media and further cultured, with daily assessment until Day 6. Those that develop to blastocysts on Days 5 or 6 can also be cryopreserved.

Embryo transfer procedure

Materials

1. Pre-equilibrated, warmed culture medium
2. 1 ml disposable syringe
3. Embryo transfer catheter
4. Sterile disposable gloves (nonpowdered)
5. Clean Petri dish
6. Fire-polished Pasteur pipette and glass probe
7. Dissecting microscope with warm stage.

Although it may seem obvious that correct identification of patient and embryos is vital, errors in communication do happen and can lead to a disastrous mistake, especially should there be patients with similar names undergoing treatment at the same time. Therefore, a routine discipline of identification should be followed to ensure that there is no possibility of mistaken identity:

1. Ensure that medical notes always accompany a patient who is being prepared for embryo transfer.
2. Name and medical numbers on medical notes and patient identity bracelet should be checked by two people, i.e. the clinician in charge of the procedure and the assisting nurse.
3. The doctor should also check name and number verbally with the patient, and doctor, nurse and patient may sign an appropriate form confirming that the details are correct.
4. The duty embryologist should check the same details with the embryology records, and also sign the same form in the presence of the doctor.

Preparation of embryos for transfer

The rate of multiple gestation resulting from IVF/ET is unacceptably high, and legislation in the UK and a few other European countries now prohibits the transfer of more than three embryos in a treatment cycle. The transfer of two embryos is recommended for patients with a good prognosis, i.e. young age, tubal infertility only, previous history of pregnancy and/or delivery. However, patients who are older than 40 years, and those whose infertility is due to multiple factors, are placed at a disadvantage by this strategy, as their embryos appear to have a decreased developmental potential.

1. Prepare a droplet (or well) of fresh medium for the selected embryos (some IVF laboratories choose to add prepared maternal serum in a concentration of 50–75% at this stage).
2. When the embryos for transfer have been identified and scored, and their details recorded, place them together in the pre-equilibrated droplet or well. No more than three embryos should be selected. If medium with a higher density is used, (i.e. with 50–75% serum) this transfer should be carried out carefully, as the embryos will 'float' in the higher density medium and must be allowed to settle before aspiration into the embryo transfer catheter.
3. After gently pushing the embryos together, leave them under low power on the heated stage of the microscope, in focus.
4. Turn off the microscope light.
5. Wash your hands with a surgical scrub preparation, and don sterile gloves.
6. Fill a 1 ml sterile syringe with warm medium, and eject any air bubbles.

7. Check that the catheter to be used moves freely though its outer sheath, attach it to the syringe and eject the medium from the syringe through the catheter, discarding the medium.
8. Draw up warm medium through the catheter into the syringe, and then push the piston down to the 10 μl mark, ejecting excess medium and again discarding it.
9. Pour some clean warm medium into the warm Petri dish on the microscope stage (for rinsing the catheter tip).
10. Place the end of the catheter into the drop or well, away from the embryos, and inject a small amount of medium to break the boundary of surface tension that may appear at the end of the catheter. Aspirate the embryos into the catheter, so that the volume to be transferred is 15–20 μl.
11. If the embryos have been loaded from a droplet under oil, rinse the tip of the catheter in the Petri dish containing clean warm medium.

Hand the catheter and syringe to the clinician for transfer to the patient. When the catheter is returned after the procedure, carefully inspect it, rotating under the microscope. It is especially important to ensure that no embryo is buried in any mucus present; note and record the presence of mucus and/or blood. Loosen the Lueur fitting, and allow the fluid in the catheter to drain into the clean Petri dish while continuing to observe through the microscope. Inform the doctor and patient as soon as you have confirmed that no embryos have been returned. If any embryos have been returned, they should be reloaded into a clean catheter, and the transfer procedure repeated. If difficulties arise during the transfer procedure causing delay, return the embryos to the culture drop in the interim, until the physician is confident that they can be safely transferred to the uterus of the patient.

There is no doubt that the technique of embryo transfer, although apparently a simple and straightforward procedure, is absolutely critical in safe delivery of the embryos to the site of their potential implantation. Studies repeatedly show that pregnancy rates can vary in the hands of different operators, and with the use of different embryo transfer catheters. In a study of embryo transfer procedures under ultrasound-guided control, Woolcott and Stanger (1998) observed guiding cannula and transfer catheter placement in relation to the endometrial surface and uterine fundus during embryo transfer. Their results indicated that tactile assessment of embryo transfer catheter was unreliable, in that the cannula and the catheter could be seen to abut the fundal endometrium, and indent or embed in the endometrium in a significant number of cases. Endometrial movement due to sub-endometrial myometrial contraction was obvious in 36% of cases, and this movement was associated

---

Luteal phase support

- Utrogestan capsules (Besins-Iscovesco)
    100 mg tds or 200 mg tds pv
- or Cyclogest pessaries (Hoechst)
    200 mg bd or 400 mg bd pv
- or Gestone (Ferring)
    50 mg or 100 mg daily by im injection

Luteal phase support continues until Day 77 post OCR, then is gradually withdrawn

---

with a reduced pregnancy rate. Their studies highlight the fact that 'blind' ET procedures may often lead to an unsatisfactory outcome, and they recommend the use of ultrasound guidance as a routine during ET. Historically, patients remained supine for several hours after ET, sometimes with legs elevated: an additional part of the above study examined fluid/air bubble movement within the uterus when the patient was asked to stand up immediately after the procedure. Repeat ultrasound examination then showed that standing up immediately had no effect on embryo movement within the uterus, reinforcing the idea that bed rest following ET is unnecessary.

Gamete intrafallopian transfer (GIFT)

The World Collaborative Report on Assisted Reproduction published in 1993 summarized the results of 99 314 IVF transfer cycles, with a clinical pregnancy rate of 17.9% and live birth rate of 12.9%. Although GIFT represented only 10% of the total number of cycles compared with IVF, the clinical pregnancy rate for this procedure was 29.3%, with a live birth rate of 20.8%. Discussion continues as to the relative merits of intrauterine versus intratubal transfer, but it may be that intratubal transfer of gametes does have advantages: embryo development in a beneficial tubal microenvironment avoids the possible hazards of in vitro culture, especially if optimal laboratory conditions are not available. In addition, the embryo undergoes physiological passage into the uterus for implantation, avoiding endometrial trauma, and there is a diminished possibility of embryo expulsion from the uterus immediately after transfer. The gametes may be transferred to the fallopian tubes via the fimbrial end, under laparoscopic guidance, or intracervically under ultrasound-guided control. In either case, the dynamics of the injection procedure are critical, and gametes should be transferred in less than 50 μl of fluid, at a very slow injection rate of 1 μl per second. The catheter must of course be precisely located using ultrasound guidance for transcervical procedures.

GIFT procedure

1. Obtain the semen sample at least 2 hours prior to the start of the procedure, and prepare as for IVF to a final concentration of 3–5 million motile sperm per ml (so that 100 000–200 000 sperm are transferred to the fallopian tube).
2. Warm the sperm preparation, medium, and 2 × 35 mm Petri dishes at 37 °C.
3. At the end of the oocyte retrieval procedure, select good-quality mature eggs for transfer, and wash them in a small amount of medium in a warmed dish or test tube.
4. Place a droplet (50–100 μl) of sperm suspension in a warmed Petri dish, and transfer the selected washed oocytes into this droplet.
5. Rinse a 0.5 ml Hamilton syringe and GIFT catheter with warm medium, and then load the catheter:
   (i) 20 μl air
   (ii) 30–40 μl oocytes + sperm
   (iii) 10–20 μl air
6. Transfer the oocytes and sperm to the fallopian tube with minimum delay, to prevent exposing them to temperature fluctuations.
7. After transfer, expel medium remaining in the catheter and examine the droplet and the catheter carefully to ensure that no oocytes have been returned. If there is an insufficient volume of adequately prepared sperm, the sperm and oocytes can be loaded separately:
   (i) 20 μl air
   (ii) 10–15 μl sperm
   (iii) 10 μl oocytes in culture medium
   (iv) 10–15 μl sperm
   (v) 20 μl air.
   This method is also preferred by some couples for religious or philosophical reasons, as it theoretically avoids in vitro mixing of the gametes – oocytes and sperm come into contact after being expelled into the fallopian tube, where the process of fertilization may occur as in natural conception.
8. Surplus oocytes remaining after the GIFT procedure may be cultured for IVF – in cases of male infertility, confirmation that fertilization may take place is a useful diagnostic test. Resulting embryos can be cryopreserved if they fulfil the required criteria for cryopreservation.

Transport IVF and transport ICSI

The facilities of a central expert IVF laboratory can be used to offer treatment in hospitals which do not have the necessary laboratory space and personnel. Carefully selected patients undergo ovarian stimulation, monitoring and oocyte retrieval under the care and management of a gynaecologist who has a close liaison with an IVF laboratory team in a location which can be reached within 2 hours of the hospital or clinic where the oocyte retrieval procedure takes place. It is an advantage to select patients with simple, uncomplicated infertility and good ovarian response, and close communication and co-ordination between the patient, physician and IVF laboratory team is essential. A successful system of transport IVF at the Royal Liverpool University Hospital in the UK (C.R. Kingsland and M.M. Biljan, personal communication) recommends that strict patient inclusion criteria should be adhered to, as follows:

1.   Women 35 years of age or less
2.   Tubal damage as the sole cause of subfertility

Patients who do not satisfy these criteria should be referred for specialized treatment in the Central Unit.
   Exclusion criteria:

1.   Women over 35 years of age
2.   Patients with LH:FSH ratio higher than 3:1
3.   Patients with laparoscopically proven moderate or severe endometriosis
4.   Patients requesting oocyte donation or donor insemination
5.   Three previously unsuccessful IVF treatment cycles.

A GnRH-agonist/FSH long protocol is used for superovulation so that a simplified monitoring regimen can be used (ultrasound assessment and optional serum oestradiol levels) and to allow scheduled admission of patients into the stimulation phase. This protocol also allows latitude in the administration of hCG, so that the timing of oocyte retrieval can be scheduled in a routine operating list. Profasi (hCG) 5000 IU is administered 36 hours prior to the planned follicular aspiration.

   The couple under treatment must visit the central unit before hCG is given, both to receive detailed information and consent forms, and to familiarize themselves with the journey and the facilities. The husband will return to the central unit on the morning of oocyte retrieval to produce a semen sample and to collect a prewarmed portable incubator. The portable incubator, plugged into a car cigarette lighter, is then used to transport the follicular aspirates which have been collected in the peripheral hospital or clinic. Follicular aspirates are collected under ultrasound-guided control into sterile test-tubes (without flushing). It is essential that each test-tube is *filled completely* and tightly capped in order to prevent pH fluctuations. A heated test-tube rack during aspiration must be used to prevent temperature fluctuations in the aspirates. The presence of blood in the aspirates has not been found to adversely affect the outcome of fertilization, embryo development and success rates. At the end of the oocyte retrieval procedure, the partner transports the follicular aspirates, together with the treatment records, to the central laboratory for oocyte identification and subsequent insemination and culture.

The embryo transfer procedure is carried out 48 hours later at the central unit. Patient follow-up is carried out by the physician at the peripheral unit.

Provided that the instructions and inclusion criteria are strictly adhered to, a highly motivated, well-coordinated team working in close liaison can achieve success rates comparable to those obtained in the specialist centre, and IVF treatment can thus be offered to couples to whom it might otherwise be unavailable. Transport ICSI can also be successfully offered on a similar basis (see chapter 12).

Coculture systems

Homologous and autologous coculture systems which culture embryos in the presence of a layer of 'feeder' cells have been used to improve embryo development in vitro, and to try to overcome the phenomenon of developmental arrest which commonly occurs in routine in vitro culture. For the same developmental stage, cocultured embryos have higher numbers of cells and a fully cohesive inner cell mass when compared with embryos cultured in simple media. It is postulated that improved development occurs as a result of four different possible mechanisms:

1. 'Metabolic locks': coculture cell layers can provide a supply of small molecular weight metabolites which simpler culture media lack. This supply may assist continued cell metabolism required for genome activation, and divert the potential for abnormal metabolic processes which may lead to cleavage arrest.
2. Growth factors essential for development may be supplied by the feeder cell layer.
3. Toxic compounds resulting from cell metabolism can be removed: heavy metal ions may be chelated by glycine produced by feeder cells, and ammonium and urea may be recycled through feeder cell metabolic cycles.
4. Feeder cells can synthesize reducing agents which prevent the formation of free radicals.

Weimer et al. (1998) suggest that there may be subpopulations of infertile patients who require a different culture environment for their embryos to develop, and in their experience the application of coculture improves the prognosis for certain patients:

1. Repeated IVF failure
2. High basal day 3 FSH levels (> 7.5 mIU.ml)
3. Advanced reproductive age (> 39)
4. Poor stimulation with unexpected poor follicular response
5. History of poor embryonic development/ovulatory disorder.

Coculture systems used include fetal calf endometrial fibroblasts, human ampullary and endometrial cell lines, granulosa cells and a commercially produced cell line of Vero (African Green Monkey Kidney) cells. The ability of a coculture system to promote embryonic development is only as good as the cell population that makes up the supporting monolayer, and before making the decision to use coculture as a clinical tool in IVF, the disadvantages of the system must be carefully considered:

1. The establishment of cell monolayers is laborious and time consuming: explants must be subcultured, with the establishment of appropriate culture conditions; cell morphology and growth patterns change with length of time and number of passages in culture.
2. Feeder cell medium is very rapidly metabolized, and medium pH can rapidly change to a level which embryos will not tolerate.
3. Reproducible conditions can be difficult to maintain.
4. Cell layers are very susceptible to bacterial, viral and mycoplasmal contamination. Screening is essential: there is a risk of disease transmission to the embryo, and both cells and medium must be rigorously checked for viruses, bacteria, fungi and mycoplasma.

Vero cell lines, used in vaccine preparation, are commercially available from the WHO library: reference Vero 6758, at passage 134, nonhazardous to human (Public Health Laboratory Service, European Collection of Animal Cell Culture, Salisbury, UK). These cells are not tumorigenic before passage 162, contain no extraneous viruses and can be used to set up a well-organized coculture system. However, the morphological appearance of the cells does not necessary indicate the general health of the cell population nor its ability to support embryonic development, and it is essential to incorporate stringent cell culture schemes as a routine. Frozen cells are thawed and seeded in culture flasks at 2–3 million cells per flask. Confluence is reached within 4 days, normally at a cell density of 6–8 million cells per flask. These first passage flasks are subcultured after trypsinization into three samples:

1. Freeze one sample for future use, as cells must not be repeatedly passaged from flasks.
2. Seed a new flask.
3. Seed culture wells at a density of 100 000 cells per well – these wells reach confluence within three days.

    Note: Do not trypsinize cells more than seven times
    Do not use them after passage 142
    After four subcultures, screen the cells for chlamydia and mycoplasma (Bio-Mérieux Kits 5532/1 and 4240/2)

Wells seeded on a Friday can be used during the whole of the following week, and are rinsed only once. Each patient has her own plates, regardless of the number of embryos to be cocultured, and plates are discarded immediately after use. Wells must never be reused for different patients. The wells are rinsed with fresh medium 1 hour before adding embryos, which may be cocultured either at the pronucleate zygote stage on Day 1, or at an early cleavage stage on Day 2. Using this culture system, Ménézo et al. (1995) improved their blastocyst development rate from 20% without coculture to 48–60%, and obtained an overall pregnancy rate per transfer of 42%, with an implantation rate per blastocyst of 20%.

Trypsinization

1. Wash monolayer with 5 ml Hank's balanced salt solution
2. Add 1.5 ml of 0.25% Trypsin + 0.2% EDTA in Ca/Mg free phosphate buffered saline
3. Incubate for 5 mins at 37 °C
4. Add 5 ml culture medium + 5% serum and resuspend cells
5. Centrifuge, 800 g 10 minutes
6. Resuspend cells in 5 ml culture medium and count with a haemocytometer
7. Seed 4-well dishes at a seeding density of 100 000 cells/well, in 1 ml of medium
8. Incubate for 3 days before using for coculture.

Coculture systems played an important role in research into embryo metabolism and preimplantation development, and the observations and data learned were instrumental in helping to develop more appropriate stage-specific culture media and systems. Current results with sequential media are such that the use of coculture systems is no longer warranted in routine clinical IVF. However, our knowledge to date regarding embryo development and interactions with media in vitro probably represents no more than 5–10% of the overall picture, and coculture systems may continue to play an important role in helping to elucidate the mechanisms and factors involved in the miraculous events of early embryo development which still remain largely unknown.

Further reading

Alikani, M. & Cohen, J. (1995) Patterns of cell fragmentation in the human embryo in vitro. *Journal of Assisted Reproduction and Genetics* **12**, Suppl.:28s.

Alikani, M. & Weimer, K. (1997) Embryo number for transfer should not be strictly regulated. *Fertility and Sterility* **68**:782–4.

Alikani, M., Palermo, G., Adler, A., Bertoli, M., Blake, M. & Cohen, J. (1995) Intracytoplasmic sperm injection in dysmorphic human oocytes. *Zygote* **3**:283–8.

Almeida, P.A. & Bolton, V.N. (1993) Immaturity and chromosomal abnormalities in oocytes that fail to develop pronuclei following insemination in vitro. *Human Reproduction* **8**:229–32.

Almeida, P.A. & Bolton, V.N. (1995) The effect of temperature fluctuations on the cytoskeletal organisation and chromosomal constitution of the human oocyte. *Zygote* **3**:357–65.

Angell, R.R., Templeton, A.A. & Aitken, R.J. (1986) Chromosome studies in human in vitro fertilization. *Human Genetics* **72**:333.

Asch, R.H., Balmaceda, J.P., Ellsworth, L.R. & Wong, P.C. (1985) Gamete Intrafallopian Transfer (GIFT): a new treatment for infertility. *International Journal of Fertility* **30**:41.

Ashwood-Smith, M.J., Hollands, P. & Edwards, R.G. (1989) The use of Albuminar (TM) as a medium supplement in clinical IVF. *Human Reproduction* **4**:702–5.

Belaisch-Allart, J. (1991) Delayed embryo transfer in an in-vitro fertilization programme: how to avoid working on Sunday. *Human Reproduction* **6**: 541–3.

Bolton, V.N. (1991) Pregnancies after in vitro fertilization and transfer of human blastocysts. *Fertility and Sterility* **55**:830–2.

Bolton, V.N., Hawes, S.M., Taylor, C.T. & Parsons, J.H. (1989) Development of spare human preimplantation embryos in vitro: an analysis of the correlations among gross morphology, cleavage rates, and development to the blastocyst. *Journal of In Vitro Fertilization and Embryo Transfer* **7**:186.

Bongso, A., Ng, S.C. & Ratnam, S. (1990) Cocultures: their relevance to assisted reproduction. *Human Reproduction* **5**:893–900.

Brenner, C., Exley, G., Alikani, M. et al. (1997) Expression of bax mRNA associated with apoptosis in human oocytes and embryos. *Proceedings of the* 10th *World Congress of In Vitro Fertilization and Assisted Reproduction*. Monduzzi Editore, pp. 627–32.

Brinsden, P.R. (1994) Clinical experience with highly purified FSH. *Newsletter: Gonadotrophin for the 90s* **1(1)**, Excerpta Medica Asia Ltd.

Caro, C. & Trounson, A. (1986) Successful fertilization and embryo development, and pregnancy in human in vitro fertilization (IVF) using a chemically defined culture medium containing no protein. *Journal of In Vitro Fertilization Embryo Transfer* **3**: 215–17.

Cohen, J. (1991) Assisted hatching of human embryos. *Journal of In Vitro Fertilization and Embryo Transfer* **8(4)**:179–89.

Cohen, J. (1999) Ooplasmic transfer in mature human oocytes. *Human Reproduction* **13(Suppl. 3)**.

Cohen, J., Alikani, M., Trowbridge, J. & Rosenwaks, Z. (1992) Implantation enhancement by selective assisted hatching using zona drilling of embryos with poor prognosis. *Human Reproduction* **7**:685–91.

Cohen, J., Alikani, M., Garrisi, J.G. & Willadsen, S. (1998) Micromanipulation of human gametes and embryos: ooplasmic donation at fertilization (Video). *Human Reproduction Update* **4(2)**:95–6.

Cohen, J., Inge, K.L., Suzman, M., Wiker, S.R. & Wright, G. (1989) Videocinematography of fresh and cryopreserved embryos: a retrospective analysis of embryonic morphology and implantation. *Fertility and Sterility* **51**:820.

Coonen, E., Harper, J.C., Ramaekers, F.C.S., Delhanty, J.D.A., Hopman, A.H.N., Garaedts, J.P.M. & Handyside, A.H. (1994) Presence of chromosomal mosaicism in abnormal preimplantation embryos detected by fluorescent in situ hybridisation. *Human Genetics* **54**:609–15.

Critchlow, J.D. (1989) Quality control in an in-vitro fertilization laboratory: use of human sperm survival studies. *Human Reproduction* **4(5)**:545–9.

Dale, B. Tosti, E. & Iaccarino, M. (1995). Is the plasma membrane of the human oocyte re-organized following fertilization and early cleavage? *Zygote.* **3**:31—7.

Dale, B., Fiorentino, A., De Stefano, R.D., Matteo, L., Wilding M. & Zullo F. (1999) Pregnancies after activated oocyte transfer: a new alternative for infertility treatment. *Human Reproduction.* **14**:1771–2.

Danforth, R.A., Piana, S.D. & Smith, M. (1987) High purity water: an important component for success in in vitro fertilization. *American Biotechnology Laboratory* **5**:58–60.

Delhanty, J.D.A., Harper, J.C., Ao, A., Handyside, A.H. & Winston, R.M.L. (1997) Multicolour FISH detects frequent chromosomal mosaicism and chaotic division in normal preimplantation embryos from fertile patients. *Human Genetics* **99**:755–60.

Edwards, R.G. & Purdy, J.M. (1982) *Human Conception In Vitro*, Academic Press, London, New York.

Elder, K.T. & Elliott, T. (1998) Problem solving and troubleshooting in IVF. *Worldwide Conferences in Reproductive Medicine*, vol. 3. Ladybrook Publishing, Australia.

Elder, K. & Elliott, T. (1999) *Blastocyst Update*. Worldwide Conferences in Reproductive Biology, Ladybrook Publications, Australia.

Felderbaum, R.E., Ludwig, M. & Diedrich, K. (1998) Are we on the verge of a new era in ART? *Human Reproduction* **13(7)**:1778–80.

Fishel, S. & Symonds, E.M. (1986) *IVF – Past, Present, & Future*. IRL Press, Oxford, Washington DC.

Gardner, D.K. (1999) Development of serum-free media for the culture and transfer of human blastocysts. *Human Reproduction* **13**, **Suppl. 4**:218–25.

Gardner, D.K. & Schoolcraft, W.B. (1999) In vitro culture of human blastocysts. In: (Jansen, R. & Mortimer, D. eds.), *Towards Reproductive Certainty: Infertility and Genetics beyond* 1999, The Parthenon Publishing Group, UK.

Gianaroli, L., Magli, C., Ferraretti, A., Fiorentino, A., Panzella, S., Tosti, E., & Dale, B. (1996) Reducing the time of sperm-oocyute interaction in human IVF improves the implantation rate. *Human Reproduction* **11**: 166–71.

Gott, A.L., Hardy, K., Winston, R.M.L. & Leese, H.J. (1990) Noninvasive measurement of pyruvate and glucose uptake and lactate production by single human preimplantation embryos. *Human Reproduction* **5**:104–10.

Gregory, L. (1998) Ovarian markers of implantation potential in assisted reproduction. *Human Reproduction Supplement* **13**, **4**: 117–32.

Gregory, L. & Leese, H.J. (1996) Determinants of oocyte and pre-implantation embryo quality metabolic requirements and the potential role of cumulus cells. *Journal of the British Fertility Society* **1(2)**, *Human Reproduction* **11**, **Natl Suppl.**:96–102.

Grifo, J.A., Boyle, A. & Fischer, E. (1990) Preembryo biopsy and analysis of blastomeres by in situ hybridisation. *American Journal of Obstetrics and Gynecology* **163**: 2013–19.

Hamberger, L., Nilsson, L. & Sjögren, A. (1998) Microscopic imaging techniques: practical aspects. *Human Reproduction* **13**, Abstract book 1:15.

Hammitt, D.G., Walker, D.L. & Syrop, C.H. (1990) Improved methods for preparation of culture media for in-vitro fertilization and gamete intra-fallopian transfer. *Human Reproduction* **5(4)**:457–63.

Handyside, A.H., Kontogianni, E.H., Hardy, K. & Winston, R.M.L. (1990) Pregnancies from biopsied human preimplantation embryos sexed by Y-specific DNA amplification. *Nature* **344**:768–70.

Harper, J.C. & Handyside, A.H. (1994) The current status of preimplantation diagnosis. *Current Obstetrics and Gynaecology* **4**:143–9.

Harper, J.C., Coonan, E. & Ramaekers, F.C.S. (1994) Identification of the sex of human preimplantation embryos in two hours using an improved spreading method and fluorescent in-situ hybridization (FISH) using directly labelled probes. *Human Reproduction* **9**:721–4.

Harper, J.C., Coonan, E., Handyside, A.H., Winston, R.M., Hopman, A.H. & Delhanty, J.D. (1995) Mosaicism of autosomes and sex chromosomes in morphologically normal, monospermic preimplantation human embryos. *Prenatal Diagnosis* **15**:41–9.

Harrison, K., Wilson, L., Breen, T., Pope, A., Cummins, J. & Hennessey J. (1988) Fertilization of human oocytes in relation to varying delay before insemination. *Fertility and Sterility* **50(2)**:294–7.

Holst, N. (1990) Optimization and simplification of culture conditions in human in Vitro Fertilization (IVF) and preembryo replacement by serum-free media. *Journal of In Vitro Fertilization and Embryo Transfer* **7(1)**:47–53.

Homburg, R. & Shelef, M. (1995) Factors affecting oocyte quality. In: (Grudzinskao, J.G. & Yorich, J.L., eds.), *Gamets: the Oocyte.* Cambridge University Press, pp. 227–91.

Howles, C.M., Macnamee, M.C. & Edwards, R.G. (1987) Follicular development and early luteal function of conception and non-conceptual cycles after human in vitro fertilization. *Human Reproduction* **2**:17–21.

James, R.M. & West, J.D. (1994) A chimaeric animal model for confined placental mosaicism. *Human Genetics* **93**:603–4.

Kermann, E. (1998) Creutzfeld-Jacob disease (CJD) and assisted reproductive technology (ART). *Human Reproduction* **13(7)**:1777.

Khan, I., Staessen, C., Van den Abbeel, E., Camus, M., Wisanro, A., Smith, J., Devroey, P. & Van Steirteghem, A.C. (1989) Time of insemination and its effect on in vitro fertilization, cleavage and pregnancy rates in GnRH agonist/HMG-stimulated cycles. *Human Reproduction* **4(5)**:531–5.

Kruger, T.F., Stander, F.S.H., Smith, K., Van Der Merue, J.P. & Lombard, C.J. (1987) The effect of serum supplementation on the cleavage of human embryos. *Journal of In Vitro Fertilization and Embryo Transfer* **4**:10.

Leese, H.J. (1987) Analysis of embryos by noninvasive methods. *Human Reproduction* **2**:37–40.

Leese, H.J., Donnay, I. & Thompson, J.G. (1998) Human assisted conception: a cautionary tale. Lessons from domestic animals. *Human Reproduction* **13, Suppl. 4**:184–202.

Leung, P., Gronow, M., Kellow, G., Lopata, A., Spiers, A., McBain, J., du Plessis, Y. & Johnston, I. (1984) Serum supplement in human in vitro fertilisation and embryo development. *Fertility and Sterility* **41**:36–917.

Levron, J., Munné, S., Willadsen, S., Rosenwaks, Z. & Cohen, J. (1995) Male and female genomes associated in a single pronucleus in human zygotes. *Journal of Assisted Reproduction and Genetics* **12, Suppl.**:27s.

Lopata, A., Johnston, I.W.H., Hoult, I.J. & Speins, A.L. (1980) Pregnancy following intrauterine implantation of an embryo obtained by in vitro fertilization of a preovulatory egg. *Fertility and Sterility* **33**:117.

Manamee, M.C., Howles, C.M. & Edwards, R.G. et al. (1989) Short term luteinising hormone agonist treatment, prospective trial of a novel ovarian stimulation regimen for in vitro fertilisation. *Fertility and Sterility* **52**:264–9.

Marrs, R.P., Saito, H., Yee, B., Sato, F. and Brown, J. (1984) Effect of variation of in vitro culture techniques upon oocyte fertilization and embryo development in human in vitro fertilization procedures. *Fertility and Sterility* 41:519–23.

Ménézo, Y., Dumont, M., Hazout, A., Nicollet, B., Pouly, J.L. & Janny, L. (1995) Culture and co-culture techniques. In: (Hedon, B., Bringer, J. & Mares, P. eds.), *Fertility and Sterility*, IFFS-95, The Parthenon Publishing Group, pp. 413–18.

Ménézo, Y., Guerin, J.F. & Czyba, J.C. (1990) Improvement of human early embryo development in vitro by co-culture on monolayers of Vero cells. *Biological Reproduction* **42**:301–5.

Ménézo, Y., Hazout, A., Dumont, M., Herbaut, N. & Nicollet, B. (1992) Coculture of embryos on Vero cells and transfer of blastocyst in human. *Human Reproduction* **7**:101–6.

Ménézo, Y., Testart, J. & Perrone, D. (1984) Serum is not necessary in human in vitro fertilization, early embryo culture, and transfer. *Fertility and Sterility* **42**:750.

Ménézo, Y., Veiga, A. & Benkhalifa, M. (1998) Improved methods for blastocyst formation and culture. *Human Reproduction Supplement* **13, Suppl. 4**:256–65.

Muggleton-Harris, A.L., Findlay, I. & Whittingham, D.G. (1990) Improvement of the culture conditions for the development of human preimplantation embryos. *Human Reproduction* **5**:217–20.

Munné, S., Alikani, M., Levron, J., Tomkin, G., Palermo, G., Grifo, J. & Cohen, J. (1995a) Fluorescent in situ hybridisation in human blastomeres. In: (Hedon, B., Bringer, J. & Mares, P. eds.), *Fertility and Sterility*. IFFS-95, The Parthenon Publishing Group, pp. 425–38.

Munné, S., Alikani, M. Tomkin, G., Grifo, J. & Cohen, J. (1995b) Embryo morphology, developmental rates, and maternal age are correlated with chromosomal abnormalities. *Fertility and Sterility* **64**:382–91.

Munné, S., Lee, A., Rosenwaks, Z., Grifo, J. & Cohen, J. (1993) Diagnosis of major chromosome aneuploidies in human preimplantation embryos. *Human Reproduction* **8**:2185–91.

Oehninger, S., Acosta, A.A., Veeck, L.L., Simonetti, S. & Muasher, S.J. (1989) Delayed fertilisation during in vitro fertilization and embryo transfer cycles: analysis of cause and impact of overall results. *Fertility and Sterility* **52**, 991–7.

Pampiglione, J.S., Mills, C., Campbell, S., Steer, C., Kingsland, C. & Mason, B.A. (1990) The clinical outcome of reinsemination of human oocytes fertilized in vitro. *Fertility and Sterility* **53**:306–10.

Parinaud, J., Vieitez, G., Milhet, P. & Richoilley, G. (1998) Use of a plant enzyme preparation (Coronase) instead of hyaluronidase for cumulus cell removal before intracytoplasmic sperm injection. *Human Reproduction* **13**:1933–45.

Pickering, S.J., Braude, P.R., Johnson, M.H., Cant, A. & Currie, J. (1990) Transient cooling to room temperature can cause irreversible disruption of the meiotic spindle in the human oocyte. *Fertility and Sterility* **54**:102–8.

Plachot, M. & Mandelbaum, J. (1990) Oocyte maturation, fertilization and embryonic growth in vitro. *British Medical Bulletin* **46**:675–94.

Plachot, M., de Grouchy, J., Montagut, J., Lepetre, S., Carle, E., Veiga, A., Calderon, G. & Santalo, J. (1987) Multi-centric study of chromosome analysis in human oocytes and embryos in an IVF programme. *Human Reproduction* **2**:29.

Plachot, M., Mandelbaum, J., Junca, A.M., Cohen, J. & Salat-Baroux, J. (1993) Coculture of human embryo with granulosa cells. *Contraception, Fertility and Sex* **19**:632–4.

Plachot, M., Veiga, A., Montagut, J. et al. (1988) Are clinical and biological IVF parameters correlated with chromosomal disorders in early life: a multicentric study. *Human Reproduction* **3**:627–35.

Purdy, J.M. (1982) Methods for fertilization and embryo culture in vitro, In: (Edwards, R.G. & Purdy, J.M. eds.) *Human Conception In Vitro.* Academic Press, London, p. 135.

Quinn, P., Warner, G.M., Klein, J.E. & Kirby, C. (1985) Culture factors affecting the success rate of in vitro fertilization and embryo transfer. *Annals of the New York Academy of Sciences* **412**:195.

Regan, L., Owen, E.J. & Jacobs, H.S. (1990) Hypersecretion of luteinising hormone, infertility, and miscarriage. *Lancet* **336**:1141–4.

Rinehart, J.S., Bavister, B.D. & Gerrity, M. (1988) Quality control in the in vitro fertilization laboratgory: comparison of bioassay systems for water quality. *Journal of In Vitro Fertilization and Embryo Transfer* **5**:335–425.

Roert, J., Verhoeff, A., van Lent, M., Hisman, G.J. & Zeilmaker, G.H. (1995) Results of decentralised in vitro fertilization treatment with transport and satellite clinics. *Human Reproduction* **10**:563–7.

Saito, H., Berger, T., Mishell, D.R. Jr & Marrs, R.P. (1984) The effect of serum fractions on embryo growth. *Fertility and Sterility* **41**:761–5.

Salha, O., Nugent, D., Dada, T., Kaufmann, S., Levett, S., Jenner, L., Lui, S. & Sharma, V. (1998) The relationship between follicular fluid aspirate volume and oocyte maturity in in vitro fertilization cycles. *Human Reproduction* **13(7)**:1901–6.

Shaw, J., Harrison, K., Wilson, L., Breen, T., Shaw, G., Cummins, J. & Hennessey, J. (1987) Results using medium supplemented with either fresh or frozen serum in human in vitro fertilization. *Journal of In Vitro Fertilization Embryo Transfer* **3**:215–17.

Schmutzler, A.G., Rieckmann, O., Sushma, V., Kupka, M., Montag, M., Prietl, G., Krebs, D. & Van der Ven, H.H. (1998). Ideal oocyte morphology depends on estradiol level. *Human Reproduction* **13**, Abstract book 1 (from 13th annual meeting of ESHRE, Göthenburg, Sweden, 1997), 184–202.

Scott, L. & Smith, S. (1998) The successful use of pronuclear embryo transfers the day following oocyte retrieval. *Human Reproduction* **13**: 1003–13.

Staessen, C., Van den Abbeel, E., Carle, Ml, Khan, I., Devroey, P. & Van Steirteghem, A.C. (1990) Comparison between human serum and Albuminar-20 (TM) supplement for in vitro fertilization. *Human Reproduction* **5**: 336–41.

Van Blerkom, J. (1996) The influence of intrinsic and extrinsic factors on the developmental potential of chromosomal normality of the human oocyte. *Journal of the Society of Gynecological Investigation* **3**:3–11.

Van Blerkom, J. & Henry, G. (1992) Oocyte dysmorphism and aneuploidy in meiotically mature human oocytes after ovarian stimulation. *Human Reproduction* **7**:379–90.

Van Blerkom, J., Atczak, M. & Schrader R. (1997) The developmental potential of the human oocyte is related to the dissolved oxygen content of follicular fluid: association with vascular endothelial growth factor concentrations and perifollicular blood flow characteristics. *Human Reproduction* **12**:1047–55.

Veeck, L.L. (1986) Insemination and fertilization. In: (Jones, H.W. Jr, Jones, G.S., Hodgen, G.D. & Rosenwaks, Z. eds.), *In Vitro Fertilization – Norfolk.* Williams & Wilkins, Baltimore, p. 183.

Veeck, L.L. (1988) Oocyte assessment and biological performance. *Annals of the New York Academy of Sciences of the USA* **541**:259–62.

Verlinsky, Y., Cieslak, J., Freidine, M., Ivakhnenko, V., Wolf, G., Kovalinskaya, L., Verlinsky White, M., Lifchez, A., Kaplan, B., Moise, J., Valle, J., Ginsberg, N., Strom, C. & Kulliev, A. (1995) Pregnancies following pre-conception diagnosis of common aneuploidies by fluorescent in situ hybridisation. *Molecular Human Reproduction* **10**:1927–34.

Verlinsky, Y., Strom, C., Cieslak, J., Kuliev, A., Ivakhnenko, V. & Lifchez, A. (1996) Birth of healthy children after preimplantation diagnosis of common aneuploidies by polar body fluorescent in situ hybridisation analysis. *Fertility and Sterility* **66**:126–9.

Weimer, K.E., Cohen, J., Tucker, M.J. & Godke, A. (1998) The application of co-culture in assisted reproduction: 10 years of experience with human embryos. *Human Reproduction supplement* **13, Suppl. 4**:226–38.

Weimer, K.E., Hoffman, D.I., Maxon, W.S., Eager, S., Muhlberger, R., Fior, I. & Cuervo, M. (1993) Embryonic morphology and rate of implantation of human embryos following co-culture on bovine oviductal epithelial cells. *Human Reproduction* **8**:97–101.

Woolcott, R. & Stanger, J. (1997) Potentially important variables identified by trans-vaginal ultrasound guided embryo transfer. *Human Reproduction* **12**:963–6.

Woolcott, R. & Stanger, J. (1998) Ultrasound tracking of the movement of embryo associated air bubbles on standing after transfer. *Human Reproduction* **13**:2107–9.

10

Cryopreservation

Benefits and concerns of an embryo cryopreservation programme

Following fresh embryo transfer in a stimulated IVF cycle, supernumerary embryos suitable for cryopreservation are available in a large number of cycles. In a routine IVF practice, 60% of stimulated in vitro fertilization (IVF) cycles may yield surplus embryos suitable for cryopreservation. Successful cryopreservation of zygotes and embryos has greatly enhanced the clinical benefits and cumulative conception rate possible for a couple following a single cycle of ovarian stimulation and IVF. Other clear benefits include the possibility of avoiding fresh embryo transfer in stimulated cycles with a potential for ovarian hyperstimulation syndrome, or in which factors that may jeopardize implantation are apparent (e.g. bleeding, unfavourable endometrium, polyps or extremely difficult embryo transfer).

However, a unit that offers embryo cryopreservation must also be aware of logistic, legal, moral and ethical problems which can arise, and ensure that all patients are fully informed and counselled. Both partners must sign comprehensive consent forms which indicate how long the embryos are to be stored, and define legal ownership in case of divorce or separation, death of one of the partners, or loss of contact between the Unit and the couple. At Bourn Hall Clinic, all couples with cryopreserved embryos in storage are contacted annually, and asked to return a signed form indicating whether they wish to

1. Continue storage
2. Return for frozen embryo transfer
3. Donate their embryos for research projects approved by the independent Ethics Committee and the Human Fertilization and Embryology Authority (HFEA)
4. Donate their embryos for 'adoption' by another infertile couple
5. Have the embryos thawed and disposed of.

Legislation in the UK which stated that embryos could remain in storage for more than five years only if further signed consent was obtained from both partners resulted in the destruction of more than 3000 embryos during 1996. Although in some cases the clinics were simply unable to contact patients who had changed address, it also became evident that many couples were unwilling to take responsibility for making decisions regarding the disposal of their embryos. Problems also arose when one of the partners refused consent for either further storage or transfer of 'custody' to the other partner. The overall result was not only a scandalous waste of a valuable resource, but a great deal of wasted laboratory and administrative time in checking and cross-checking all records and consents, and trying to trace patients lost to follow-up. All IVF units are urged to avoid a similar problem by investing the time and effort in ensuring that all patients are adequately informed, and that consent forms are clear and comprehensive.

A further potential problem arising from embryo storage has recently been raised: in 1995 Teddar et al. reported Hepatitis B transmission between frozen bone marrow samples in a liquid nitrogen storage tank. This has led to widespread discussion and concern regarding the possibility of pathogen transmission between samples in ART laboratories (see below).

Principles of cryobiology
John Morris

The first live births following frozen-thawed embryo transfer were reported in 1984 and 1985 by groups in Australia, The Netherlands and the UK. Since that time, the original protocols have been modified and simplified such that cryopreservation as an adjunct to a routine IVF programme may lead to successful survival of up to 80% of the embryos frozen, with subsequent pregnancy and live birth rates of 28% and 22% respectively (at Bourn Hall Clinic). Although the routine protocols required are simple and easily undertaken, an understanding of the basic principles of cryobiology involved is essential to ensure that the methodology is correctly and successfully applied to minimize cell damage during the processes of freezing and thawing. There are two major classes of physical stresses that cells are exposed to during freezing:

> Direct effects of reduced temperature
> Physical changes associated with ice formation.

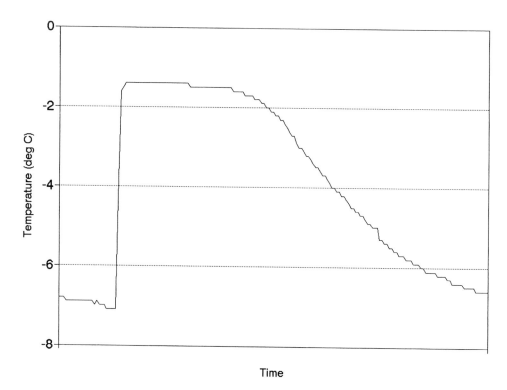

Figure 10.1   Temperature changes during the freezing of an aqueous solution of glycerol (5% w/v).

Direct effects of reduced temperatures

Cold shock injury (damage to cell structure and function arising from a sudden reduction in temperature) is species specific and well documented for spermatozoa (cattle, pig), oocytes and embryos (pig). This phenomenon is associated with modifications in membrane permeability and changes in the cytoskeletal structure (reviewed by Watson & Morris, 1987). This phenomenon is not evident following conventional cooling of human sperm and embryos. However, when freezing oocytes, ovarian tissue and testicular tissue, the possibility of sublethal injuries does exist, particularly those associated with breakdown of mitotic spindles.

Physical changes associated with ice formation

The temperature changes observed during the freezing of an aqueous solution are illustrated in Figure 10.1. Water and aqueous solutions have a strong tendency to cool below their melting point before nucleation of ice occurs: this phenomenon is referred to as supercooling, or more correctly undercooling. For example, whilst $0\,°C$ is the melting point of ice, the temperature of water may be reduced significantly below $0\,°C$ before ice formation occurs, and in carefully controlled conditions water may be cooled to approximately $-40\,°C$ before ice nucleation becomes inevitable (homogeneous nucleation temperature). Following ice nucleation and initial crystal growth the temperature rises to its melting point and remains relatively constant at that temperature during the subsequent phase change to ice ('latent heat plateau'), when the temperature then changes more rapidly to the environment temperature.

The tendency of a system to supercool is related to a number of factors including temperature, rate of cooling, volume, exclusion of atmospheric ice nuclei and purity of particulates. In cryopreservation of cells and tissues in IVF systems, there is thus a strong tendency for supercooling to occur. To avoid the damaging effects of supercooling on cells and in particular embryos (see below) ice formation is initiated in a controlled manner. This is commonly referred to as 'seeding' – although, strictly speaking, this term refers to the introduction of a crystal to an undercooled solution. 'Nucleation' is the initiation of ice other than by seeding, and this is the process generally practised in IVF.

Ice crystallization in an aqueous solution effectively removes some water from solution. The remaining aqueous phase becomes more concentrated, and a two-phase system of ice and concentrated solution coexist. As the temperature is reduced, more ice forms and the residual nonfrozen phase becomes increasingly concentrated. For example in glycerol and water a two-phase system occurs at all temperatures to $-45\,°C$. At $-45\,°C$ the non-frozen phase solidifies, with a glycerol concentration of 64% w/v; this is the eutectic temperature.

In dilute aqueous solutions such as culture media, there is a dramatic increase in ionic composition following ice formation and by $-10\,°C$ the salt concentration reaches *c.* 3 molal – not surprisingly, this is lethal to cells. A number of additives, known as cryoprotective additives, reduce cellular damage during freezing and thawing by simply increasing the volume of the residual unfrozen phase. This reduces the ionic composition of the solution at any subzero temperature. It must also be noted that all other physical parameters of the solution change following the formation of ice, including gas content, viscosity and pH.

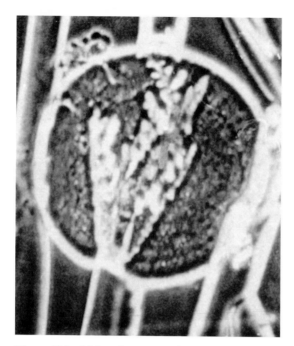

Figure 10.2   Light microscopy of a human oocyte
following ice nucleation in the extracellular medium.

The effects of freezing on cells

Cells in suspension are not punctured by ice crystals (Figure 10.2), nor are they
mechanically damaged by ice. Cells partition into the unfrozen fraction and
are exposed to increasing hypertonic solutions (Figure 10.3). Varying amounts
of water may be removed osmotically from the cell, dependent on the rate of
cooling. At 'slow' rates of cooling, cells may remain essentially in equilibrium
with the external solutions. As the rate of cooling is increased, there is less time
for water to move from the cell, which becomes increasingly supercooled until
eventually intracellular ice is formed. An optimum rate of cooling results from
the balance of these two phenomena. At rates of cooling slower than the
optimum, cell death is due to long periods of exposure to hypertonic conditions. At rates of cooling faster than the optimum, cell death is associated with
intracellular ice formation, which is inevitably lethal. The actual value of the
optimum rate is determined by a number of biophysical factors:

1.   Cell volume and surface area
2.   Permeability to water (Lp for human sperm 2.4 μm/min/atm cf. oocyte Lp of
     0.44 μm/min/atm)

(a)

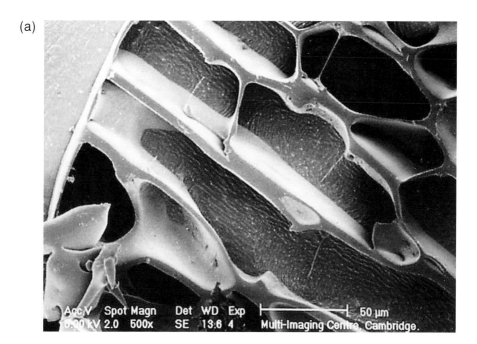

(b)

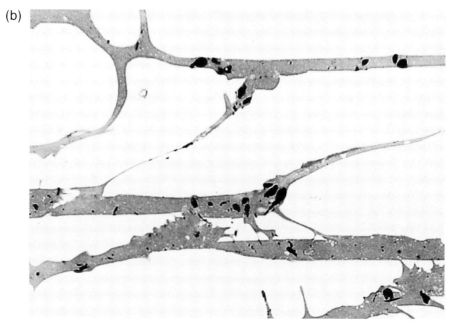

Figure 10.3   Ultrastructure of human sperm following freezing in a 0.25 ml straw, cells were suspended in glycerol (10%). (a) Freeze fracture followed by etching reveals the structure of ice crystals, cells are entrapped within the freeze concentrated material and few cell structures are evident. (b) Freeze substitution followed by sectioning shows cells entrapped within the freeze concentrated matrix.

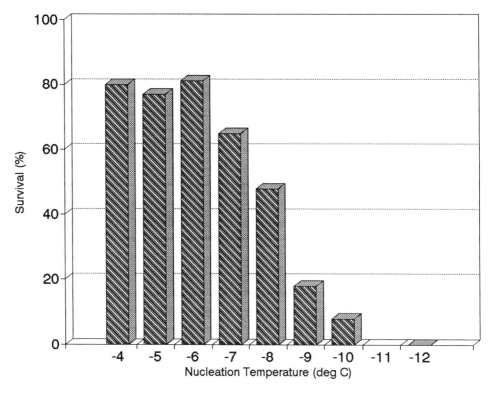

Figure 10.4   The survival of mouse cell embryos after seeding at various subzero temperatures. Redrawn from Whittingham (1977).

3. Arrhenius activation energy (EA is 3.9 Kcal mol for both human sperm and oocytes)
4. Type and concentration of cryoprotective additives.

Embryos with a large surface area and low water permeability have an optimum rate of cooling which is much slower than that observed with sperm. Computer models can predict the osmotic behaviour of cells during freezing, and this can be used to predict the influence of cooling rates on the recovery of many cell types. Computer modelling has been used to predict cell behaviour for oocytes and embryos. However, the predicted results with sperm have not been in agreement with experimental observations. For example, although conventional models have suggested that human sperm cells should equally survive cooling rates up to 10000 °C/min, experimentally the survival rate begins to decline beyond 100 °C/min.

Approaches to cryopreservation have generally utilized linear rates of cool-

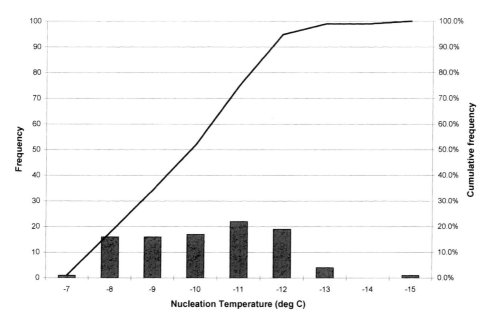

Figure 10.5   The measured nucleation temperatures within 0.25 ml straws cooling at $0.3\,^{\circ}\mathrm{C}\,\mathrm{min}^{-1}$.

ing. Morris et al. (1999) reported an alternative approach, which is based on the fact that the majority of physical parameters which the cells are exposed to during freezing vary in a nonlinear manner with temperature. Modification of the freezing process to take into account what the cell encounters and responds to has been demonstrated to give better recovery on thawing than linear rates of cooling.

Supercooling and cell survival

Controlled ice formation during freezing is recognized to be a key factor in determining the viability of embryos following freezing and thawing (see Whittingham, 1977). In a carefully controlled series of experiments, samples which were nucleated below $-9\,^{\circ}\mathrm{C}$ had a low viability, whilst nucleation at higher subzero temperatures of $-5\,^{\circ}\mathrm{C}$ to $-7.5\,^{\circ}\mathrm{C}$ resulted in much higher viability (Figure 10.4). An analysis of the spontaneous nucleation behaviour of straws (Figure 10.5) clearly demonstrates that if nucleation is not controlled the recovery of embryos would be expected to be very low. The physical basis of this injury is clear from examination of the thermal histories of supercooled straws (Figure 10.6). Normal practice is to cool straws to a temperature of approximately $-7\,^{\circ}\mathrm{C}$, hold at this temperature for thermal equilibration, and

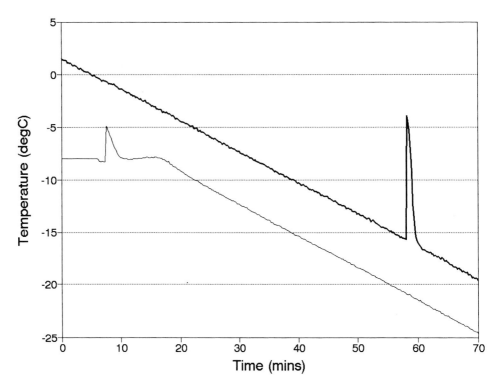

Figure 10.6   Measured temperatures within straws. During conventional cryopreservation the straws are held at a temperature of −7°C and nucleated, the resultant rise in temperature following ice nucleation is small. In the absence of induced nucleation the straws may reach very low temperatures before spontaneous nucleation occurs. A large rise in temperature to the melting point of the suspending medium then occurs followed by a rapid reduction in temperature; this will inevitably result in intracellular ice formation within embryos or oocytes.

then initiate ice formation in the straw by touching the outside of the straw with cold forceps etc. The temperature of the straw rises to the melting point of the solution, and then following ice formation the temperature returns at a rate of 2.5°C/min to −7°C. Cellular dehydration then occurs during subsequent slow cooling. By contrast, in a straw supercooled to −15°C spontaneous ice formation again results in a temperature rise followed by a rapid rate of cooling at 10°C/min to −15°C. The combination of a rapid rate of cooling and the large reduction in temperature does not permit cellular dehydration, and lethal intracellular ice formation is then inevitable. This has been observed by direct cryomicroscopy.

Ice nucleation

Ice nucleation must be controlled in order to obtain high viability of embryos in a cryopreservation programme. The differences between those laboratories which achieve good results and those which are less successful can often be attributed to this practical step. Straws can be frozen horizontally or vertically – this has no effect on viability or ease of ice nucleation. Embryos sink in the cryoprotective additive and will always be found at the wall of the straw when frozen horizontally, or at the bottom of the column of liquid when frozen vertically. Following thermal equilibration at the nucleation temperature $(-7°C)$, ice formation is initiated by touching the outside of the straw or ampoule with a liquid nitrogen cooled spatula, forceps, cotton bud etc., at the level of the meniscus. This causes a local cold spot on the vessel wall, which leads to ice nucleation. Immediately following ice nucleation the temperature will rise rapidly (cf. Figure 10.1) and the ice front will propagate through the sample. Practical difficulties may arise from a number of points:

1. Because straws have a large surface area, small diameter and a thin wall, very rapid warming occurs when they are removed from a cold environment. Measured temperature excursions that occur at different points of the cryopreservation procedure are illustrated in Figure 10.7. If straws are removed from the controlled rate freezing apparatus for excessive times during the nucleation procedure, they can warm to a temperature which is too high for ice nucleation to occur. Ice nucleation may occur because of the local cooling induced by the nucleating tool, but it is possible that the bulk temperature of the fluid may not allow ice crystal growth to propagate through the sample. In some laboratories, it is common practice to check that ice propagation has occurred throughout the sample. If straws are removed from the controlled rate cooling equipment, this in itself may cause melting of the nucleated ice.

2. The thermal control of the freezing apparatus may not be sufficiently accurate or stable at the nucleation temperature. The temperature achieved may allow nucleation to occur because of the thermal mass of the nucleating tool, but may not be sufficiently low to allow subsequent ice propagation. Any thermal fluctuations within the freezing apparatus may also lead to melting of ice.

3. Within straws, nucleation of ice at temperatures very close to the melting point results in a very slow propagation of ice through the sample. In some cases, the ice propagation can actually become blocked, and embryos are then effectively supercooled. In this case the embryos would not be expected to survive further cooling.

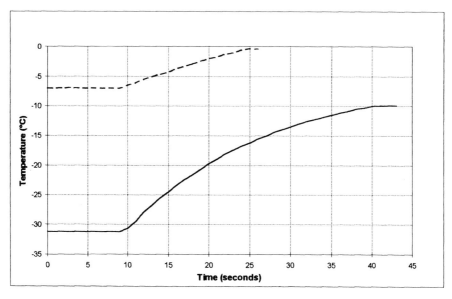

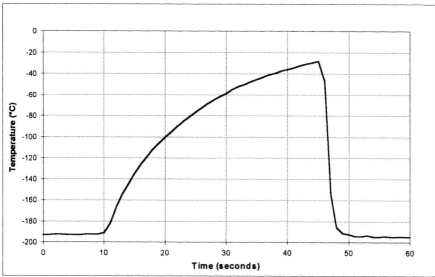

Figure 10.7   Measured temperatures within straws following removal from a controlled rate freezer or from a liquid nitrogen vessel at various points during the freezing cycle. Prior to nucleation the temperature rise within 5 seconds is sufficient to prevent ice nucleation. At $-30\,°C$ the sample temperature may rise very quickly and if transfer to liquid nitrogen is carried out at this point of the cycle care must be taken to ensure that the increase in temperature is minimized. Following liquid nitrogen immersion the temperature of straws may rise by $130\,°C$ within 20 seconds.

Vitrification

An alternative approach to cryopreservation is by vitrification. Conventional methods of cryopreservation have been developed to accommodate the consequences of ice formation, and vitrification is a process which combines the use of concentrated solutions with rapid cooling in order to avoid the formation of ice. Samples reach low temperatures in a glassy state which has the molecular structure of a viscous liquid and is not crystalline. This method has the potential advantages of being rapid to carry out and does not require a controlled rate cooling apparatus. Good survival of mammalian embryos has been demonstrated by vitrification in a number of laboratories, but this approach is still experimental. The high levels of additives that are necessary to achieve vitrification are potentially cytotoxic.

Storage of cryopreserved samples

Recently there has been a clear demonstration of Hepatitis B transmission between frozen bone marrow samples in a liquid nitrogen storage tank. This raises the possibility of pathogen transmission between samples in ART laboratories. Potential sources of contamination include:

1. *Within the freezing apparatus*
Vapour phase controlled rate freezers spray nonsterile liquid nitrogen directly onto the samples. This may be further compounded by liquid condensation that may accumulate within ducting between freezing runs. Ideally, a freezing apparatus should have the capability of being sterilized between freezing runs.

2. *During storage*
Straws may be contaminated on the outside, or seals and plugs may leak. Particulates may then transfer via the liquid nitrogen within the storage vessel.

3. *From liquid nitrogen*
Generally, liquid nitrogen has a very low microbial count when it is manufactured. However, contamination may occur during storage and distribution. Any part of the distribution chain that periodically warms up, in particular transfer Dewars, may become heavily contaminated. The microbial quality of the liquid nitrogen when delivered from the manufacturer varies widely with geographical region and more extreme reports of microbial contamination may reflect local industrial practices.

The HFEA in the UK has prepared a consultation document with guidelines for safe storage of human gametes in liquid nitrogen; basic recommendations include patient screening for Hepatitis and HIV viruses, careful hygiene throughout, double containment of storage straws or the use of sealed ampoules

Embryo freezing and thawing

Embryo selection for cryopreservation

Using 1,2-propanediol as cryoprotectant, embryos can be frozen at either the pronucleate or early cleavage stages. Careful selection of viable embryos with a good prognosis for survival is paramount in achieving acceptable success rates.

1. *Pronucleate*: The cell must have an intact zona pellucida, and healthy cytoplasm with two distinct pronuclei clearly visible. Accurate timing of zygote freezing is essential to avoid periods of the cell cycle which are highly sensitive to cooling. During the period when pronuclei start to migrate before syngamy, with DNA synthesis and formation of the mitotic spindle, the microtubular system is highly vulnerable to temperature fluctuation leading to possible scattering of the chromosomes. Zygotes processed for freezing at this stage will no longer survive cryopreservation. The timing of pronucleate freezing is crucial, and the process must be initiated while the pronuclei are still distinctly apparent: normally from 20 to 22 hours after insemination.
2. *Cleavage*: 2–8 cell embryos must be of good quality, Grade 1 or 2, with less than 20% cytoplasmic fragments. Uneven blastomeres and a high degree of fragmentation jeopardize survival potential.

Media preparation

Ready-to-use media for freezing and thawing embryos are now available from the majority of companies who supply culture media; individual methods and protocols vary slightly with the different preparations, and manufacturers' instructions should be followed for each. The protocol outlined below has been used at Bourn Hall Clinic from 1986 to the present time.

MATERIALS
Phosphate buffered saline (PBS) – Gibco Ltd, PO Box 35, Paisley, Scotland.
1,2-Propanediol (PROH) – Sigma (propylene glycol)
Sucrose

Freezing solutions

1. 100 ml PBS (Gibco)
2. 1.5 M PROH
   86.3 ml PBS
   13.7 ml PROH (agitate gently as you add)
3. 1.5 M PROH/0.1 M sucrose
   86.3 ml PBS
   13.7 ml PROH (agitate gently)
   4.1 g sucrose (allow to dissolve)

Thawing solutions

1. 1.0 M PROH + 0.2 M Sucrose
   90.9 ml PBS
   9.1 ml PROH (agitate gently)
   8.2 g sucrose (allow to dissolve)
2. 0.5 M PROH + 0.2 M sucrose
   Use a 1:1 mixture of (1) & (3)
3. 0.2 M Sucrose
   100 ml PBS
   8.2 g sucrose
4. PBS

Optional: Phenol red may be added to each as a colourant:
0.2 ml Phenol red to each 100 ml of solution.

After preparation the solutions are filtered through a 0.22 μm Millipore filter, labelled, and stored in 10 ml sterile aliquots at room temperature in the dark.

Working solutions: + 20% serum. Add 0.2 ml human serum albumin to each 1 ml of solution immediately before use.

Method

Details of each patient and embryos must be carefully recorded on appropriate data sheets. Meticulous and complete record keeping is crucial, and must include the patient's date of birth, medical number, date of oocyte retrieval (OCR), date of cryopreservation, number and type of embryos frozen, together with clear and accurate identification of storage vessel and location within the storage vessel. The data sheets should also confirm that both partners have signed consent forms. Both ampoules and straws have been successfully used for embryo storage, and each has advantages and disadvantages. The choice between them is a matter of individual preference, as well as availability of storage space and laboratory time to prepare and sterilize ampoules. When straws are used, they must be handled with care to avoid external contamination, and to avoid inadvertent temperature fluctuations during seeding or transfer to the storage Dewar. The measured temperature excursions within straws can be very dramatic (Figure 10.7). It is likely that in straws frozen horizontally the embryos will be adjacent to the wall, where they will be exposed to the highest thermal gradient; great care must be taken in handling cryopreserved material. Plastic cryovials are not recommended for embryo freezing. Handle the preselected embryos with fire-polished clean sterile Pasteur pipettes, using a different pipette for each patient. Fine glass probes may also be required, to help in locating the embryos within their dishes or wells.

1. Use 1 ml aliquots of each solution per patient, and add 20% human serum albumin just before use to make the working solutions
2. Warm the solutions to 37°C
3. Prepare labelled dishes, either 3 × 35 mm Petri dishes per patient, or one 4-well Nunc plate per patient
4. Transfer embryos and warmed solutions to room temperature: the embryos are transferred initially to the first solution at 37°C, and thereafter allowed to cool gradually to room temperature. Pipette the embryos:
1. F1 (PBS + 20% serum): wash to remove traces of medium, then pipette into
2. F2 (PBS + serum + 1.5 mM PROH): leave to equilibrate at room temperature, 15 minutes
3. F3 (PBS + serum + PROH + 0.1 M sucrose): leave for 10–15 minutes at room temperature
4. Load into prelabelled straws or ampoules.
   Straws: IMV BP 81 L'Aigle, France. Paillette Cristal 91, Ref.ZA 180.
   Distributed by Rocket-Medical, Imperial Way, Watford, WD2 4XX, UK.

Loading into straws

Label the straws with a pen or wire marker (patient's initials).
Label the plastic plug with patient's name, hospital number, date and straw number.
Insert a plug a short way into the straw.

With a marker pen make 3 marks on each straw:

1. At 2 cm from the plug
2. 0.7 cm from the first mark away from the plug
3. A further 0.5 cm away from the second mark.

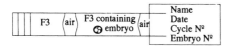

Figure 10.8   Loading embryos into a cryostraw before freezing.

Attach a 1 ml syringe with appropriate silicone tubing adapter to the straw, and fill as follows:

1. Aspirate F3 to the first mark
2. Aspirate air so that this F3 reaches the second mark
3. Aspirate F3 + embryos so that the first F3 fraction reaches the third mark
4. Apirate air so that the first F3 fraction almost reaches the cotton plug
5. Aspirate a small volume of F3 so that the first fraction reaches the plug and wets the PVA
6. Insert the plug.

NB: It is essential that the plug is surrounded by medium – this freezes and forms a vapour-tight seal. If in doubt, wet the inside of the straw with F3 using a needle/syringe before inserting the plastic plug. Each straw must be clearly identifiable with precise patient details including name, date of birth, record number and date of freezing (Figure 10.8).

Straws which are improperly loaded can lead to problems: if the proportion of air to liquid is too great, rapid air expansion on thawing will cause the plug to 'blow' out of the straw, with a danger of losing the embryo.

Ampoules

Tissue-culture washed borosilicate glass ampoules with a fine-drawn neck can be used. First fill the ampoule with approximately 0.4 ml of the sucrose/PROH solution using a needle and syringe, then carefully transfer the embryos using a fine-drawn Pasteur pipette. Using a high-intensity flame, carefully heat-seal the neck of the ampoule. It is important to ensure (under the microscope) that the seal is complete, without leaks: leakage of liquid nitrogen into the ampoule during freezing will cause it to explode immediately upon thawing! It is often impossible to detect whether the glass neck is completely sealed, and the possibility of explosion can be avoided by opening the ampoule under liquid nitrogen before thawing.

Care must be taken to ensure that no air bubbles are trapped within the freezing medium after the sample has been loaded, into either ampoules or straws. Air bubbles can sometimes be seen in both vessels on thawing, and these present a hazard to the fragile dehydrated embryo. Warming solutions to 37°C before starting the procedure may effectively act as a 'degassing' mechanism.

The Edinburgh Assisted Conception Unit recommend the use of glass ampoules which can be sealed using silicone rubber bungs (John Keith, personal communication). These consist of Durham tubes (code TTD 03, Camlab; manufactured by SAMCO, resistance glass, 35 × 8 mm, supplied in boxes of 250). The ampoules are robust, pack easily and conveniently into a visitube, and are used without preparing a fine-drawn neck. They are easy to load, with good visualization, and seeding is easy to perform, as the ice can be readily seen and ampoules do not warm up as easily as do straws. Handling during thawing is simplified, as the bung can be removed and contents pipetted with no risk of exploding ampoules. They can also be contained within a plastic cryovial for storage as a means of potential contamination control. Stoppers: silicone rubber, top diameter 7 mm, bottom diameter 5 mm, sold by most lab suppliers (e.g. ESCO, code no. TSR BGE 005). Using this system, their figures show survival of 80% of embryos thawed, and a clinical pregnancy rate of 20% per transfer of two thawed embryos.

Preparation: Tubes and stoppers are soaked for 1 hour and rinsed thoroughly three times in water for irrigation. The tubes should be individually rinsed once during the washing to remove debris. Pack the tubes into a Pyrex beaker, cover with aluminium foil, and heat-sterilize at 180°C for one hour. Stoppers are dried using lint-free paper tissues, and sterilized by autoclaving.

Freezing programme

A variety of programmable and programmed controlled-rate freezers are now available (Planer, Cryologic, Biotronics, Asymptote). The basic programme used to freeze pronucleate or cleavage stage embryos includes the following steps:

Cool at 1°C/min to starting temperature of approximately 20°C, and hold for 5 minutes to complete loading of samples

Cool at 2°C/min to − 7°C

Hold at − 7°C for 5 to 10 minutes, to allow equilibration of all samples

Perform manual seeding at − 6.5°C to − 7°C

Slow cool at − 0.3°C/min to − 30°C

Cool rapidly to below − 100°C

Plunge into liquid nitrogen, and transfer to storage Dewar.

With human embryos it is common practice to cool within the controlled rate freezing apparatus down to below $-100\,^\circ$C after the slow cooling to $-30\,^\circ$C, before transfer to liquid nitrogen. With embryos in veterinary IVF cryopreservation, straws are often transferred to liquid nitrogen directly from $-30\,^\circ$C. This procedure would give equally good results for human embryos and is indeed used by some laboratories with no reduction in viability. It is essential that the transfer is carried out rapidly because the temperature of the straws may rise very rapidly when they are removed from the controlled rate device (see Figure 10.7).

Embryo cryopreservation: method

- Wash in phosphate buffered saline $+$ 20% serum
- Transfer to 1 ml of 1.5 M Propanediol (PROH) $+$ 20% serum
- Leave for 15 minutes at room temperature
- Transfer to 1 ml of 1.5 M PROH $+$ 0.1 M sucrose $+$ 20% serum
- Leave for 10–15 minutes at room temperature
- Load into ampoules or straws, transfer to programmed cell freezer.

Thawing

Prepare:

1. $30\,^\circ$C water bath for straws, or $37\,^\circ$C water bath for ampoules
2. Labelled Petri dishes or Nunc plate
3. Thawing solutions at room temperature
4. Fire-polished sterile Pasteur pipettes and probe
5. Patient freeze/thaw data sheet.

The thawing protocol is carried out at room temperature, and the embryos placed in equilibrated culture medium at room temperature before being allowed to warm gradually to $37\,^\circ$C in the incubator.

1. Remove straws or ampoules from liquid nitrogen.
2. (a) Straws: hold at room temperature 40 seconds
   Wipe with a dry tissue to remove excess ice
   Plunge into $30\,^\circ$C water bath for 1 minute
   Remove the plug from the straw(s) and release the embryos into the first thawing solution (1.0 M PROH, 0.2 M sucrose)

(b) Ampoules: thaw in 37 °C waterbath

Using a fine-drawn pipette, aspirate and decant the contents of the ampoule into the Petri dish or well.

3. Identify the embryo(s) under the microscope, and transfer to solution T1. This solution is dense, and the embryos will rise and float, making them difficult to find and susceptible to damage. Use a probe to carefully move and direct them down into the solution.

4. Leave for 5 minutes.

5. Transfer to T2 (PBS + 20% serum + 0.5 M PROH + 0.2 M sucrose), 5 minutes.

6. Transfer to T3 (PBS + 20% serum + 0.2 M sucrose), 5 minutes.

7. Wash in PBS (T4) and then transfer through two wash drops or wells of culture medium before placing the embryos in their final culture drop or well. Observe the embryos for evidence of damage: fractured zona, lysed blastomeres, yellow grainy appearance of the cytoplasm.

8. Incubate at 37 °C in the CO_2 incubator until the time of embryo transfer.

Pronucleate embryos may be cultured overnight to confirm continued development, and cleavage stage embryos are incubated for a minimum of 1 hour before transfer.

Embryo thawing
- Rapid thaw to 30 °C
- Incubate at room temperature in

1.0 M PROH/0.2 M sucrose + 20% serum	5 minutes
0.5 M PROH/0.2 M sucrose + 20% serum	5 minutes
0.2 M sucrose + 20% serum	5 minutes

- Wash through 3 drops of culture medium
- Incubate at 37 °C:

Pronucleate: incubate overnight to assess cleavage
Cleaved: incubate at least 1 hour

Blastocyst freezing

Although the same propanediol protocol has recently been applied to the freezing of blastocysts, they can also be successfully frozen using glycerol at a final concentration of 9%. Prepare culture dishes containing two drops of each glycerol dilution under a layer of equilibrated oil (or four-well plates containing two aliquots of each glycerol dilution), and equilibrate the dishes to 37 °C in the CO$_2$ incubator.

Make dilutions to final concentrations of:

(a) Freezing:
1. 5% glycerol (v/v) in culture medium, 10 minutes.
2. 9% glycerol (v/v) in culture medium containing 0.2 M sucrose, 10 minutes
(b) Thawing:
1. 0.5 M sucrose in culture medium, 10 minutes
2. 0.2 M sucrose in culture medium, 10 minutes.
3. Wash through 2–3 drops or aliquots of culture medium and replace in culture.

The basic programme used to freeze blastocysts includes the following steps:
   Start temperature 20 °C

1. Cool at 1 °C/min to − 7 °C
2. Hold at − 7 °C for 5 to 10 minutes to allow equilibration of all samples
3. Perform manual seeding
4. Slow cool at 0.3 °C/min to − 30 °C
5. Hold for 5–10 minutes
6. Plunge directly into liquid nitrogen

Planer Kryo 10 operation

1. Ensure that there is an adequate level of liquid nitrogen in the Dewar, leaving an air space. The container should not be more than two-thirds full. Immerse the probe and attach the pressure gauge securely. Close the red toggle switch on the pressure gauge.
2. Switch power on, and pressurize the system by pressing the white switch on the platform. An orange indicator light should appear and extinguishes automatically when the correct pressure is reached (5–7.5 psi).
3. Press RUN/HOLD. The display will prompt 'Enter access level 1'
4. Enter password: 3333
5. Display prompts: 'Which programme?' Use arrow keys to alter, select programme and press ENTER.
6. Display reads 'Programme Start 20 °C'
7. Press RUN. Ramp 1 will lead to starting temperature, and alarm will sound when it is reached. Display reads 'Load Samples'.
8. Load samples and press RUN.
9. When seeding temperature is reached, the alarm sounds and the machine will hold the temperature at −6.5 °C. SEED all the samples, then press RUN. The machine continues the programme to Ramp 5.

10. Before the end of the programme, prepare a small vessel of liquid nitrogen containing prelabelled plastic goblets, held under the nitrogen with artery forceps. At the end of the programme, remove all the samples and plunge them directly into the liquid nitrogen filled goblets.

11. Transfer the samples to their preselected storage space, and confirm the recorded position on appropriate embryo storage records.

IMPORTANT: Seeding must be performed whilst the chamber is at -6.5 *to* $-7\,^{\circ}C$. *Use a liquid nitrogen cooled spatula or forceps to touch the meniscus at the top of the column of liquid, and replace the sample in the chamber immediately.*

12. To switch off, or abort a run:
     Press 5: display prompts 'ENTER to confirm', press ENTER.
     Display reads 'Run, chamber temp = ... °C'
     Press RUN
     Display reads 'Do not switch off'
     When ambient temperature is reached, display reads 'ready to restart'
     Switch power off
     Open the toggle switch on the Dewar to release the pressure

During a run, the display can be altered using arrow keys to show: time left for that segment, demand temperature, ramp end temperature, ramp rate, name and no. of programme, chamber temperature.

Clinical aspects of frozen embryo transfer

Freeze-thawed embryos must be transferred to a uterus that is optimally receptive for implantation, postovulation. Patients with regular ovulatory cycles and an adequate luteal phase may have their embryos transferred in a natural cycle, monitored by ultrasound and blood or urine luteinizing hormone (LH) levels in order to pinpoint ovulation. Embryo transfer is routinely carried out three days after the onset of the LH surge, i.e. 2 days postovulation. Older patients, or those with irregular cycles may have their embryos transferred in an artificial cycle with the administration of hormone replacement therapy using exogenous steroids after creating an artificial menopause by downregulation with a GnRH agonist.

Transfer in a natural menstrual cycle

1. Patient selection
       regular cycles, 28 ± 3 days

previously assay luteal phase progesterone to confirm ovulation. An ovulation 'kit' such as Clearplan can also be used in a previous cycle to confirm that the patient has regular ovulatory cycles.

2. Cycle monitoring
   from Day 10 until ovulation is confirmed, by:
   daily ultrasound scan
   daily plasma LH (± oestradiol, progesterone)

3. Be prepared to cancel if:
   peak oestradiol is <650 pmol/L
   endometrial thickness is <8 mm at the time of LH surge

4. Timing of the embryo transfer

   Pronucleate embryos
   thaw on Day 1 after ovulation (LH + 3)
   culture overnight before transfer.

   Cleavage stage embryos
   Thaw and transfer on Day 2 after ovulation (LH + 4)

   Blastocysts
   Thaw and transfer on Day 4 after ovulation (LH + 6)

Patients with irregular cycles may be induced to ovulate using clomiphene citrate or gonadotrophins, and embryo transfer timed in relation either to the endogenous LH surge or following administration of human chorionic gonadotrophin (hCG). Although it is possible to estimate embryo transfer time using an ovulation 'kit' to detect the LH surge, this is far less accurate, and does present a risk of inappropriate timing.

Transfer in an artificial cycle

1. Patient selection: oligomenorrhoea/irregular cycles, Age > 38 years
2. Downregulate with GnRH analogue (buserelin or nafarelin) for at least 14 days, continue downregulation until the time of embryo transfer.
3. Oestradiol valerate

days	1–5	2 mg
	6–9	4 mg
	10–13	6 mg
	14 onwards	4 mg

4. Progesterone
   Day 15–16 Gestone 50 mg intramuscular (Ferring)
   or cyclogest pessaries 200 mg twice daily (Cyclogest, Hoechst)
   or utrogestan pessaries 100 mg three times daily (Utrogestan, Besins-Iscovesco)

and double dose from Day 17 onwards (100 mg Gestone, 400 mg twice daily cyclogest, 200 mg three times daily utrogestan).
5. Embryo transfer
    (a) Pronucleate: thaw on Day 16 of the artificial cycle, culture overnight before transfer on Day 17.
    (b) Cleavage stage embryos: thaw and replace on Day 17.
6. If pregnancy is established, continue hormone replacement (HRT) therapy:
    8 mg oestradiol valerate
    Higher dose of progesterone supplement daily until Day 77 after embryo transfer; then gradually withdraw the drugs with monitoring of blood P4 (progesterone) levels.

This protocol is also successfully used for the treatment of agonadal women who require ovum or embryo donation. In combination with prior gonadotrophin releasing hormone (GnRH) pituitary suppression, the artificial cycle can be timed to a prescheduled programme according to the patients (or clinic's) convenience.

Results

In a series of 1009 FER cycles at Bourn Hall Clinic from 1991 to 1994, the clinical pregnancy rates using the different transfer regimens can be seen in Table 10.1:

Table 10.1

	Number	No. pregnant (%)
All cycles	1009	259 (26)
Natural cycles	421	35 (32)
HRT cycles	588	124 (21)
Freeze all embryos	290	110 (38)
Surplus embryos only	719	149 (21)
Cleaving embryos	241	44 (18)
Pronucleate embryos	768	215 (28)

Notes:
HRT: Hormone replacement therapy.
Clinical pregnancy rates (viable gestation sacs per embryo transfer procedure) after frozen-thawed embryo transfer at Bourn Hall Clinic from 1991 to 1994.

Oocyte cryopreservation

Prior to 1997, the options for preserving a young woman's fertility after treatment for malignant disease were very limited: a full IVF treatment cycle with cryopreservation of embryos prior to the initiation of chemotherapy, or oocyte or embryo donation following recovery from the malignant disease. The first option is available only to women with partners to provide a semen sample for fertilization of the harvested oocytes. However, the success of frozen embryo cryopreservation in a competent IVF programme is such that these patients maintain a very good chance of achieving a pregnancy after transfer of frozen–thawed embryos following recovery from their disease. On the other hand, this strategy also raises the risk of creating embryos with a higher than average chance of being orphaned.

Many of the legal and ethical problems created by the cryopreservation and storage of embryos might be overcome by preserving oocytes, especially for young women about to undergo treatment for malignant disease which will result in loss of ovarian function. A few pregnancies after oocyte freeze–thawing and fertilization were reported in the mid-1980s, but low oocyte survival rates prevented the technique from being adopted clinically. Progress in the field remained static until the mid-1990s, when promising reports began to appear.

Human oocytes are particularly susceptible to freeze-thaw damage due to their size and complexity. Cryopreserved mouse oocytes showed high rates of aneuploidy after thawing, thought to arise from abnormalities of the spindle apparatus, which is highly temperature sensitive and depolymerizes with temperature reduction. Abnormal spindle organization after thawing resulted in the presence of 'stray' chromosomes in the cytoplasm. Premature cortical granule release with subsequent zona hardening and parthenogenetic activation were also observed. However, in 1993–94, Gook et al. used propanediol/sucrose as cryoprotectant and were able to successfully recover up to 64% of human oocytes cryopreserved, with normal meiotic spindle and chromosome configuration after thawing. They further demonstrated that the frozen-thawed oocytes could be fertilized by intracytoplasmic sperm injection, and 50% produced embryos of normal karyotypes without stray chromosomes. Oocyte cryopreservation is now offered in their clinic to patients risking loss of ovarian function.

In February 1997, an Italian clinic reported the birth of a healthy baby girl following oocyte freeze–thawing and intracytoplasmic injection, and some of the factors influencing the survival rate and fertilization of human oocytes after cryopreservation have been evaluated (Fabbri et al., 1998). Their results showed:

Better survival rates with cumulus enclosed compared with denuded oocytes
Better survival using 0.2 M sucrose as compared with 0.1 M sucrose
Exposure to 1.5 M propanediol for a period of at least 15 minutes gave optimal survival
Embryos resulting from normal insemination had a significantly reduced cleavage rate compared with ICSI generated embryos.

The above conditions yielded an average oocyte survival rate of 60%, with 64% fertilization after ICSI. To date, the same group have reported a further 6 deliveries and 2 ongoing pregnancies (Porcu et al., 1997). The protocol used is similar to that for embryo cryopreservation, with mechanical partial removal of oocyte cumulus. The oocytes are washed with warm PBS + 30% HSA, transferred to 1.5 M propanediol + 0.2 M sucrose, and equilibrated for 15 minutes before loading into cryostraws. The freezing programme is identical to that for embryos, with manual seeding at $-8\,°C$.

For oocyte thawing, straws were rapidly thawed in a $30\,°C$ water bath for 40 seconds, and cryoprotectant removed by stepwise dilution at room temperature:

1.0 M propanediol + 0.2 M sucrose, 5 minutes
0.5 M propanediol + 0.2 M sucrose, 5 minutes
0.2 M sucrose, 10 minutes
PBS solution: 10 minutes at room temperature minutes at $37\,°C$
Transfer into culture medium at $37\,°C$.

The cumulus is removed after one hour of culture, and oocytes checked for signs of survival (intact zona pellucida and plasma membrane, clear perivitelline space of normal size, no evidence of cytoplasmic leakage or oocyte shrinkage).

Oocytes which survive and demonstrate an extruded polar body after 2–3 hours of culture can be inseminated by ICSI.

Research in animal systems suggests that freezing of immature oocytes may provide an alternative approach in the future: meiosis is arrested in Prophase I of the dictyate stage, with chromosomes located within a membrane bound nucleus or germinal vesicle, eliminating the risk of damaging the microtubules of the meiotic spindle. Nevertheless, there is still risk of zona hardening and damage to the cytoskeleton., and the GV oocytes must be matured in vitro. Although human GV oocytes have been successfully recovered, matured, and fertilized after freezing, no pregnancies have as yet been reported.

Recently, Stachecki et al. (1999) have demonstrated that the high concentration of sodium in conventional freezing media is detrimental to oocyte cryopreservation and that improved survival of mouse oocytes may be achieved by replacing the sodium in the freezing medium with choline.

Ovarian tissue cryopreservation

Cryopreservation and banking of ovarian tissue is an attractive strategy for fertility conservation: ovarian biopsy/oophorectomy can be carried out rapidly, at any stage of the menstrual cycle, before cancer treatment is begun, and tissue can be stored for children as well as for young adults. Small pieces (1 mm^3) of ovarian cortex contain large numbers of primordial follicles, which theoretically can either be later returned to the patient by grafting, or cultured in vitro to generate oocytes for in vitro fertilization.

Oocytes in primordial follicles are small (approx. 1% of the volume of a ripe metaphase II oocyte), and less differentiated, with fewer organelles and no zona pellucida or cortical granules. As they are arrested in prophase, theoretically they should carry a lower risk of carrying cytogenetic errors.

High rates of follicle survival after freeze-thawing tissue have already been reported in mice, sheep and human ovaries. When isolated primordial follicles are transferred in the mouse, or ovarian tissue slices are grafted into sheep, it is possible to obtain follicular survival with subsequent maturation, oestrogen secretion and restoration of fertility to the hosts. Following this success, many patients throughout the world now have ovarian tissue cryopreserved, awaiting further research that will hopefully allow the future restoration of their fertility after chemotherapy or radiotherapy. During 1999, promising results of a preliminary study carried out at the University of Leeds were reported: ovarian biopsies were taken from healthy volunteers undergoing laparoscopic assessment for reversal of sterilization, and one of the biopsies sutured to a heterotopic site, the anterior surface of the uterus. Other pieces of the biopsy tissue were studied for assessment and survival of follicles after freeze-thawing. During reversal of sterilization three months later, the heterotopic grafts were recovered and sectioned for quantitative follicle counting and stained for granulosa cell mitotic activity. In this first study of follicle survival after human ovarian heterotopic autografting, follicles were identified in all of the grafts, with a survival rate of 27%.

These techniques open a new and very optimistic vista for the preservation of ovarian function after treatment for malignant disease. The protocol used for cryopreserving ovarian tissue is as yet tentative, as many permutations are yet to be tested and studied (Nugent et al., 1998, Newton et al., 1996).

1. Equilibrate thin slices of ovarian cortex for 30 minutes on ice in buffered medium containing cryoprotectant (e.g. 1.5 ml/l DMSO), serum (5–10%) and 0.1 mM of sucrose/mannitol.
2. Load the tissue in cryovials into an automated freezer starting at 0 °C, and cool at 2 °C/min to −7 °C.
3. Soak for 10 minutes before seeding.
4. Continue to cool at 0.3 °C/min to −40 °C
5. Cool at faster rate of 10 °C/min to −140 °C
6. Transfer to liquid nitrogen Dewar for storage.
7. When required, thaw rapidly at approximately 100 °C/min
8. Wash tissues stepwise in progressively lower concentrations of medium.

Semen cryopreservation

Semen can be successfully cryopreserved using either glycerol alone, or a complex cryoprotective medium as cryoprotectant. Cooling and freezing can be carried out by using a programmed cell freezer, or by simply suspending the prepared specimens in liquid nitrogen vapour for a period of 30 minutes. Cryopreserved semen has long been used successfully for artificial insemination, intrauterine insemination and IVF. When it is to be used for intrauterine insemination or IVF, the sample must be carefully washed or prepared by density gradient centrifugation to remove all traces of cryoprotectant medium. Although freeze-thawing does produce damage to the cells with loss of up to 50% of prefreeze motility, the large numbers of cells available can still achieve successful fertilization even with low cryosurvival rates. There is, however, a noticeable difference in cryosurvival rates between normal semen and semen with abnormal parameters such as low count and motility; and samples from men who require sperm cryopreservation prior to chemotherapy treatment for malignant disease frequently show very poor cryosurvival rates. The now routine introduction of ICSI into IVF practice has overcome this problem, so that successful fertilization using ICSI is possible even with extremely poor cryosurvival of suboptimal samples.

Sample preparation

Samples should be prepared and frozen within 1–2 hours of ejaculation.

1. Perform semen analysis according to standard laboratory technique, and

label two plastic conical tubes and an appropriate number of 0.5 ml freezing straws or ampoules for each specimen. Record all details on appropriate record sheets.
2. Add small aliquots of cryoprotectant medium (CPM) to the semen at room temperature over a period of 2 minutes, to a ratio of 1:1.
   If the ejaculated volume is greater than 5 ml, divide the sample into two aliquots before mixing with CPM.
3. Aliquot the diluted sample into straws or ampoules, labelling aliquots for assessment of post-thaw count and motility.
4. Dilute specimens with CPM according to count.

60 million/ml	dilute 1:1 semen:/CPM
20–60 million/ml	dilute 2:1 semen:/CPM
20 million/ml	dilute 4:1 semen:/CPM

5. Reassess the number of motile sperm/ml, which should ideally be 10 million or above.
6. Aliquot into prelabelled straws.

Manual freezing

1. Place the ampoules or straws (in goblets) on a metal cane.
2. Refrigerate at 4 °C for 15 minutes.
3. Place into liquid nitrogen vapour for 25 minutes.
4. Plunge into liquid nitrogen for storage, and record storage details.

Kryo-10 semen freezing programme

1. Start temperature 24 °C (room temperature).
2. Cooling: -2 °C per minute to 0 °C
   -10.0 °C. per minute to -100 °C.
4. HOLD: 10 minutes (total programme time = 37 minutes)
5. Transfer to liquid nitrogen flask for temporary storage before placing in liquid phase of cryostorage tank.
6. Record all storage details appropriately.
7. Assess post-thaw motility: thaw straws at 34 °C. Wipe the outside to remove debris and condensation, snip both ends with scissors, discard one or two drops of the sample and assess the sample for count and motility.
   %Crysosurvival = (post-thaw motility/pre-freeze motility) × 100

Insemination

Intracervical: after thawing, aspirate the semen with a 2 ml syringe and a Kwill five-inch filling tube. Insemination should be carried out immediately, as frozen-thawed sperm do not remain active for as long as fresh sperm.

Intrauterine: process the thawed sample on a discontinuous density gradient, wash, and resuspend in 0.5–1 ml of culture medium before loading into the appropriate catheter for insemination.

Cryoprotective medium (CPM)

Primary stock solutions

1. Sodium Citrate ($Na_3(C_6H_5O)2H_2O$) 0.1 N
    Primary buffer (PB)
    Dissolve 8.82 g sodium citrate in 300 ml distilled water.
2. Glucose ($C_6H_2O_6$) 0.33 M
    Primary glucose (PG)
    Dissolve 5.46 g glucose in 100 ml distilled water.
3. Fructose ($C_6H_{12}O_6$) 0.33 M
    Primary fructose (PF)
    Dissolve 5.4 g fructose in 100 ml distilled water.

Filter through a 0.22 µm Millipore filter and store in sterile containers at 4 °C.

Secondary buffer (KSB)

KSB buffer is used in the final preparation of CPM and has a 1 month storage life at +5 °C.

It is composed of 3 parts PB:1 part PG:1 part PF, i.e. 300 ml PB:100 ml PG:100 ml PF.
Mix thoroughly.

Storage

Aliquots of KSB can be frozen with glycerol added:
    13ml KSB +3ml glycerol.
Store in sterile containers (e.g. 50 ml Falcon flasks) at − 20 °C.

Final CPM preparation

KSB	13 ml	65% by volume
Glycerol	3 ml	15% by volume
Egg yolk	4 ml	20% by volume

1. Thaw frozen KSB/glycerol mixture.
2. Obtain the yolk from a fresh free-range egg and separate it from the white by carefully rolling the isolated yolk on filter paper.
   Using a sterile disposable syringe and needle, withdraw the required volume from the yolk sac.
   It is important to ensure that the aliquot of egg yolk is free of egg white albumin.
3. Add egg yolk to KSB and glycerol and mix thoroughly.
4. Heat inactivate at $56\,°C$ for 30 minutes and then cool.
5. Add glycine: 200 mg/20 ml CPM.
6. Adjust pH of CPM to pH 7.2–3 using 0.1 M NaOH or 1.3% $NaHCO_3$ solution.
7. CPM can be stored at $4\,°C$ for 10 days.

Freezing of testicular and epididymal samples

Whereas the relatively poor survival rates (50%) obtained after freeze–thawing sperm samples have not in the past presented a major problem due to the abundance of cells in the original specimens, the current use of suboptimal ejaculate, epididymal and testicular samples in combination with ICSI now demands a different approach in order to recover as many sperm cells as possible from each sample. Sample cryopreservation in cases of epididymal and testicular aspiration or biopsy has considerable advantages both to the patient and to the clinical and laboratory staff, in that sperm and oocyte retrieval procedures may be carried out on separate occasions; this strategy is now a successful routine in the majority of ART programmes offering this form of treatment. Generally epididymal and testicular samples are cryopreserved using protocols developed for ejaculated sperm: this may not be optimal. Many changes to the membranes of sperm occur during maturation, and it is likely that the water permeability of testicular sperm, a major factor in determining the cellular response to freezing, is very different from that of ejaculated sperm.

In a recent experimental approach to sperm cell cryobiology, it has been demonstrated that the standard linear cooling rates previously applied are not necessarily the best approach, as recovery of sperm is determined by the manner in which the cells encounter physical gradients. A new type of cell freezer has been developed which controls the physical parameters of solidification to take into account what the cell actually encounters and responds to. Clinical results of this new approach to sperm cryopreservation are awaited.

In cases where prolonged washing and searching yield only very few sperm, sperm can be frozen individually or in small groups by injecting them into empty zona pellucida 'shells', using a crude freezing solution with 8% glycerol in PBI supplemented with 3% HSA. Samples are recovered after washing the zonae through droplets, and more than 70% of sperm survive using this procedure with resulting successful pregnancy rates (Walmsley et al. 1999).

The criteria for sperm freezing have now changed, in that even the most inadequate samples can be frozen/thawed for successful ICSI. It is no longer necessary to do TESA/MESA on the same day as the oocyte retrieval – numerous groups report success with frozen/thawed testicular and epididymal samples. All biopsy samples can be successfully frozen.

The use of cryopreservation buffers without egg yolk is recommended for testicular and epididymal samples:

For 1 litre of medium

Water for cell culture	830 ml
Sodium chloride NaCl	5.8 g
Potasssium chloride KCl	0.4 g
Calcium lactate	0.76 g
Magnesium sulphate $MgSO_4.7H_2O$	0.12 g
Sodium dihydrogen orthophosphate $NaH_2PO_4.2H_2O$	0.05 g
Sodium bicarbonate $NaHCO_3$	2.6 g
HEPES	4.77 g
Glucose	8.59 g
Fructose	8.59 g
Glycine	10.0 g
Penicillin	50 KIU
Streptomycin	50 mg
Human serum albumin (immuno 20% solution)	20 ml
Glycerol	150 ml

Method

- Dissolve all the chemicals in the water with gentle shaking, then add the serum albumin. Add glycerol and mix thoroughly.
- Filter through 0.22 μm Millipore filter into sterile flasks or tubes, and store in aliquots at $-20\,°C$.

Sample processing

Freezing whole biopsy samples without prior processing is not recommended, as cryoprotectant solution will not equilibrate evenly throughout the tissue. Pieces of macerated tissue can however be frozen with some success. It has also been reported that a higher proportion of testicular sperm retain their motility on thawing if they have been incubated 24–48 hours before freezing, and Van den Berg (1998) suggests that incubation at 32 °C may be beneficial. If there is doubt about sperm viability after thawing, a simple HOS test will identify viable sperm before injection.

Cryopreservation of semen for cancer patients

Patients who are to be treated with combined chemotherapy for various types of cancer, such as Hodgkin's disease and testicular tumours, are frequently young or even adolescent. Recent progress in oncology has given these patients a greatly improved prognosis for successful recovery, and cryopreservation of spermatozoa before treatment is begun can preserve fertility for the majority of patients.

All treatment regimes are toxic to spermatogenesis, and the majority of patients will be azoospermic after 7 to 8 weeks of treatment. In some cases spermatogenesis is restored after some years, but in others there is minimal recovery even after a decade.

Animal studies have indicated that spermatogenesis may be protected from the adverse effects of chemotherapy by inhibiting pituitary control of spermatogenesis with GnRH agonists, androgens or male contraceptive regimens. Similar protective regimens in humans are currently ineffective, and the strategy is still under trial.

Currently, there are no pretreatment parameters which can predict a patient's prognosis for recovery of fertility; the possibility of erectile dysfunction after treatment should also be borne in mind. Patients should be given general advice about the need for contraception when recovery is unpredictable, and advised to seek medical help early if fertility is required. Informed consent forms should be signed after discussion and counselling.

Ideally, three sperm samples are collected before chemotherapy is initiated; animal studies suggest that chemotherapy may have a mutagenic effect on late-stage germinal cells, but, in the absence of a known clinical significance in humans, on balance, sample collection after the start of treatment is preferable to no storage at all. Patients should, of course, receive appropriate counselling in such cases. Spermatogenesis is often already impaired due to the effects of the disease: many demonstrate hypothalamic dysfunction, and in severe cases pituitary gonadotropin secretion is altered. The tremendous stress caused by cancer reduces fertility potential by the action of stress hormones in the brain, leading to altered catecholamine secretion, rise in prolactin and corticotrophin-releasing factor, which in turn suppress the release of GnRH. However, in the light of the dramatic success of ICSI treatment, semen samples should be frozen regardless of their quality. Prior to sample collection for storage, patients should be screened for Hepatitis and HIV viruses.

Patients are naturally concerned that their cancer treatment might cause an increased risk of congenital malformation in a subsequent pregnancy: the results of studies to date are reassuring, although we have not yet accumulated enough data for each cancer or treatment regimen. There are now several published reports of successful treatment for couples using sperm stored prior to treatment; type of treatment depends upon the quality of the sample, but pregnancies and live births are reported after AI, IUI, IVF and ICSI.

In the future, autotransplantation of cryopreserved testicular tissue may become an alternative option for young men who are not yet producing sperm, or who are unable to produce an ejaculate. This strategy has already been employed at the Christie Hospital in Manchester, where testicular tissue from 11 patients has been frozen prior to chemotherapy for Hodgkin's disease. Histological assessment revealed normal spermatogenesis in 9 cases and varying degrees of degenerative/atrophic changes in 2 cases. So far, 7 men have completed chemotherapy, and reinjection of thawed testicular cells into the seminiferous tubules is planned in due course. Recent research has shown that gonocytes from immature mice injected into the tubules of sterilized hosts restore spermatogenesis and produce fertile spermatozoa – hopefully, this strategy may provide another option for cancer patients, especially for children.

Further reading

Al-Hasani, S., Ludwig, M., Diedrich, K., Bauer, O., Kipker, W., Diedrich, Ch., Sturm, R. & Yilmaz, A. (1996) Preliminary results on the incidence of polyploidy in cryopreserved human oocytes after ICSI. *Human Reproduction* **11**:Abstract book 1, 50–1.

Ashwood-Smith, M.J. (1986) The cryopreservation of human embryos. *Human Reproduction* **1**:319–32.

Avery, S.M., Spillane, S., Marcus, S., Macnamee, M. & Brinsden, P. (1995) Factors affecting the outcome of frozen embryo replacement – experience of 1009 cycles. Presented at 15th World Congress on Fertility and Sterility, Montpelier. Abstract no. S6/0C.023.

Cohen, J., Devane, G.W., Elsner, C.W., Fehilly, C.B., Kort, H.I., Massey, J.B. & Turner, T.G. (1988) Cryopreservation of zygotes and early cleaved human embryos. *Fertility and Sterility* **49**:2.

Cohen, J., Simons, R.F., Edwards, R.G., Fehilly, C.B. & Fishel, S.B. (1985) Pregnancies following the frozen storage of expanding human blastocysts. *Journal of In Vitro Fertilization and Embryo Transfer* **2**: 59–64.

ESHRE Capri workshop group (1998) Male infertility update. *Human Reproduction* **13**:2025–32.

Fabbri, R., Porcu, E., Marsella, T., Primavera, M.R., Fabbro, L., Ciotti, P.M., Magrini, O., Venturoli, S. & Flamigni, C. (1998) Oocyte cryopreservation. *Human Reproduction* **13 Suppl.** **4**:109–16.

Fehilly, C.B., Cohen, J., Simons, R.F., Fishel, S.B. & Edwards, R.G. (1985) Cryopreservation of cleaving embryos and expanded blastocysts in the human: a comparative study. *Fertility and Sterility* **44**:638–44.

Gook, D.A. (1996) Oocyte time-travel … can eggs arrive safely? *Alpha Newsletter*, vol. 6, June 1996.

Gook, D.A., Osborn, S.M., Bourne, H. & Johnston, W.I.H. (1994) Fertilization of human oocytes following cryopreservation: normal karyotypes and absence of stray chromosomes. *Human Reduction* **9**:684–91.

Gook, D.A., Osborn, S.M. & Johnston, W.I.H. (1993) Cryopreservation of mouse and human oocytes using 1,2-propanediol and the configuration of the meiotic spindle. *Human Reproduction* **8**:1101–9.

Gook, D.A., Osborn, S.M. & Johnston, W.I.H. (1995a) Parthenogenetic activation of human oocytes following cryopreservation using 1,2-propanediol. *Human Reproduction* **10**:654–8.

Gook, D.A., Schiewe, M.C., Osborn, S.M., Asch, R.H., Jansen, R.P.S. & Johnston, W.I.H. (1995b) Intracytoplasmic sperm injection and embryo development of human oocytes cryopreserved using 1,2-propanediol. *Human Reproduction* **10**:2637–41.

Gosden, R.G., Oktay, K., Radford, J.A. et al. (1997) Ovarian tissue banking. *Human Reproduction Update* **3**, CD-ROM, item 1, video.

Hammerstedt, R.H., Graham, J.K. & Nolan, J.P. (1990) Cryopreservation of human sperm. *Journal of Andrology* **11(1)**:73–88.

Hartshorne, G.M., Elder, K., Crow, J., Dyson, H. & Edwards, R.G. (1991) The influence of in vitro development upon post-thaw survival and implantation of cryopreserved human blastocycts. *Human Reproduction* **6**:136–41.

Hartshorne, G.M., Wick, K., Elder, K. & Dyson, H. (1990) Effect of cell number at freezing upon survival and viability of cleaving embryos generated from stimulated IVF cycles. *Human Reproduction* **5**:857–61.

Lassalle, B., Testart, J., Renard, J.P. (1985) Human embryo features that influence the success of cryopreservation with the use of 1, 2, propanediol. *Fertility and Sterility* **44**:645–51.

Lutjen, P., Trouson, A., Leeton, J., Findlay, J., Wood, C. & Renou, P. (1984) The establishment and the maintenance of pregnancy using in vitro fertilization and embryo donation in a patient with primary ovarian failure. *Nature* **307**:174.

McLaughlin, E.A., Ford, W.C.L. & Hill, M.G.R. (1990) A comparison of the freezing of human semen in the uncirculated vapour above liquid nitrogen and in a commercial semi-programmable freezer. *Human Reproduction* **5**:734–8.

Mahadevan, M. & Trounson, A. (1983) Effects of CPM and dilution methods on the preservation of human spermatozoa. *Andrologia* **15**:355–66.

Mazur, P. (1970) Cryobiology: the freezing of living systems. *Science* **168**:93–4.

Mazur, P. (1984) Freezing of living cells: mechanisms and implications. *American Journal of Physiology* **247**:125–42.

Meirow, D. & Schenker, J.G. (1995) Cancer and male infertility. *Human Reproduction* **10**:2017–2022.

Morris, G.J., Acton, E. & Avery S. (1999) A new approach to sperm cryopreservation. *Human Reproduction* **14**:1013–21.

Newton, H., Aubard, Y., Rutherford, A; Sharma, V. & Gosden, R.G. (1996) Low temperature storage and grafting of human ovarian tissue. *Human Reproduction* **11**:487–91.

Nugent, D., Meirow,.D., Brook, P.F., Aubard, Y. & Gosden, R.G. (1997) Transplantation in reproductive medicine: previous experience, present knowledge, and future prospects. *Human Reproduction Update* **3**:267–80.

Nugent, D., Newton, H., Gosden, R.G. & Rutherford, A.J. (1998) Investigation of follicle survival after human heterotopic grafting. *Human Reproduction* **13(1)**:22–3.

Oktay, K., Nugent, D. & Newton, H. (1997) Isolation and characterisation of primordial follicles from fresh and cryopreserved human ovarian tissue. *Fertility and Sterility* **67**:481–6.

Oktay, K., Newton, H., Aubard, Y., Salha, O. & Gosden, R.G. (1998) Cryptopreservation of immature human oocytes and ovarian tissue: an emerging technology? *Fertility and Sterility* **69**:1–7.

Pickering, S.J., Braude, P.R., Johnson, M.H., Cant, A. & Currie, J. (1990) Transient cooling to room temperature can cause irreversible disruption of the meiotic spindle in the human oocyte. *Fertility and Sterility* **54**:102–8.

Porcu, E., Fabbri, R., Seracchioli, R., Ciotti, P.M., Magrini, O. & Flamigni, C. (1997) Birth of a healthy female after intracytoplasmic sperm injection of cryopreserved human oocytes. *Fertility and Sterility* **68**:724–6.

Ragni, G. & Vegetti, W. (1995) Cryopreservation of Semen. In: (Hedon, B., Bringer, J. & Mares, P. eds.), *Fertility and Sterility: a Current Overview*. The Parthenon Publishing Group, UK.

Salat-Baroux, J., Cornet, D., Alvarez, S., Antoine, J.M., Tibi, C., Mandelbaum, J. & Plachot, M. (1988) Pregnancies after replacement of frozen-thawed embryos in a donation program. *Fertility and Sterility* **49**:817–21.

Sathanandan, M., Macnamee, M.C., Wick, K. & Matthews, C.D. (1991) Clinical aspects of human embryo cryopreservation. In: (Brinsden, P. & Rainsbury, P. eds.), *A Textbook of In Vitro Fertilization and Assisted Reproduction*. The Parthenon Publishing Group, UK.

Schmidt, C.L., Taney, F.H., de Ziegler, D., Kuhar, M.J., Gagliardi, C.L., Colon, J.M., Mellon, R.W. & Weiss, G. (1989) Transfer of cryopreserved-thawed embryos: the natural cycle versus controlled preparation of the endometrium with gonadotropin-releasing hormone agonist and exogenous estradiol and progesterone (GEEP). *Fertility and Sterility* **52**:1609–16.

Shaw, J., Diotavelli, L. & Trounson, A. (1991) A simple rapid dimethylsulfoxide freezing technique for the cryopreservation of one-cell to blastocyst stage premplantation mouse embryos. *Reproduction, Fertility and Development* **3**:621–6.

Smith, A.U. (1952) Behaviour of fertilized rabbit eggs exposed to glycerol and to low temperatures. *Nature* **170**:373.

Stachecki, J.J., Cohen J. & Willadsen, S.M. (1999) Cryopreservation of mouse oocytes: The effect of replacing sodium with choline in the freezing medium. *Cryobiology* **37**:346–54.

Testart, J., Belaisch Allart, J., Lassalle, B., Hazout, A., Foreman, R., Rainhorn, J-D., Gazengel, A. & Frydman, R. (1987) Factors influencing the success rate of human embryo freezing in an in vitro fertilization and embryo transfer program. *Fertility and Sterility* **48**:107–12.

Trounson, A. & Mohr, L. (1983) Human pregnancy following cryopreservation, thawing, and transfer of an eight-cell embryo. *Nature* **305**:707–9.

Van den Berg, M. (1998) In: (Elder, K. & Elliott, T. eds.), *The Use of Epididymal and Testicular Sperm in IVF*. World Wide Conferences on Reproduction Biology, Ladybrook Publishing, Australia.

Walmsley, R., Cohen, J., Ferrara-Congedo, T., Reing, A. & Garrisi, J. (1999) The first births and ongoing pregnancies associated with sperm cryopreservation within evacuated egg zonae. *Human Reproduction* **13**:61–70.

Watson P.F. & Morris, G.J. (1987) Cold shock injury in animal cells. In: (Bowler, P. & Fuller, J. eds.), *Temperature and Animal Cells.* Symposia of the Society for Experimental Biology no. 41, Company of Biologists, Cambridge, UK.

Whittingham, D.G. (1977) Some factors affecting embryo storage in laboratory animals. In: *The Freezing of Mammamilian Embryos, Ciba Foundation Symposium* **52**:97–108.

Whittingham, D.G., Leibo, S.P. & Mazur, P. (1972) Survival of mouse embryos frozen to $-196\,°C$ and $-269\,°C$. *Science* **178**:411–14.

11

Micromanipulation techniques

Introduction

Micromanipulation of cells dates from the turn of the last century when biologists and physiologists used a variety of manipulator systems to dissect or record from cells. Experiments in which sperm were injected into eggs around the mid-1960s were primarily designed to investigate the early events of fertilization, i.e. the role of membrane fusion, activation of the oocyte and the formation of the pronuclei. Two series of early experiments by independent groups demonstrated major species differences. Hiramoto showed in the 1960s that microinjection of spermatozoa into unfertilized sea urchin oocytes did not induce activation of the oocyte or condensation of the sperm nucleus, whereas others demonstrated the opposite in frog oocytes. Ryuzo Yanagimachi and his group later demonstrated that isolated hamster nuclei could develop into pronuclei after microinjection into homologous eggs, and a similar result was obtained when freeze-dried human spermatozoa were injected into a hamster egg. These experiments indicated that, during activation of mammalian oocytes, membrane fusion events may be bypassed without compromising the initiation of development. The experiments not only provided information on the mechanism of fertilization, but also led to a new technique in clinical embryology.

The first clinical application of microinsemination techniques was partial zona dissection (PZD) developed by Jacques Cohen and colleagues to aid fertilization in human oocytes (Figure 11.1). This mechanical technique involves breaching a slit in the zona pellucida with a sharp glass micropipette and subsequently placing the dissected oocyte into a suspension of spermatozoa, on the assumption that sperm entry is facilitated by the slit. In the same year, S.C. NG and colleagues in Singapore reported the first pregnancy from subzonal sperm injection (SUZI), where several spermatozoa are inserted into

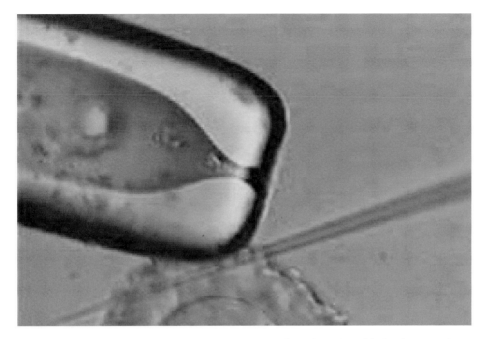

Figure 11.1   The last stages of partial zona dissection where friction between the inserted needle and the holding pipette results in a slit in the zona pellucida.

the perivitelline space (Figure 11.2). In 1990, the same group reported activation of human oocytes following intracytoplasmic injection of human spermatozoa, and in 1992 Palermo and colleagues in Brussels reported the first pregnancies from this technique of ICSI. Since the time of these pioneering reports, many thousands of healthy and normal ICSI babies have been born world-wide (Figure 11.3).

Jacques Cohen and colleagues developed a second micromanipulation technique that has proved to be useful in improving the outcome of ART in humans in 1990. They demonstrated that assisted hatching (AH), cutting a slit in the zona pellucida or dissolving a hole in the zona with an acid solution, facilitated implantation of the human embryo in selected cases (see later in this chapter).

Intracytoplasmic sperm injection

Patient selection: indications for treatment

Prior to 1992, the majority of cases of severe male factor infertility were virtually untreatable, and failure of fertilization was observed in up to 30% of

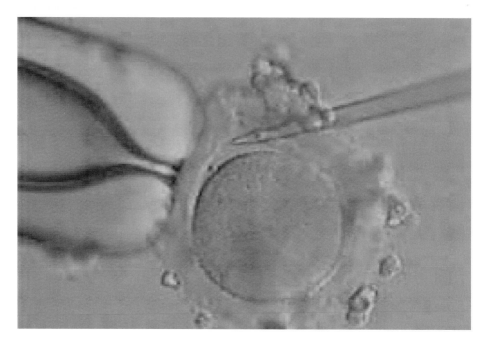

Figure 11.2   Injection of a spermatozoon into the perivitelline space of a human oocyte (SUZI).

in vitro fertilization–embryo transfer (IVF–ET) treatments for male infertility. The introduction of micromanipulation techniques such as zona drilling (ZD), partial zona dissection (PZD) and subzonal sperm injection (SUZI) raised the hopes of a better prognosis for these cases, but did not overall provide a substantial improvement in success rates. The introduction and successful application of intracytoplasmic sperm injection by the team led by Professor Van Steirteghem at The Free University in Brussels, Belgium, has produced a dramatic improvement in the treatment of severe male infertility by assisted reproductive technology.

The establishment of ICSI as a routine technique was quickly followed by the introduction of techniques for collecting sperm samples from the epididymis and directly from the testis, so that it is now possible to treat the whole spectrum of male infertility: from suboptimal ejaculate samples or ejaculatory failure, to obstructive and nonobstructive causes of azoospermia. However, an increasing list of genetic defects have been found to be associated with male infertility: a higher incidence of numerical and structural chromosomal aberrations are found in infertile and subfertile men than in the neonatal population, in particular karyotypes 47XXY, 47XYY, 46XX, 46X,derY, Robertsonian translocations, reciprocal translocations, inversions and additional marker

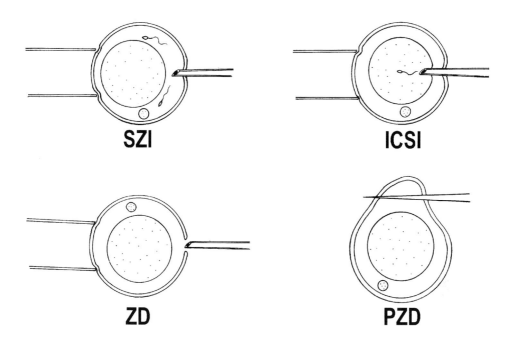

Figure 11.3   Microinsemination techniques include subzonal injection (SZI), intracytoplasmic sperm injection (ICSI), zona drilling (ZD) and partial zona dissection (PZD).

chromosomes. Between 12 and 18% of men with azoospermia or severe oligospermia (less than 300 000 sperm in the ejaculate) have deletions in intervals 5 and 6 on the long arm of the Y chromosome. Microdeletions of the q11 region of the Y chromosome are related to the dysfunction of Deleted in Azoospermia (DAZ) and RNA-Binding Motif (RBM) genes, and Androgen Receptor gene mutations have also been reported in infertile men. In a population of approximately 3000 infertile men, the pathological (nonpolymorphic, phenotype associated) microdeletions rate in at least 1 of 4 critical regions on the Y chromosome was found to be as high as 22%, with an additional (as yet unknown) percentage being attributed to cryptic mosaicism. Furthermore, it appears that microdeletions will be transmitted in at least 10% of unselected father/son pairs. Three to ten per cent of infertile men present with Congenital Bilateral Absence of the Vas Deferens (CBAVD), and approximately 65% of these individuals carry Cystic Fibrosis, with defects in the Cystic Fibrosis Conductance Regulator (CFTR) gene. Many are compound heterozygous for the CFTR mutation, with an increased risk of having children with CF or CBVAD.

Although the genetic risk for couples who require ICSI treatment has yet to be fully defined, karyotyping, and preferably also Y-microdeletion analysis is recommended as part of the pretreatment screening process for all men referred for ICSI. The couple should also have access to professional genetic counselling to discuss potential risks, and appropriate informed consent must be obtained before treatment.

In cases of obstructive azoospermia, samples can be aspirated from the epididymis. The 'open' microsurgical technique of microepididymal sperm aspiration (MESA) has now been largely superseded by the simpler procedure of percutaneous epididymal sperm aspiration (PESA), which can be carried out by fertility specialists without microsurgical skills, and can be performed under local anaesthetic or mild sedation as an out-patient procedure. Aspiration is carried out using a 25 g butterfly needle connected to a syringe. If no sperm can be aspirated from the epididymis, a modification of the technique using wide-bore needle aspiration of the testis (TESA or TEFNA) often harvests sufficient testicular spermatozoa to carry out an ICSI procedure.

In nonobstructive azoospermia, spermatogenesis is impaired. The epididymis is devoid of sperm, but the testis usually contains focal areas of spermatogenesis. Multiple biopsies may be required in order to identify these areas. The focal nature of spermatogenesis in such patients makes diagnosis based upon a single biopsy unrealistic, but prepared testicular samples can also be cryopreserved for a future ICSI procedure at the time of diagnostic testicular biopsy.

Immature sperm cells can be identified not only from testicular biopsies, but also occasionally from ejaculates of men with nonobstructive azoospermia. Fertilization and pregnancies can be achieved by microinjection of spermatids in the elongating phase of maturation; although fertilization, pregnancies and live births have been reported following injection of round spermatids, the results are disappointingly low, probably influenced not only by technical features, but also by the pathology involved. More intensive research is required to improve the selection and handling of these cells, and to ascertain the genomic imprinting and gene expression required for the development of viable embryos. When using immature cells for in vitro conception, careful patient screening, genetic counselling and follow-up of pregnancies and babies are mandatory.

Testicular biopsy is carried out either by multiple needle aspirations (TEFNA or TESA) or by open biopsy (TESE), and both procedures may be safely carried out with local anaesthetic/mild sedation.

The ICSI (intracytoplasmic sperm injection) procedure involves the injection of a single sperm cell directly into an oocyte, and it therefore can be used not only for cases in which there are extremely low numbers of sperm, but in bypassing gamete interaction at the level of the zona pellucida and the vitelline membrane; it can also be used in the treatment of qualitative or functional sperm disorders.

1. Couples who have suffered recurrent failure of fertilization after IVF–ET may have one or more disorders of gamete dysfunction in which there is a barrier to fertilization at the level of the acrosome reaction, zona pellucida binding or interaction, zona penetration, or fusion with the oolemma. ICSI is always indicated for patients who have unexplained failure of fertilization in two or more IVF–ET cycles.

2. Severe oligospermia can be treated with ICSI; if as many normal vital sperm can be recovered as there are oocytes to be inseminated, fertilization can be achieved in approximately 90% of these patients. In extreme cases of crypto-zoospermia, where no sperm cells can be seen by standard microscopy, centrifugation of the neat sample at a higher than usual centrifugal force (1800 g, 5 minutes) may result in the recovery of an adequate number of sperm cells.

3. Severe asthenozoospermia, including patients with sperm ultrastructural abnormalities such as Kartagener's syndrome, or '9 + 0' axoneme disorders can be treated by ICSI.

4. Teratozoospermia, including absolute teratozoospermia or globozoospermia.

5. In cases of congenital absence of the vas deferens, vasectomy or postinflammatory obstruction of the vas, sperm samples can be retrieved by percutaneous epididymal sperm aspiration (PESA), testicular sperm aspiration (TESA) or testicular biopsy (TESE).

6. Samples can be recovered by needle or open biopsy of the testis in cases of nonobstructive azoospermia.

7. With ejaculatory dysfunction, such as retrograde ejaculation – a sufficient number of sperm cells can usually be recovered from the urine.

8. Paraplegic males have been given the chance of biological fatherhood using electroejaculation and IVF; they may also be successfully treated using a combination of TESE and ICSI.

9. Immunological factors – couples in whom there may be antisperm antibodies in female sera/follicular fluid, or antisperm antibodies in seminal plasma following vasectomy reversal or genital tract infection can be successfully treated by ICSI.

10. Oncology – male patients starting chemotherapy or radiotherapy should have semen samples frozen for use in the future. Although the sperm quality of the frozen-thawed sperm may be grossly impaired. ICSI offers the patient an excellent chance of eventually achieving fertilization. Testicular biopsy speci-

mens may also be cryopreserved for these patients as a further backup when the quality of the ejaculate is inadequate for freezing.

11. For preimplantation genetic diagnosis where PCR is used, ICSI should be used as the means of fertilization to prevent sperm contamination of the sample.

Analysis of overall pregnancy rates achieved after gamete intrafallopian transfer (GIFT), standard IVF and ICSI in the treatment of male factor infertility suggests the following indications for treatment, based upon parameters of semen assessment:

	ICSI	*Standard IVF*
Total sperm count	$< 1 \times 10^6$ per ml	$> 5 \times 10^6$ per ml
Motility	$< 20\%$	$> 30\%$
Progression	< 1	> 2
Motile concentration	$< 100\,000$ per ml	$> 5 \times 10^6$ per ml
Normal Motile Conc.	$< 100\,000$ per ml	$> 5 \times 10^6$ per ml

A consensus suggests that cases with the following semen parameters should have either a trial of standard IVF first, or treatment in which the eggs are divided 50:50 for IVF and ICSI.

Total sperm count	Between 1 and 5×10^6
Motility	20–30%
Progression	1.5–2.0
Motile concentration	100 000 to 5×10^6
Normal motile concentration	100 000 to 5×10^6

ICSI now has a confirmed place not only in the treatment of male factor infertility, but also in cases of idiopathic infertility where the barrier to fertilization may include factors in the female partner which affect or involve the oocyte. To date, published fertilization rates for most categories of patients reach 67%, with a clinical pregnancy rate of 36% and an ongoing/delivery rate of 28%.

Practical aspects

When scheduling patients for ICSI, unless the laboratory is fortunate in having a scientist dedicated entirely to carrying out each ICSI procedure, it is important that the whole IVF team should appreciate the extra dimension of time and effort which every case involves, and make an effort to schedule the entire laboratory workload accordingly. ICSI requires the same meticulous attention to detail required in all IVF manipulations, but the number of details requiring attention is dramatically increased. Successful results with ICSI can only be achieved with the dedication of concentrated time, effort and patience.

Important considerations regarding the location of micromanipulation facilities

The laboratory should be on a ground floor, near a structural frame or wall to minimize vibration interference, and must be kept dust-free. The equipment must be installed on a substantial bench top, away from traffic of people or trolleys, etc. Any vibration will seriously interfere with the injection procedure, and it is essential to make sure that the equipment is completely stable, using anti-vibration material if necessary. Subdued lighting is helpful for microscopy. Well in advance of any ICSI procedure, ensure that the microscope is set up optically and checked. Check that the tool holders and all other parts of the micromanipulation system are correctly fitted and adjusted for optimal range of movement, and that the microtools can be accurately aligned.

Microtools

Two types of microtools are used: the holding pipette (a blunt-ended tube with constricted lumen) which is used to hold and immobilize the oocyte, and the injection pipette which will be used to aspirate and inject the sperm cell. Holding pipettes have an outer diameter of 0.080 to 0.150 mm and an inner diameter of 0.018 to 0.025 mm; injection pipettes have outer diameters of 0.0068 to 0.0078 mm and inner diameters of 0.0048 to 0.0056 mm. Both types of microtool are bent to an angle of approximately 30° at the distal end in order to facilitate horizontal positioning and manipulation adjustment within culture dishes. Aspiration pipettes (of different diameters) may also be used to aspirate anucleate fragments, or for blastomere biopsy for preimplantation diagnosis. A third type of microtool may be used for piercing or cutting the zona pellucida in assisted zona hatching techniques or partial zona drilling.

Specifically tooled, sterile, ready-to-use holding and injection pipettes are now commercially available. For groups who are initiating an ICSI programme, ready-made pipettes provide a means of bypassing significant capital expenditure in obtaining equipment for their manufacture, and overcoming the hurdle of dedicating personnel and time to acquire the expertise involved in making them proficiently. However, the design and manufacture of the microtools is extremely important, and uniform microtool quality is crucial for consistent results. A blunt injection pipette can damage the oocyte by compression, whereas a pipette with too large a diameter will result in the injection of an excessive amount of fluid with resulting damage.

Materials

1. A viscous solution of 10% Polyvinyl pyrrolidine (PVP) is used to impair sperm motility prior to immobilization and aspiration into the injection pipette. Experienced operators can carry out the procedure without the use of PVP, but it is helpful in the initial stages of learning and practice. Although questions have been raised about the wisdom/safety of injecting this artificial agent directly into ooplasm, no adverse effects have as yet been reported.
2. Hyaluronidase is used to enzymatically disperse cells of the cumulus and corona, prior to their removal from the oocyte by dissection. Preparations in current use are of animal (sheep or bovine) origin; an enzyme of plant origin has recently become available.
3. Equilibrated mineral oil.
4. HEPES-buffered culture medium.
5. Shallow Falcon dish (type 1006), or the lid of a standard 60 mm Petri dish.

Companies that supply culture medium now also provide ICSI 'kits', with ready-to-use PVP and Hyalase solutions, as well as equilibrated mineral oil.

PVP preparation

Dissolve 1 g PVP-K90 (molecular weight 360 000 ICN Flow) in 10 ml culture grade water.

   Dialyse the solution at 4 °C versus culture grade water for 2 days, changing the water seven times each day.

   Dialysis tubing = Viskin size 9–36/32″ (Medicell International Ltd, London, UK).

   Lyophilize the dialysate, and store at room temperature until further use.
PVP (polyvinyl pyrrolidone) stock solution: 1 g lyophilized PVP dissolved in 10 ml HEPES buffered culture medium containing 0.5% human serum albumin. Filter through an 8 μm Millipore filter, and store at 4 °C for a maximum of 3 weeks.

Oocyte preparation and handling

Patients for ICSI have a scheduled oocyte retrieval after programmed superovulation, according to protocols described previously (see Preparation for oocyte retrieval, chapter 9).

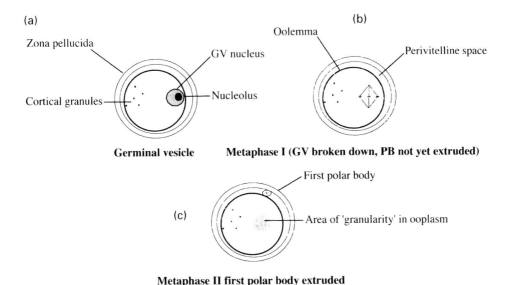

Germinal vesicle   **Metaphase I (GV broken down, PB not yet extruded)**

Metaphase II first polar body extruded

Figure 11.4   Variations in egg maturity found after hyalase treatment and corona dissection. (a) Germinal vesicle; (b) metaphase I; (c) metaphase II.

Oocyte identification is carried out immediately after follicle aspiration, using a dissecting microscope with heated stage. Take care to maintain stable temperature and pH of the aspirates at all times. At the end of the oocyte retrieval, note quality and maturity assessment of the oocytes, and then pre-incubate them for approximately 2–3 hours at 37 °C in an atmosphere of 5% CO_2 in air.

Preparation for injection: cumulus–corona removal

1. Hyaluronidase solution, 80 IU/ml: dissolve 1 mg of Hyalase (Type VIII, Sigma, cat. no. H3757) in 4 ml protein-free Earle's balanced salt solution (EBS), filter, and warm to 37 °C. Prepare the hyaluronidase solution fresh daily, at least 1 hour before use.
2. Prepare a culture dish containing one drop of hyalase solution and 5 wash drops of culture medium, covered with an overlay of equilibrated mineral oil (denudation may also be carried out in Nunc 4-well dishes). Incubate at 37 °C in the CO_2 incubator for 30–60 minutes.
3. Prepare a thin glass probe and some hand-drawn and fire-polished Pasteur pipettes, with the lumen ranging down to approximately 200 μm (denudation pipettes are also commercially available).

4. Remove the oocyte and hyalase dishes from the incubator, group the oocytes together in small batches (4–8 eggs per drop) and then wash the groups of oocytes through the hyalase drop, agitating gently until the cells start to dissociate (approximately 1 minute). Carefully aspirate the oocytes, leaving as much cumulus as possible behind. Wash by transferring them through at least 5 drops of culture medium, and change to a fine-bore pipette for aspiration in order to finally remove all of the coronal cells. All corona cells must be removed, as they will hinder the injection process by blocking the needle or obscuring clear observation of the cytoplasm and sperm.

5. Assess the quality and maturity of each oocyte under an inverted microscope. Use the glass probe to roll the oocytes around gently in order to identify the polar body, and examine the ooplasm for vacuoles or other abnormalities. Separate metaphase I or germinal vesicle (GV) oocytes from metaphase II oocytes, and label them.

6. Culture the dissected oocytes for a minimum of 1 hour before beginning micromanipulation.

7. Examine the oocytes again before starting the injection procedure to see if any more have extruded the first polar body. ICSI is carried out on all morphologically intact oocytes which have extruded the first polar body (Figure 11.4).

Preparation for injection

Materials
HEPES-buffered culture medium
10% PVP solution
Equilibrated mineral oil
Shallow Falcon dish (type 1006) or shallow lid of equivalent Petri dish

1. Prepare injection dishes by pipetting small (2–5 µl) droplets of HEPES-buffered culture medium for individual oocytes, a larger droplet for a sample of sperm, and a droplet of PVP for sperm immobilization prior to aspiration. The droplets can be arranged in a circle with sperm/PVP in the center, or in parallel groups, but must be positioned so that they are not too close to the edge of the dish, where manipulation will be difficult. The oocyte droplets should not be too close to the sperm/PVP, in order to avoid mixing – use an arrangement which allows quick and easy distinction between sperm and oocyte droplets, with numbers on the bottom of the dish. Small volumes of media evaporate very quickly, and they should be covered immediately with a layer of oil. Equilibrate the dishes in the incubator for at least 20–30 minutes, and keep them in the incubator until you are ready to begin the procedure.

2. At the same time, prepare and equilibrate another culture dish into which the oocytes will be transferred after injection.

Micromanipulator

1. Make sure that the heating stage on the microscope is warm, ensure that all controls can be comfortably operated, and that you are confident that all parts function smoothly before you begin. It is essential to check that you can smoothly carry out very small movements. This involves not only the equipment itself, but its position on the bench in relation to your (comfortable) seating position.
2. Insert holding and injection pipettes into the pipette holders, tighten well and make sure (again) that there are no air bubbles in the tubing system. Bubbles interfere with accuracy when attempting to control movement with fine precision.
3. Align the pipettes so that the working tips are parallel to the microscope stage. First align the holding pipette under low magnification, then again under low magnification align the injection pipette. Check the position of both under high magnification. It is important to begin with pipettes in accurate alignment, with both working tips sharply in focus. If a part of the length is out of focus, the pipette is probably not parallel to the stage, but pointing upwards or downwards.
4. Adjust the injection controls: oil should just reach the distal end of the pipette; do not try to fill the needle with oil, it won't work! Briefly touch the tips of both pipettes in oil, and then in medium, so that the ends fill by capillary action (a drop of oil behind the drop of medium will act as a buffer). The injection dish is still in the incubator, so you should be using a 'blank' dish for this!

Transfer the gametes to the injection dish

1. Carefully add a small aliquot of sperm suspension (0.3–5 μl, depending on the concentration of prepared sperm) to the edge of the central PVP or medium droplet. The viscous solution should facilitate sperm handling by slowing down their motility, and also prevents the sperm cells from sticking to the injection pipette during the procedure. Be careful of sperm density: too many sperm will make sperm selection and immobilization more difficult.
2. After the sperm droplet has been carefully examined for the presence of debris or any other factors that might cause technical difficulties, examine all the denuded oocytes again for the presence of a first polar body; wash them with HEPES-buffered medium and transfer one oocyte into each oocyte droplet on the injection dish.

   Keep the oocytes in the incubator until you are confident that the injection procedure can proceed smoothly. Until sufficient experience of the procedure has been gained, it may be advisable to keep sperm and egg dishes separate, avoiding overexposure of the oocytes while selecting and immobilizing sperm.

3. Place the injection dish with central sperm droplet on the microscope stage. Using the coarse controls of the manipulator, lower the injection pipette into the drop.

Sperm selection and immobilization

1. Try to select sperm which appear morphologically normal.
2. Motile spermatozoa are immobilized by crushing their tails: select the sperm to be aspirated, and lower the tip of the injection needle onto the midpiece of the sperm, striking down and across, and crushing the tail against the bottom of the dish. This 'tail crushing' impairs motility, and destabilizes the cell membrane; the latter may be required for sperm head decondensation. If the resulting sperm has a 'bent' tail, it will be difficult to aspirate into the needle, and will stick inside the needle. When this happens, the sperm may be abandoned and the procedure repeated with another sperm. Do not strike too hard, or the sperm will stick to the bottom of the dish, also making aspiration into the needle difficult. After some practice, sperm immobilization in routine ICSI cases can be carried out quite quickly. If the preparation contains only a few sperm with barely recognizable movement and a large amount of debris, this part of the procedure can be very tedious and require great patience!
3. Aspirate the selected immobilized sperm, tail first, into the injection pipette. Position it approximately 20 μm from the tip (Figure 11.5).
4. Lift the injection needle slightly, and move the microscope stage so that the injection pipette is positioned in the first oocyte drop. If the sperm moves up the pipette (due to the difference in density between culture medium and PVP) bring it back near the tip before beginning the injection procedure.

Injection procedure

1. Lower the holding pipette into the first oocyte droplet, and position it adjacent to the cell. Using both microtools, slowly rotate the oocyte to locate the polar body. Aspirate gently so that the cell attaches to the pipette. The pressure should be great enough to hold the oocyte in place, but not so strong that it causes the oolemma to bulge outwards.

Position the oocyte so that the polar body is at 6 or 12 o'clock, to minimize the possibility of damaging the meiotic spindle.

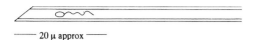

——— 20 μ approx ———

Figure 11.5   Single sperm inside microinjection needle prior to injection.

2. Move the injection pipette close to the oocyte, and check that it is in the same plane as the right outer border of the oolemma on the equatorial plane at the 3 o'clock position. Check that the sperm can be moved smoothly within the injection needle, and position it near the bevelled tip.

3. Advance the pipette through the zona, penetrating ooplasm until the needle tip almost touches the 9 o'clock position. If the pipette is in the wrong plane, entry into the cell will be difficult. The membrane may rupture spontaneously, or may require negative pressure, sucking the membrane into the pipette before expelling the sperm. When it breaks, there will be a sudden flux of cytoplasm into the pipette. Inject the sperm slowly into the oocyte with a minimal amount of fluid (1–2 picolitres).

    The sperm should be ejected past the tip of the pipette, to ensure a tight insertion among the organelles which will hold it in place while the pipette is withdrawn. Some surplus medium may be reaspirated to reduce the size of the breach created during perforation. If the ooplasm is elastic and difficult to break, it may be necessary to withdraw the pipette from the first membrane invagination and slowly repeat the procedure.

4. Gently remove the injection pipette, and examine the breach area. The membrane should be funnel-shaped, pointing in towards the centre. If the border of the oolemma is everted, cytoplasm may leak out, and the egg may subsequently cytolyze. Release the oocyte from the holding pipette.

5. Repeat the sperm aspiration and injection until all the selected metaphase II oocytes have been injected.

6. Wash all the oocytes in culture medium, transfer to the prepared, warmed culture dish, and incubate overnight in the CO_2 incubator.

Injection procedure: important points!!!

1. All conditions must be stable: temperature, pH, equipment properly set up, adjusted, aligned, and checked for leaks and air bubbles. Check everything, including secure and comfortable operating position, before you begin.

2. Correct immobilization of sperm.

3. Advance far enough into the ooplasm with the injection pipette.

4. Ensure that the plasma membrane is broken.

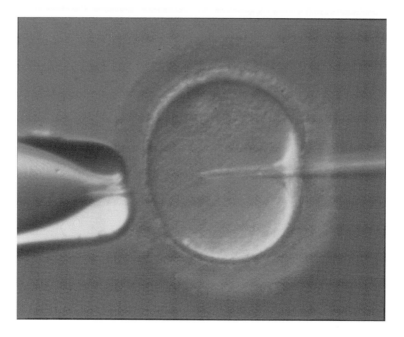

Figure 11.6   Intracytoplasmic sperm injection.

5. Inject a minimal volume.
6. If the sperm comes out of the ooplasm into the perivitelline space, reinject.

Assessment of fertilization and cleavage

Sixteen to 18 hours after injection, assess the number and morphology of pronuclei through an inverted microscope, rolling the oocyte gently with a glass probe. Polar bodies should also be counted, with reference to digynic zygotes or activated eggs; polar bodies may fragment, even in normal mono-spermic fertilization. Rapid cleavage (20–26 hours postinjection) can occur in ICSI zygotes (Figure 11.7).

Evaluate normally fertilized, cleaved embryos after a further 24 hours of culture. Embryo transfer is usually performed approximately 48 hours after microinjection. Suitable supernumerary embryos may be cryopreserved either on Day 1 (pronucleate stage) or on Day 2 (early cleavage stage).

No fertilization after ICSI

Complete failure of fertilization is rare after ICSI; most of these cases involve semen containing no motile sperm, or round-headed sperm. Some cases of

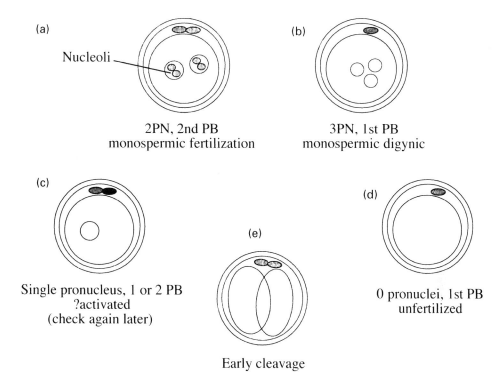

Figure 11.7   Diagrams showing variations of fertilization after ICSI. PN: pronuclei; PB: polar body; (a) 2 pronuclei, 2 polar bodies; (b) 3 pronuclei, 1 polar body; (c) 1 pronucleus, 2 polar bodies; (d) no pronuclei, 1 polar body; (e) early cleavage.

failed fertilization may be attributed to low oocyte number, abnormal morphological appearance, or fragile oocytes which are easily damaged after ICSI. Fertilization rates using epididymal and testicular sperm are equivalent to those of ejaculated sperm, but the use of immature sperm cells results in a dramatic decrease in fertilization and pregnancy rates. Round spermatid (ROS) injection has shown fertilization rates in the region of 17–27%, significantly lower than that following injection of elongated and mature spermatids. A higher proportion of single pronucleate zygotes has been observed after ROS injection (35%) than after injection of elongated forms (17.5%), and the birth of a live healthy baby has been reported after the transfer of embryos derived from single pronucleate zygotes following ROS injection. To date, overall, only 2% of embryos derived from ROS injection implant, and ethical issues surrounding this treatment remain unresolved.

Transport ICSI

In the same manner that a central IVF laboratory can be utilized to offer assisted conception treatment at nearby peripheral hospitals or clinics, a central ICSI laboratory can offer this specialized technique to peripheral hospitals which do not have the equipment or expertise. Preovulatory oocytes and prepared sperm from patients are transported from the peripheral unit by the male partner immediately after the oocyte recovery procedure. Culture tubes containing the gametes are transported in a portable incubator, as described for transport IVF. On arrival at the central unit, the oocytes can be transferred to culture dishes and prepared for the ICSI procedure, and sperm preparation assessed and adjusted if necessary. Fertilized oocytes are cultured to the early cleavage stage, and the embryos may then be transported by the male partner back to the peripheral unit for the embryo transfer procedure. Supernumerary embryos may also be cryopreserved at the central unit if appropriate.

As with transport IVF, co-operation between participating units is particularly important in order to provide an effective service. Well-planned protocols are essential for selection, consultation and counselling of patients, the handling, preparation and transport of gametes, and communication of treatment cycle details/transport arrangements between units.

Assisted hatching

Jacques Cohen postulates that an inability of blastocysts to hatch from the zona pellucida may be one of the factors involved in the high implantation failure rate of human IVF procedures. The human zona becomes more brittle and loses its elasticity after fertilization, and spontaneous hardening also occurs after in vitro and in vivo ageing. It also changes in its sensitivity to low pH (it is easier to create a hole with acid Tyrode's solution in a zygote than in an unfertilized oocyte).

Early observations from videocinematography studies suggested that embryos which show a thick, even zona pellucida on Day 2 had a poor prognosis for implantation. In addition, embryos produced as a result of microsurgical fertilization had a higher implantation rate, and when cultured in vitro hatched one day earlier than expected (Day 5 instead of Day 6). Following these observations, a series of experiments in a mouse embryo system led to the development of a clinical protocol based upon the following results:

1. Large holes are more efficient in supporting hatching than small holes: if the

hole is too small, the embryo can become 'trapped' and fail to hatch. Zona drilling using an acid Tyrode's solution prevented 'trapping' which occurred as a result of mechanical partial zona drilling, and optimal hole size is approximately half the size of a single blastomere: 15–20 μm.

2. Embryos with such large gaps in their zonae should be transferred after the onset of compaction, on Day 3: if embryo transfer is traumatic, blastomeres may escape through the gap in the zona; embryo transfer must therefore be gentle and atraumatic.

3. The artificial gap in the zona may also allow invasion of toxins into the embryo, with immune cell invasion or release of cytotoxins from neighbouring non-invasive immune cells; therefore prophylactic steroid and antibiotic treatment is recommended after embryo transfer.

4. Embryos must be preselected for assisted hatching, based upon previous IVF history (repeated failed implantation), maternal age, basal FSH levels, cleavage rates and morphology of the embryos with attention to zona thickness or variation.

Protocol

The protocol below for assisted hatching by acid drilling of the zona pellucida is adapted from J. Cohen (1992): Zona pellucida micromanipulation and consequences for embryonic development and implantation. In: *Micromanipulation of Human Gametes and Embryos*, chapter 8, J. Cohen, H.F. Malter, B.E. Talansky and J. Grifo, Raven Press, New York.

Embryo transfer after assisted hatching procedures is accompanied by immunosuppressive and antibiotic treatment for the patients two days before, and five days after transfer.

1. Perform zona drilling with acid Tyrode's (AT) solution approximately 72 hours after oocyte retrieval, with embryo transfer 5 to 7 hours later (i.e. drill before the formation of intercellular connections, but transfer after they have been established).

2. Perform the procedure in HEPES-buffered human tubal fluid (HTF) medium with 15% serum.

3. Use a straight microtool with an aperture of 7–8 μm.

4. Use mouth-controlled suction for the zona drilling procedure.

5. Embryos are contained in small microdroplets (25 μl) under mineral oil in a depression slide or shallow Falcon 1006 dish containing one droplet of AT solution and four wash droplets.

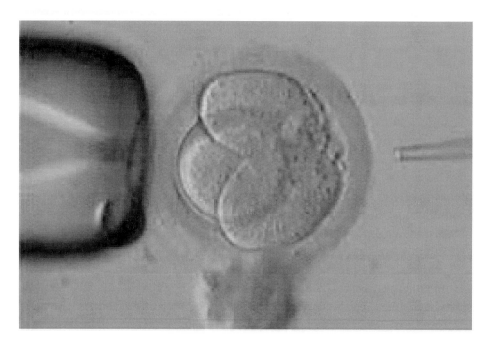

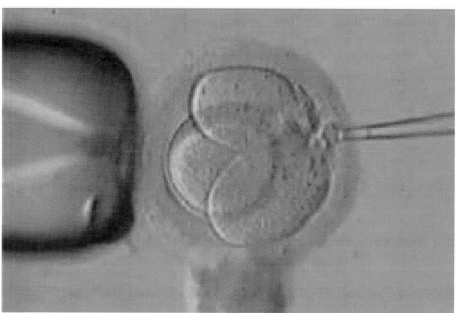

Figure 11.8   In assisted hatching, acid Tyrode's solution is forced under pressure through a blunt micropipette, dissolving a portion of the zona pellucida with a circular motion.

6. Micromanipulate each embryo individually, and immediately wash each, one to four times to remove the acidic medium (Figure 11.8).

Tyrode's solution is acidified by titrating to pH 2.3–2.5 with HCl.

Step-by-step

1. Front load the microneedle before each micromanipulation, using mouth-controlled suction.
2. Clamp the embryo onto the holding pipette (syringe suction system) so that the acidic Tyrode's filled microneedle at the 3 o'clock area is exposed to empty perivitelline space or to extracellular fragments. There should be no more than a 2 second delay from the time the hatching needle enters the drop to the initiation of hatching.
3. Expel acidic medium gently over a small (30 μm) area by holding the needle tip very close to the zona. Small circular motions can avoid excess acid in a single area.
4. The inside of the zona is more difficult to pierce, and the expulsion pressure may need to be increased. The optical system should be optimized for this part of the procedure, as the stream of acid may be relatively invisible, and the piercing of the inside of the zona may be almost imperceptible.
5. Expulsion of the acidic medium should be ceased immediately when the inside of the zona is pierced or softened. Suction is recommended at this point, to aspirate all of the expelled acid solution (the total time to breach the zona should be approximately 5–7 seconds), and move the embryo to another area of the droplet, away from the acid solution.
6. A small 'inside' hole may be widened mechanically by moving the microneedle through the opening in a tearing motion while continuing gentle suction.
7. Carefully transfer the embryo through the wash droplets, and return to culture for incubation prior to embryo transfer.

Successful assisted hatching has also been carried out with the use of a 1.48 μm diode laser (Fertilase™, MTG,Germany); a few milliseconds of laser irradiation instantly makes an opening in the zona pellucida, and apertures ranging from 3 to 25 μm can be obtained. The procedure has been shown to be safe, simple and rapid.

Equipment for ICSI

For microinjection

Dissecting microscope with heated stage
Inverted microscope with heated stage, attached to micromanipulators

$\times 4$ objective for locating eggs and drops
$\times 20$ objective for microsurgery
$\times 15$ eyepiece
Hoffman modulation or Nomarski optics
Video monitoring facility
Bilateral micromanipulators for manipulation in three dimensions
Microtool holders
Two suction devices with steel syringes (80–$100\,\mu l$) filled with light mineral oil (BDH), or appropriate alternative device for controlling holding and injection micropipettes
Incubator
Supply of 5% CO_2 in air.

For making microtools

Borosilicate glass capillary tubing
Micropipette puller
Power supply with controlled variable voltage
Power cleaner to overcome power surges in mains electricity
Microforge
Microbeveller
Oven for heat sterilization.

Supplies

Shallow Falcon Petri dishes (Type 1006)
Culture medium
Culture medium + HEPES
Human serum albumin (HSA)
Hyaluronidase solution
Mineral oil
PVP solution
Pasteur pipettes
Hand-pulled polished glass pipettes
Pipette bulbs
Holding pipettes
ICSI needles.

Adjustment of Narishige manipulators for ICSI
(with thanks to Terry Leonard)

This guide refers to Nikon/Narishige system; the same principles apply to an Olympus system, but the details are slightly different.

Before attempting to fit or adjust the micromanipulators, first adjust the microscope optically, ideally using an oocyte in the same type of Petri dish to be used for ICSI. The microscope settings will influence the working distance of the microtools. The final position of the micromanipulators on the microscope will depend upon:

(a) the angle at which the tool holder is fixed
(b) the combined length of the tool holder and needle from the point where it is held in the tool holder attachment to the centre of the light source.

Before finding the ideal position for the micromanipulators, they should be fitted correctly to the microscope, and final adjustments made later.

Micromanipulator parts

1. Mounting bar: this joins the coarse manipulator to the microscope.
2. Coarse manipulator: consists of three parts, each controlling one of the three dimensions of movement. There are two types: manually operated and motor driven.
3. Fine manipulator: consists of two parts:
    (a) the driving section: attached to the coarse manipulator, controls fine movements directed by joystick.
    (b) ball joint/tool holder attachment: attached to the driving section, used both to hold the microtool holder and to vary the angle at which it is held.
4. Joystick: links to the driving section via oil-filled tubes. The movement of the joystick is scaled down and transferred to the fine manipulator.

The mounting arrangement which attaches the coarse manipulator to the microscope is **L**-shaped. In the Nikon/Narishige system, the mounting is fitted to the illumination pillar as illustrated in Figure 11.9.

The mounting bar position is marked with a white **L**-shape.

The mounting bars have tracks into which the coarse manipulator fits, and the position of the coarse manipulator can be adjusted along these tracks. The entire mounting bar can be adjusted up and down.

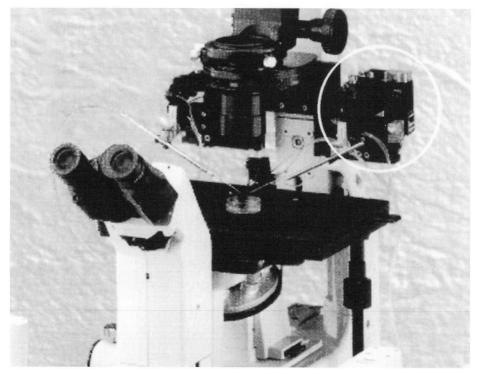

Figure 11.9   Nikon/Narishige coarse manipulator mounting.

Adjusting the coarse manipulators

1. Set the mounting bars at 90 degrees from the microscope stage or bench top.
2. Set the second part of the mounting at 90 degrees to the first, and ensure that the track is set flat.
3. Attach the coarse micromanipulator and adjust the lower section (left/right movement) so that it is parallel with the mounting bar. Set the other two sections of the coarse manipulator at right angles to each other (Figure 11.10).

Attaching the fine manipulator

The fine manipulator is attached to the coarse manipulator by a small metal rod (coupling bar). This can be screwed into one of the two holes on the driving section of the fine manipulator, depending on the side on which it is to be used. In order to fit the fine manipulator on the right hand side, find the 'R' mark on the driving section and screw the coupling bar into the hole directly behind this mark. Attach the coupling bar/driving section to the coarse manipulator and tighten. Position the driving section so that it is parallel with the microscope or 90 degrees to the bench. Attach the left hand side in the same manner, screwing

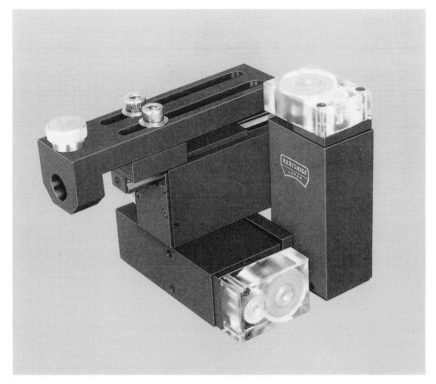

Figure 11.10 Adjusting the coarse manipulator.

the coupling bar into the hole directly behind the 'L' mark. Arrange the joysticks so that the 'R' and 'L' marks are facing the operator on the appropriate sides (Figure 11.11).

Attaching the ball joint/tool holder attachment

The ball joint/tool holder attachment has a black metal bar projecting from it. This is fitted into the **V**-groove of the driving unit. The ball joint is then rotated to an appropriate angle so that when a needle is held in it, the tip of the microtool will be parallel with the microscope stage. The extent to which it is rotated will depend upon the angle at which the microtool is bent. For example, for a microtool which is angled at 35 degrees from the plane of the needle, the ball joint must be rotated 35 degrees anticlockwise from the vertical position (Figure 11.11).

The manipulators should now be attached in the correct manner, but they may not be in the optimal working position. The ideal position will vary depending upon the angle of the needle and the combined length of the microtool and tool holder. It is therefore best to have a fixed tool angle, a fixed

Fine Micromanipulator

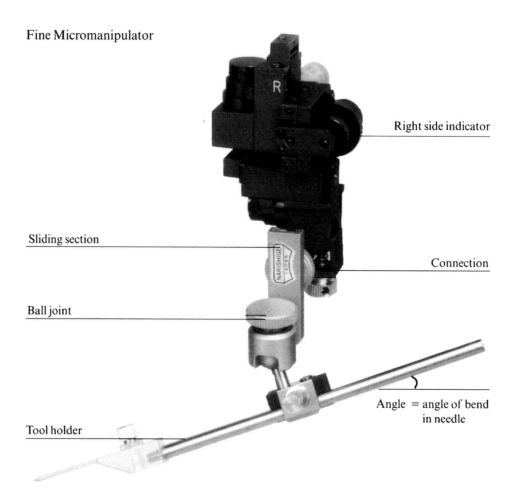

Right side indicator

Sliding section

Connection

Ball joint

Angle = angle of bend
in needle

Tool holder

Figure 11.11   Attaching the fine manipulator.

length of projection of the tool from the tool holder, and a fixed (marked) point
where the tool holder is clamped to the tool holding attachment. If any of these
three factors change, the fine adjustments will require resetting.

Finding the best position for the micromanipulators

Adjust the three coarse manipulators so that they are in the middle of their
range of movements.

Adjust the range of movements of the three fine manipulators on the joystick
so that they are in the middle of the scales.

Forward/backward movement

First ensure that the hole in the stage is positioned directly in the middle of the light path. View the micromanipulator from the side of the microscope, then align the tool holder attachment with the middle of the hole in the microscope stage. This can be adjusted by changing the position of the coupling bar on the fine manipulator, the projection from the ball joint, or the two screws (Figure 11.10) on the very top of the coarse manipulator which controls the forward/backward movement.

Left/right movement

Place a microtool holder together with a microtool in the tool holder attachment. Attach it at the very tip of the tool holder, and gently slide it along towards the light source. If it will not reach the light source, the entire manipulator should be moved to the left. Likewise, if it reaches it too soon (before the marked point) the entire manipulator should be shifted to the right. This adjustment is performed by loosening the bolts which attach the coarse micromanipulator to the mounting bar. After this adjustment, ensure that the micromanipulator is still parallel to the bar.

Up/down movement

Adjust the manipulator so that the microtool is approximately 0.5 cm from the surface of the stage. For large adjustments loosen the bolts which attach the mounting bar to the microscope and move up or down. Remember to ensure that it is still 90 degrees from the bench after adjustment. Fine up/down adjustments can be made by moving the small sliding section above the ball joint.

Alignment of the ICSI needle in the manipulator

When using a Narishige tool holder, push the needle in so that 4–5 cm of the needle is outside the holder. Place the tool holder in the right hand micromanipulator with the needle tip over the light source. The angle at which the tool holder is held should be such that the angled tip of the needle is parallel with the stage of the microscope. Under a very low power ($\times 4$ objective), place the tip of the ICSI needle in the field of vision of the microscope. Loosen the tool holder attachment and rotate the tool holder so that the bent portion of the needle appears to be straight. Ensure that you can focus on a good portion of the needle (from the tip). The portion of the needle after the bend will be out of focus. If the microscope has a graticule, make sure that the movement of the needle from right to left does not vary. Place the ICSI needle along the middle of the microscope field with the tip almost in the centre. Align the holding pipette in the same manner so that the tips of the needle and pipette are facing each other, and then raise them up away from the stage.

Perform the final adjustment of the angle at which the tool holder is held within a sperm droplet. Find a nonmotile sperm and then bring the ICSI needle into the same optical plane. Raise the ICSI needle off the surface of the Petri dish very slightly, move it over the top of the sperm, and try to touch the sperm by lowering the needle. If it is impossible to touch the sperm, the needle is not parallel with the surface. The end of the needle will be lower than the tip. To rectify this, raise the needle and rotate the ball point anticlockwise slightly, lower the needle, and try to touch the sperm again. If the tip of the needle can touch the sperm, but the rest of the needle is not in focus, the tip of the needle is lower than the bend. To rectify this, raise the needle and rotate the ball joint slightly in a clockwise direction.

Ratio of movement and joysticks

1. Focus on the tip of the microtool.
2. Loosen the two screws on the movement adjustment rings.
3. Ignore the ratios written on the side of the joystick, and rotate the adjustment rings anticlockwise until you are satisfied with the movement as observed down the microscope.

When all of the adjustments and alignments are made, the need to repeat any of these should be minimal, unless the style of the needle or tool holder is changed. When removing the tool holder from its attachment, keep the ball joint at the same angle so that when a new needle is inserted, it will be at approximately the right angle for use. Fine adjustments will be necessary for each manipulation (Figure 11.12).

Microtool preparation

The following details describe the procedures currently in use at Bourn Hall, and are intended as guidelines for reference only. Specific details will vary according to individual equipment, facilities and the personnel using them, and a significant amount of 'trial and error' adjustment is to be expected.

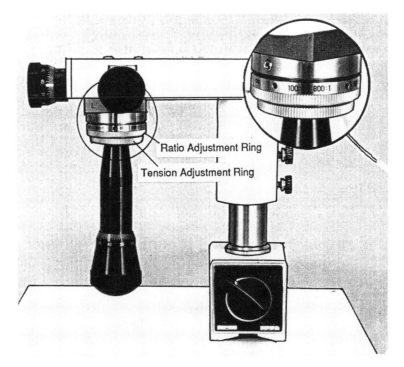

Figure 11.12   Arranging the joysticks.

Equipment

Microtools are made by applying heat and force to capillary tubing. The heat source is a filament controlled by voltage applied through an electrical resistance device and, when the glass is semi-melted, force is provided by a simple spring pulling device with adjustable settings. The tools can then be modified using a grinding wheel to grind the tip to the required size, and a microforge to cut, bend, constrict or pull the tapered sections of the micropipette.

Capillary tubing

Most microtool holders on micromanipulation equipment are designed for tubing of a specific diameter, commonly 1 mm. Tubing is available in a variety of wall thicknesses: a thin wall helps to maintain a large lumen with the smallest tip diameter possible, whereas thicker-walled tubing is better for holding pipettes.

Borosilicate glass capillary tubing, from Clark Electromedical, supplied in containers of 500 pieces can be used.

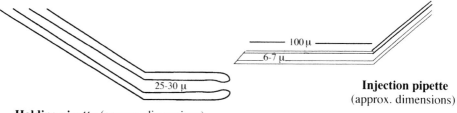

Figure 11.13   Injection and holding pipettes.

For holding pipettes: 1.00 × 0.78 mm (outer/inner diameter), 100 mm
length (GC100–10)
Injection pipettes: 1.00 × 0.58 mm, 100 mm length (GC100T-10)
(See Figure 11.13.)

PCP7 Plug board (*Research Instruments*)
Used to supply a controlled voltage which heats the pipette puller and microforge filaments. The amp-meter readings should be set before starting and,
because mains electricity varies in different locations, suggested peg settings
are approximate only.

IMMAC power cleaner
Used to stabilize the power supply to overcome power surges in mains
electricity.

Micropipette puller (*MPP11, Research Instruments*)
Can be used to draw any type of pipette, to a range of diameters. The
adjustable controls allow repeatable control over the pulling process by adjusting distance travelled with the left and right carriage stops and force of pull
with the adjustable spring force. Time is varied manually by using a stopwatch
to time the operation of the carriage release pin.
   More sophisticated pullers (e.g. Sachs-Flaming puller, Sutter Instruments)
are available, which incorporate microprocessor control over the variable
parameters. Programmes for particular tools can be entered into the machine
and stored in memory slots.

Microforge (*Research Instruments*)
Used to alter the pulled section of the capillary: the tapered sections of a
micropipette can be cut, bent, constricted, pulled or polished. It consists of a
heating filament and micromanipulators used to control the position of the
microtool in relation to the filament. It also has a magnification system (× 80)

with an eyepiece micron scale arranged to focus on the filament and micro-pipette during forging procedures. The temperature of the filament is control-led by the same plug board used for the puller.

Microbeveller or microgrinder (Research Instruments)
Used for adjusting the size of the bevel on injection pipettes. It has a $\times 20$ eye-piece incorporating 100XY graticule and $\times 20$ objective. Each small divi-sion of the graticule $= 3.5\,\mu m$ approximately.

The abrasive grinding wheel is partially immersed in a water bath, and the wheel gradually grinds the tip of the pipette to the appropriate size. The pipette is observed through the eyepiece at 1–2 minute intervals, until the required dimensions are reached.

Pipette storage containers
Pipettes may be safely stored by immobilizing them with Blu-tack inside plastic Petri dishes. Glass storage containers with Pyrex glass covers (Research Instruments) are used for heat sterilization.

Oven for heat sterilization
Glassware and pipettes are heat sterilized at 180°C for 2 hours.

Attention must also be paid to the environment for microtool preparation, and to allocating dedicated laboratory space and scientist time. Vibration will interfere with the necessary precision, and the individual units may be isolated on foam pads if necessary. Adequate lighting is very important, and the microforge should be in a position in which it can be comfortably operated. The environment should also be dust-free, free of drafts and the interruption of slamming doors, etc.

Procedure

Pulling
A pulled section of capillary tubing must be produced, which is at least 1 cm in length, and the correct diameter in the area of the tip. Different pipette shapes are obtained by different combinations of spring force, length of pull and filament temperature, and different specifications of glass have different pulling characteristics, i.e. thick-walled (holding pipette) and thin-walled (injection pipette) tubing behave differently. For thick-walled tubing, the second pull is usually at a lower temperature than the first pull, and for thin-walled tubing the second pull often has to be at a higher temperature than the first pull. The

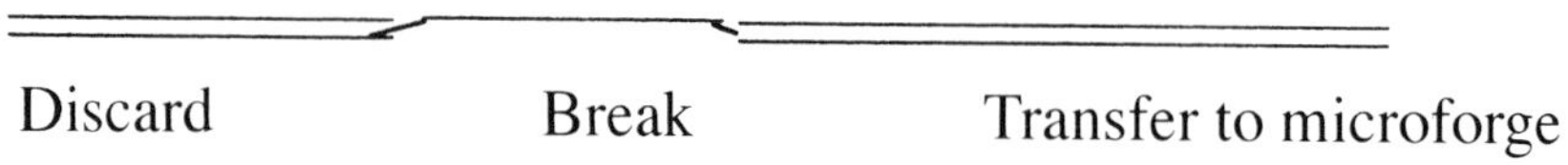

Discard   Break   Transfer to microforge

Figure 11.14   Breaking a capillary.

settings listed here are specifically for ICSI pipettes, and are for guidance only. They may require adjustment according to variables such as air temperature, electricity supply, individual variation, etc. Pipettes for other uses such as zona cutting or drilling or blastomere biopsy require different settings and procedures.

Holding pipettes
Use thick-walled tubing, 1.00 × 0.78, 100 mm length

     Setting: Puller: Left carriage stop   75
                       Traverse   10
                       Right carriage stop   0
                       Force   6

Current (PCP7 power controller) at 6.5
(Top Red 6, Bottom Red 5)

1. 'Soak' (apply the current) for 15 seconds, release the traverse pin to effect the pull, and then switch off the current. Remove the tubing, the piece on the RIGHT side will be used; break the tubing manually near the end of the tapering (Figure 11.14).
2. Transfer the pulled pipette to the microforge. Move the pipette under the glass bead, positioned tangentially to the surface of the bead at the area where a break is required. Heat the bead at a low setting, until it appears just noticeably hot (Top Black 3, Bottom Black 5), and carefully bring the needle into contact with the bead. When the two surfaces adhere, immediately turn the filament off. The pipette should break cleanly as the bead cools. Jagged or angled breaks can be avoided by keeping the two surfaces as parallel as possible. Slight angles or imperfections in the break are irrelevant, as the final 'polishing' step will melt these down. If the tip has more substantial deviations, it will have to be rebroken, provided that it is possible to do so without losing the appropriate diameter (Figure 11.15).

Injection pipettes
The tips should be long, thin, and reasonably parallel, to minimize the size of the hole created in the zona and the oolemma. The holes must be small enough to avoid the injection of too much medium at the time of injection, and to prevent loss of cytoplasm on needle withdrawal.

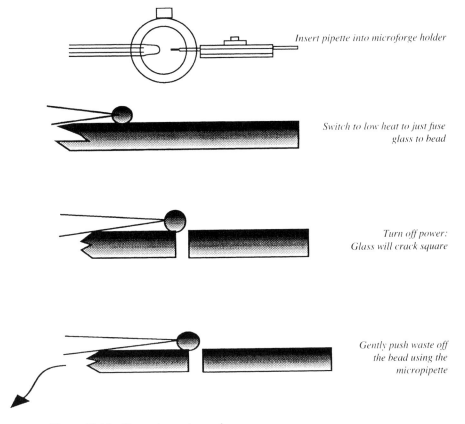

Insert pipette into microforge holder

*Switch to low heat to just fuse
glass to bead*

*Turn off power:
Glass will crack square*

*Gently push waste off
the bead using the
micropipette*

Figure 11.15   Preparing a clean edge.

Use thin-walled tubing, 1.00 × 0.58, 100 mm length
Two separate pulls are required for each needle

1. Settings: Pull (1) Left carriage stop   55
    Current   6.5
    (Top Red 6, Bottom Red 5)
    Traverse   10
    Right carriage stop   0
    Force   4

Insert the tubing, 'soak' for 10 seconds, then release the traverse pin. Switch off the
current when the pull stops.

                    Pull (2)   Left carriage stop   100
    Traverse   0
    Right carriage stop   10
    Force   4
    Current   6.5 (Red)

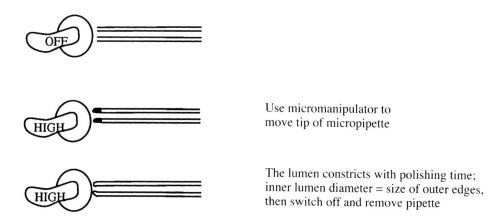

Use micromanipulator to
move tip of micropipette

The lumen constricts with polishing time;
inner lumen diameter = size of outer edges,
then switch off and remove pipette

Figure 11.16   Polishing and reducing the tip.

Switch on the current, release the pin (no 'soaking'), switch off the current
when the pull stops.
Use the tubing on the LEFT side.

2.   The beveller is then used to grind the end of the pipette so that the tip has an
outer diameter of 7 μm (2 graticules on the scale) and an angle of approximately 35 degrees (Figures 11.16 and 11.17).
Load the needle into the right hand groove of the holder, apply positive air
pressure with a syringe, and grind with the wheel set at full speed. The
grinding time will vary according to the initial tip size, and progress of the
grinding should be regularly monitored accordingly (e.g. initial size 3–4 μm,
grind for approximately 5 minutes, check every 1 or 2 minutes.
Keeping the needle in the holder, check that the bevel is suitable, and then
turn it so that the opening of the needle faces towards you. Mark the top of the
pipette with a marker pen. The grinding wheel must be kept clean, by rubbing
regularly with abrasive paper. The purified water in the water bath must also
be replaced regularly.

3.   Microforge: to add a bend, and modify the tip if necessary.
Insert the needle into the holder so that the bevel is facing towards you, i.e.
rotate the mark at the tip of the needle 90 degrees away from you.
Heat the filament: Black Top 3, Bottom Black 5 (this must be adjusted by trial
and error, so that it is neither too high nor too low!)
Add a 30 degree bend: move the angle adjuster to the sixth division, and bring
the needle towards the heated bead until the tip of the needle is horizontal;
then switch the current off (Figure 11.18).
If necessary, a spike or point can be added by gently fusing the tip of the needle
to the heated bead (same setting as for making the 30 degree bend), and then
pulling the needle away from the bead before switching the current off.

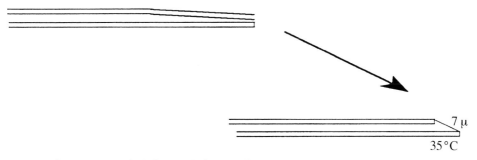

Figure 11.17   Tip before and after grinding.

NB: If the needle has a good bevel and sharp tip after adding the 30 degree angle, the last step, which can be very difficult, is not necessary.

4. Place carefully into glass pipette container, and heat sterilize at 180°C for 2 hours.

Notes on pipette pulling

First pull (*injection pipette*) *or Only pull* (holding pipette)

Pipette too thin:

1. Move the carriage stop to make the pull shorter.
2. Increase filament heat.
3. Lower spring force by 0.5, 1.0 or 2.0 divisions.

Pipette too thick:

1. Make pipette longer by moving the carriage stop.
2. Lower the filament temperature by altering the power controller settings.
3. Increase the spring force by 0.5 division or more if necessary.

Second pull

Pipette breaks before second pull (when moving the thin part back inside the filament coil):

1. Increase filament heat slightly on first pull (to make a slightly thicker pipette).

Pipette too thin:

1. Move carriage stop on the first pull, to create a shorter pull.
2. Increase filament temperature slightly, by altering power controller settings on the first pull.

Pipette too thick:

1. Move the carriage stop on the first pull to create a longer pull.

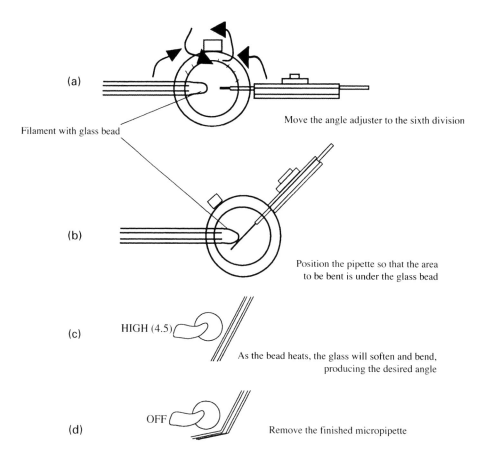

(a)

Filament with glass bead

Move the angle adjuster to the sixth division

(b)

Position the pipette so that the area
to be bent is under the glass bead

(c)   HIGH (4.5)

As the bead heats, the glass will soften and bend,
producing the desired angle

(d)   OFF

Remove the finished micropipette

Figure 11.18   Adding a bend.

2.   Lower filament temperature slightly by altering the power controller settings
on the first pull.

Profile of the pipette is incorrect:

1.   Alter the spring force, i.e.   First pull = 5, Second pull = 7, then try
First pull = 5, Second pull = 6, or 6.5

Notes on the Microforge

Setting up

Insert a preformed filament of platinum–iridium wire into the filament holder.
Using the micrometer stage, move the filament just to the left of the centre of

the field of view. A new filament's heat response to the voltage applied may vary from the old filament, and changes to the filament such as glass ball size and even the surrounding air flow can affect the heat/voltage response. As the filament heats up, it will expand in size, and this expansion will vary between different filaments. Care must be taken to monitor this expansion, so that the hot filament is not driven directly into a needle during forging! During forging procedures it is usually best to heat the filament initially at a low voltage setting, increase as necessary.

Setting a glass bead onto the filament

Pull a sharp needle on the puller, and clamp it into position on the microforge with the tip facing the filament. Heat the filament so that the glass easily melts, and bring the needle tip into contact with the hot filament so that a bead of glass melts on the filament surface. Draw the needle away and turn the heat off; a glass bead should be left attached to the surface of the filament. This may require several steps of moving the needle into and away from the filament, until an appropriate size is reached; then heat the filament to round out the mass of glass. Once set up, a bead can be used for some time. When it eventually becomes too large or misshapen, it should be removed and renewed.

Cleaning glass from the filament

When the bead acquires too much adherent glass, the size can be reduced by heating the filament until it is dull orange in colour, and then rolling the tip of a waste pipette along the filament so that glass from the filament adheres to the pipette. The section of tip used should have a diameter of approximately 70 μm.

Loading the micropipette

Clamp the micropipette into the carriage by closing the lid between finger and thumb. With the lever of the XY-positioner in the vertical, and the rotator in the horizontal position, slide the pipette so that it can be conveniently visualised. Using the lever-micromanipulator, check that the tip can be moved to touch the filament, and leave it well clear of the filament. Lightly clamp the carriage on its bar.

APPENDIX

Causes of azoospermia

The Johnsen Score scores the degree of spermatogenesis found in a biopsy: a number of tubules are assessed, and each one is given a score for the most advanced stage of spermatogenesis seen:

>   1 = no cells present in the tubule
>   2 = Sertoli cells
>   3 = spermatogonia
>   4–5 = spermatocytes
>   6–7 = spermatids
>   8–10 = spermatozoa

Mean Johnsen Score (MJS) = average of all the tubules assessed, i.e.
MJS = 2 is the Sertoli Cell Only syndrome
MJS-8–10 is normal spermatogenesis
MJS between 2 and 8 represents varying degrees of subnormal spermato-
    genesis, but a qualitative description is required.
There is a correlation between testicular size and MJS.

Pathologies

A. Pretesticular: deficient gonadotropin drive – low FSH
B. Androgen Resistance: familial pseudohermaphroditism
C. Testicular failure: no spermatogenesis – raised FSH
D. Post testicular duct obstruction: functional sperm usually present, size of testes is normal, FSH is not raised

A. Pretesticular: pathologies which result in secondary testicular failure (hypogonadotrophic hypogonadism) due to decreased gonadotropin release (low serum FSH). Testicular biopsy may show a prepubertal appearance, with precursors of Sertoli cells, prespermatogenic cells, and absence of Leydig cells.

1.	Congenital	partial or complete Kallman's syndrome: GnRH deficiency associated with agenesis of the first cranial nerve & thus anosmia. Low FSH and LH, small but potentially normal testes.

2.	Acquired	space-occupying lesions
		    pituitary tumours
		    craniophraryngioma

   trauma, meningitis, sarcoidosis
   Cushing's syndrome (adrenal hypoplasia)
   congenital adrenal hyperplasia
   haemochromatosis

B. Androgen resistance: familial incomplete male pseudohermaphroditism, type 1: partial or complete defects in amount or function of the androgen receptor. Patients fall into a wide spectrum of disorders, probably due to variable manifestations of a single gene defect. Cryptorchidism is common, and the testes remain small in size. The testes demonstrate normal Leydig cells and tubules containing both germ cells and Sertoli cells, but there is usually no maturation beyond the primary spermatocyte. Plasma testosterone and LH are high, suggesting that there is a defect in the feedback control of testosterone on the hypothalamus.

Four (phenotypically) separate clinical disorders:

1. Rosewater's syndrome (mildest form)
2. Reinfenstein's syndrome
3. Gilbert–Dreyfus syndrome
4. Lub's syndrome (most severe) – phenotypic females with partial Wolffian duct development and masculine skeletal development.

C. Testicular failure: testicular biopsy can show a wide variation in appearance, e.g.:

   sclerosing tubular degeneration is seen in Klinefelter's syndrome,
   disorganization with extensive hyalinization and tubular atrophy is seen
   after orchitis.

1. Congenital Klinefelter's syndrome (XXY)
      autosomal abnormalities
      torsion (maturation arrest)
      cryptorchidism, anorchia
      sickle-cell disease
      myotonic muscular dystrophy
      Noonan's syndrome (male Turner's)
2. Acquired mumps orchitis
      epididymo-orchitis
      testicular trauma
      inguinal/scrotal surgery
      radiotherapy

D. Post-testicular: obstructive causes of azoospermia. Testicular biopsy shows well preserved normal spermatogenesis, and there may be sloughing of superficial layers of the seminiferous epithelium. The upper epididymis is the most common site of genital tract obstruction (2/3 of lesions), and multifocal sites of obstruction may be present. Obstructive lesions can be caused by specific or nonspecific infection, and oedema and/or haematoma as a result of trauma can lead to epididymal or vasal obstruction.

1. Congenital   congenital absence of the vas deferens (CAVD)
                  cystic fibrosis
                  Young's syndrome
                  Zinner's syndrome: congenital absence of the vas deferens, cor-
                  pus and cauda epididymis, seminal vesicle, ampulla and ejacula-
                  tory duct – may be bilateral or unilateral and can be associated
                  with ipsilateral renal agenesis – due to failure of the Wolffian
                  (mesonephric) duct
2. Acquired   TB
                  Gonococcal or chlamydial infection
                  surgical trauma
                  smallpox
                  bilharziasis
                  filariasis
                  vasectomy

E. Other causes of spermatogenic failure or disorder: may be associated with defective testosterone synthesis, decreased metabolic clearance rates, increased binding of testosterone to plasma proteins, increased plasma oestradiol and low, normal or moderately elevated serum FSH levels.

1. Systemic illness
        fevers, burns, head trauma
        chronic renal failure
        thyrotoxicosis, diabetes
        male anorexia nervosa
        surgery, general anaesthesia.
2. Drugs/industrial toxins
        (a) Therapeutic: sulphasalazine, nitrofurantoin, cimetidine, niridazole, col-
            chicine, spironolactone, testosterone injections, cytotoxic agents
        (b) Occupational: carbon disulphide (rayon), lead, dibromochlorpropane,
            radiation
        (c) Recreational abuse: alcohol, opiates, anabolic steroids.
3. Absent spermatogenesis
        Germinal Aplasia or Hypoplasia – Sertoli cell only (del Castillo) syndrome.
        Only Sertoli cells are present in the tubular epithelium, none of the spermato-

genic elements remain. In germinal cell hypoplasia, there is a generalized reduction in the numbers of germ cells of all stages. The numbers of more mature cells are greatly reduced, and the germinal epithelium has a loose, poorly populated appearance. There are two forms:

    (a) serum FSH is grossly elevated, Sertoli cells show severe abnormalities on EM – no inhibin production

    (b) serum FSH is normal – normal inhibin production

Testis size is often not markedly reduced, and this may lead to diagnostic difficulties. These patients are frequently misdiagnosed as having an obstructive lesion, and biopsy is the only means of making a correct diagnosis.

4. Leydig cell failure leads to low testosterone levels, and raised serum FSH and LH. In this situation the testis is atrophied, with gross reduction in size.

5. Immotile sperm – Kartagener's immotile cilia syndrome
    Normal numbers of sperm are present in the semen, but they are all immotile. Transmission electron microscopy shows that the central filaments of the tails are absent, and this anomaly may be present in cilia throughout the body, resulting in chronic sinusitis and bronchiectasis.

6. Retrograde ejaculation: diabetes, multiple sclerosis, sympathectomy, prostatectomy, funnel bladder neck.

7. Ejaculatory failure: spinal cord injury, multiple sclerosis, diabetes, abdominal aortic surgery, A–P resection, psychomimetic/antihypertensive drugs, hypogonadism.

Chromosomal anomalies

Klinefelter's syndrome

Bilateral testicular atrophy, signs of hypogonadism with a greater span than height, often with gynecomastia. FSH and LH are extremely high, often with low testosterone. Diagnosis can be made on clinical and biochemical grounds, and confirmed by buccal smear or karyotype (XXY). Affects 1 in 400 live-born males, and are found in around 7% of infertile men. Testicular histology: obvious and gross spermatogenic failure with disappearance of all the spermatogenic elements in all the tubules. Marked hyperplasia of the Leydig cells.

46 XX Klinefelter's

Patients are phenotypically male, with same clinical and endocrinological features as the XXY patient. H-Y antigen has been demonstrated – this karyotype exhibits Y chromosome expression despite its apparent absence.

46 XX (Noonan's syndrome)

Male equivalent of Turner's (XO). They have normal male phenotype, but are usually cryptorchid and show varying degrees of hypoandrogenization. Testicular atrophy, raised FSH and LH, reduced testosterone.

Robertsonian translocation

A form of chromosomal aberration which involves the fusion of long arms of acrocentric chromosomes at the centromere. Breaks occur at the extreme ends of the short arms of two nonhomologous acrocentric chromosomes; these small segments are lost, and the larger segments fuse at their centromeric region, producing a new, large submetacentric or metacentric chromosome.

'Balanced translocations' may produce only minor deficiencies, but translocation heterozygotes have reduced frequencies of crossing over and are usually subfertile through the production of abnormal gametes.

Until the mid-1990s, virtually all of the above pathologies resulted in untreatable male sterility; this situation was completely reversed by the ability to combine surgical techniques to recover samples from the epididymis and directly from the testis, with intracytoplasmic injection of single sperm cells.

Further reading

Barak, Y. Spermatid injection: pregnancy after transfer of single pronucleate embryos (1997) *Alpha Newsletter* **10**:1–3.

Bonduelle, M. et al. (1994) Prospective follow-up study of 55 children born after subzonal insemination and intracytoplasmic sperm injection *Human Reproduction* **9(9)**:1765–9.

Cohen, J. (1991) Assisted hatching of human embryos. *Journal of In Vitro Fertilization and Embryo Transfer* **8(4)**:179–89.

Cohen, J. (1992) Zona pellucida micromanipulation and consequences for embryonic development and implantation. In: (Cohen, J., Malter, H.F., Talansky, B.E. & Grifo, J., eds.), *Micromanipulation of Human gametes and Embryos.* Raven Press, New York.

Cohen, J., Alikani, M., Trowbridge, J. & Rosenwaks, Z. (1992) Implantation enhancement by selective assisted hatching using zona drilling of embryos with poor prognosis. *Human Reproduction* **7**: 685–91.

Cohen, J., Alikani, M., Garrisi, J.G., & Willadsen, S. (1998) Micromanipulation of human gametes and embryos: ooplasmic donation at fertilization (Video). *Human Reproduction Update* **4(2)**:195–6.

DeFelici, M. & Siracusa, G. (1982) "Spontaneous" hardening of the zona pellucida of mouse oocytes during in vitro culture. *Gamete Research* **6**:107–12.

Downs, S.M., Schroeder, A.C. & Eppig, J.J. (1986) Serum maintains the fertilizability of mouse oocytes matured in vitro by preventing hardening of the zona pellucida. *Gamete Research* **15**:115–22.

Germond, M., Nocera, D., Senn, A., Rink, K., Delacrétaz, G. & Fakan, S. (1995) Microdissection of mouse and human zona pellucida using a 1.48 µ diode laser beam: efficiency and safety of the procedure. *Fertility and Sterility* **25**:604–11.

Grifo, J.A., Boyle, A. & Fischer, E. (1990) Preembryo biopsy and analysis of blastomeres by in situ hybridisation. *American Journal of Obstetrics and Gynaecology* **163**:2013–19.

Hamberger, L., Sjögren, A. & Lundin, K. (1995) Microfertilization techniques: choice of correct indications. In: (Hedon, B., Bringer, J. & Mares, P. eds.), *Fertility and Sterility: A Current Overview.* IFFS-95, The Parthenon Publishing Groups, New York, London, pp. 405–8.

Handyside, A. (1991) Pre-implantation diagnosis by DNA amplification. In: C. Chapman, M., Grudzinskas, G., Chard, T. & Maxwell, A. eds.), *The Embryo.* Springer Verlag, Amsterdam.

Handyside, A.H., Kontogianni, E.H., Hardy, K. & Winston, R.M.L. (1990) Pregnancies from biopsied human preimplantation embryos sexed by Y-specific DNA amplification. *Nature* **344**, 768–70.

Harper, J.C. & Handyside, A.H. (1994) The current status of preimplantation diagnosis. *Current Obstetrics and Gynaecology* **4**:143–9.

Harper, J.C., Coonan, E. & Ramaekers, F.C.S. (1994) Identification of the sex of human preimplantation embryos in two hours using an improved spreading method and fluorescent in-situ hybridization (FISH) using directly labelled probes. *Human Reproduction* **9**:721–4.

Hirsch, A. (1992) The investigation and treatment of the infertile male: pathophysiology and principles of treatment. In: (Brinsden, P. & Ramsbury, P. eds.), *A Textbook of In Vitro Fertilization and Assisted Reproduction.* Parthenon Publishing Group, London.

Jequier, A.M. (1986) *Infertility in the Male: Current Reviews in Obstetrics and Gynaecology,* Churchill LIvingstone, UK.

Kent-First, M. (1996) A genetic aetiology for male infertility: new questions for the infertile couple. *Alpha Newsletter* **5**:1–3.

Kent-First, M., Kol, S. & Muallem, A. (1996) Infertility in intracytoplasmic sperm injection derived sons. *The Lancet* **348**:332.

Kobayashi, K., Mizuno, K. & Hida, A. (1994) PCR analysis of the Y chromosome long arm in azoospermic patients: evidence for a second locus required for spermatogenesis. *Human Molecular Genetics* **3**:1965–7.

Longo, F.J. (1981) Changes in the zonae pellucidae and plasmalemmae of ageing mouse eggs. *Biological Reproduction* **25**:299–411.

Munné, S., Alikani, M., Levron, J., Tomkin, G., Palermo, G., Grifo, J. & Cohen, J. (1995) Fluorescent in situ hybridisation in human blastomeres. In: (Hedon, B., Bringer, J. & Mares, P. eds.), *Fertility and Sterility.* IFFS-95, The Parthenon Publishing Groups, New York, London, pp. 425–38.

Nagy, Z.P., Janssenswillen, C., Silber, S., Devroey, P. & Van Steirteghem, A.C. (1995) Using ejaculated, fresh, and frozen-thawed epididymal and testicular spermatozoa gives rise to comparable results after intracytoplasmic injection. *Human Reproduction* **9**:1743–8.

Nagy, Z.P., Liu, J., Joris, H., Devroey, P. & Van Steirteghem, A. (1993a) Intracytoplasmic single sperm injection of 1-day old unfertilized human oocytes *Human Reproduction* **8**:2180–4.

Nagy, Z.P., Liu, J., Joris, H., Devroey, P. & Van Steirteghem, A. (1993b) Time-course of oocyte activation, pronucleus formation and cleavage in human oocytes fertilized by intracytoplasmic sperm injection. *Human Reproduction* **9**:1743–8.

Nijs, M. & Vanderzwalmen, P. (1998) ICSI with immature sperm. *British Fertility Society, Sheffield,* April 1998. **Abstract S5,** p. 19.

Oates, R.D., Cobl, S.M., Harns, D.H., Pang, S. Burgess, C.M. & Carson, R.S. (1996) Efficiency of ICSI using intentionally cryopreserved edipidymal sperm. *Human Reproduction* **600**:133–8.

Palermo, G., Joris, H., Devroey, P. & Van Steirteghem, A.C. (1992). Pregnancies after in-tracytoplasmic injection of single spermatozoon into an oocyte. *Lancet* **340**: 17–18.

Palermo, G., Joris, H., Derde, M.-P., Camus, M., Devroey, P. & Van Steirteghem, A.C. (1993) Sperm characteristics and outcome of human assisted fertilization by subzonal insemination and intracytoplasmic sperm injection. *Fertility and Sterility* **59**:826–35.

Qureshi, S.J., Ross, A.R., Ma, K., Cooke, H.J., McIntyre, M.A., Chandley, A.C. & Hargreave,

T.B. (1996) Polymerase chain reaction screening for Y chromosome microdeletions: a first step towards the diagnosis of genetically-determined spermatogenic failure in men. *Molecular Human Reproduction* **2(10)**:775–9.

Safran, A., Reubinoff, E., Porat-Katz, A. & Lewin, A. (1998) Assisted reproduction for the treatment of azoospermia. *Human Reproduction,* **13, Suppl. 4**: 41–60.

Silber, S.J., Van Steirteghem, A.C., Liu, J., Nagy, Z., Tournaye, H. & Devroey, P. (1995) High fertilization and pregnancy rate after intracytoplasmic sperm injection with spermatozoa obtained from testicle biopsy. *Human Reproduction* **10**:148–52.

Simoni, M., Kamischke, A. & Nieschlag, E. (1998) The current status of the molecular diagnosis of Y-chromosomal microdeletions in the work-up of male infertility. *Human Reproduction* **13(7)**:1764–8.

Svalander, P., Forsberg, A.-S., Jakobsson, A.-H. & Wikland, M. (1995) Factors of importance for the establishment of a successful program of intracytoplasmic sperm injection treatment for male infertility. *Fertility and Sterility* **65**:828–37.

Twigg, J.P., Irvine, D.S. & Aitken R.J. (1998) Oxidative damage to DNA in human spermatozoa does not preclude pronucleus formation at intracytoplasmic sperm injection. *Human Reproduction* **13(7)**:1864–71.

Van Assche, E., Bonduelle, M. & Tournaye, H. (1996) Cytogenetics of male infertility. *Human Reproduction* **11, (Suppl. 4)**:1–26.

Vanderzwalmen, P., Nijs, M., Stecher, A., Zech, H., Bertin, G., Lejeune, B., Vandamme, B., Chatziparasidou, A., Prapas, Y. & Schoysman, R. (1998) Is there a future for spermatid injection? *Human Reproduction* **13, Suppl. 4**:71–84.

Van Steirteghem, A.C., Liu, J., Joris, H., Nagy, Z.P., Janssenswillen, C., Tournaye, H., Derde, M.-P., Van Assche, E. & Devroey, P. (1993) Higher success rate by intracytoplasmic sperm injection than by subzonal insemination. Report of a second series of 300 consecutive treatment cycles. *Human Reproduction* **8**:1055–60.

Van Steirteghem, A., Liu, J., Nagy, P., Joris, H., Staessen, C., Smitz, J., Tournaye, H., Camus, M., Liebaers, I. & Devroey, P. (1995) Microinsemination. In: (Hebon, B., Bringer, J. & Mares, P. eds.), *Fertility and Sterility: A Current Overview.* IFFS-95, The Parthenon Publishing Groups, New York, London, pp. 295–404.

12

Preimplantation genetic diagnosis

JOYCE HARPER

Preimplantation genetic diagnosis (PGD) is an early form of prenatal diagnosis, developed in the late 1980s to help couples who are at risk of transmitting an inherited disease to their offspring. If such couples wish to have a healthy family, the only option open to them apart from PGD is prenatal diagnosis by amniocentesis or chorionic villus sampling (CVS). The main disadvantage of prenatal diagnosis is that if the diagnosis shows the fetus to be affected, the couple have to decide whether they wish to terminate the pregnancy or carry on with the knowledge that their child is going to be affected by the genetic disease. PGD offers some of these couples an alternative, as the diagnosis is performed on the preimplantation embryo and only unaffected embryos are transferred to the patient. The pregnancy is therefore initiated with the knowledge that the fetus is free from the disease.

When PGD was first developed, the main referral group consisted of patients who had already experienced several terminations of affected pregnancies, or those with moral or religious objections to termination. However, in recent years PGD has been used to help patients who have experienced repeated miscarriages due to unbalanced chromosome arrangements in the fetus. In addition, some infertility patients, mainly those treated for severe male infertility by intracytoplasmic sperm injection (ICSI), have been found to carry chromosomal translocations; PGD can be performed for these couples so that normal embryos are replaced.

PGD covers several fields: IVF, genetics, embryo biopsy and single cell diagnosis. Before discussing embryo biopsy and single cell diagnosis, it is important to outline the inheritance of genetic disease and principles of prenatal diagnosis.

The genetics of inherited disease

There are three main groups of inherited disease that can be diagnosed by PGD:

1. Single gene defects
2. Triplet repeat disorders
3. Chromosomal abnormalities.

Single gene defects may affect the autosomes (chromosomes 1–22) or the sex chromosomes (X and Y). Single gene defects are inherited by autosomal recessive, autosomal dominant and X-linked (sex-linked) modes. The triplet repeat disorders are a recently identified group of diseases caused by an expansion of a triplet repeat of bases on a chromosome. Chromosomal abnormalities, such as translocations and inversions, can lead to a fetus with an unbalanced chromosome complement.

Since chromosomes exist in pairs (one of each pair inherited from each parent), genes are present in two copies, with the exception of those carried on the sex chromosomes in males: they have only one X and one Y chromosome. The majority of genetically inherited diseases are caused by a mutation within a specific gene which causes the gene to be inactive or faulty. Whether the disease is expressed when both or only a single copy of the gene carries a mutation depends upon the mode of inheritance. The mutations that lead to a disease can be caused by a single change, or by more complicated changes in the bases within the gene. This change may be a deletion, substitution or insertion in the base sequence. Within a single gene, there are 'hot spots' prone to mutation. For example, over 800 cystic fibrosis (CF) mutations have been identified, but, in the UK, 70% of individuals who carry CF have the same mutation, ΔF508, caused by a deletion of three base pairs in exon 10 of the CF gene.

Age-related aneuploidy is also an important factor that may lead to chromosomally abnormal offspring. This is not an inherited disease, and it can occur in any pregnancy.

Autosomal recessive disease

The inheritance of autosomal recessive disease is shown in Figure 12.1. Autosomal recessive inheritance accounts for the majority of genetic disease. If an individual has one normal gene and one abnormal gene, he or she is a carrier of the disease and will be unaffected. The individual will be affected by the disease if the genes inherited from both the mother and the father carry the

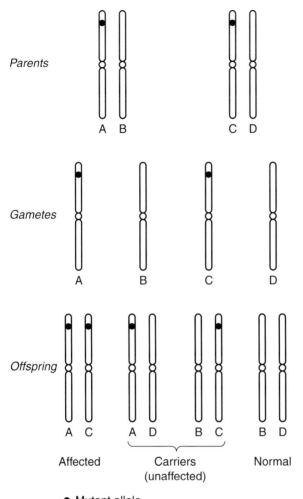

Figure 12.1   Autosomal recessive inheritance.

mutation. For example, if both the mother and the father are carriers of CF, the offspring have a 1:4 chance of being affected, 1:4 chance of being unaffected, and a 2:4 chance of being a carrier.

The most common autosomal recessive single gene defect is β-thalassemia, which is caused by a mutation in the β-globin gene. PGD for β-thalassemia has been slow to develop, and to date only a few cycles have been performed. This is due to the fact that there are many different mutations for β-thalassemia, especially between different ethnic groups. The majority of couples carry different mutations (compound heterozygotes) and this complicates PGD (see section on PCR diagnosis).

Table 12.1. *PGD for autosomal recessive diseases*

Cystic fibrosis (various mutations)
Sickle-cell anaemia
Tay Sach's disease
Spinal muscular atrophy
β-thalassemia
Adrenogenital syndrome
Hypophosphatemia

Cystic fibrosis is the most common autosomal recessive single gene defect for which PGD has been applied. Since ΔF508 is such a common mutation, there are many couples in whom both partners carry this mutation, making PGD relatively simple.

Table 12.1 shows the major autosomal single gene defects that have been diagnosed by PGD.

Autosomal dominant disorders

A single copy of the mutated gene will lead to the disease in disorders that are dominant in their inheritance (Figure 12.2). These diseases are not as life-threatening as some recessive diseases, and therefore affected individuals can still reproduce and transmit the disease to their offspring. Many dominant disorders are late in onset, such as Huntington's disease and some inherited cancers.

PGD has been developed for a few dominant diseases, such as Marfan's syndrome, Polyposis Coli and Huntington's Disease (Table 12.2).

X-linked diseases

X-linked diseases affect genes which are carried on the X chromosome, and more than 400 such diseases have been identified. They can be inherited in a recessive or dominant manner, but almost all severe types have recessive inheritance. Males inherit the X chromosome from their mother, and if this inherited X chromosome is abnormal they will be affected with the disease (Figure 12.3). Therefore, carrier mothers transmit the disease to half of their male offspring, and half of her daughters will be carriers. The gene involved has been characterized for some X-linked diseases, so that a specific diagnosis can be made at the prenatal stage. However, for some X-linked diseases the gene

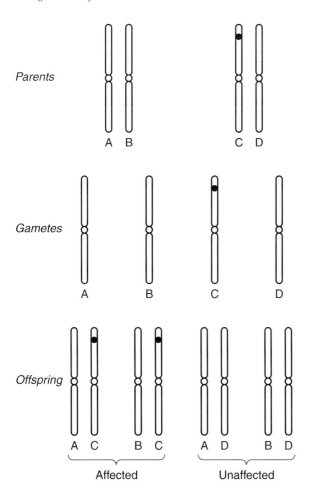

• Mutant allele

Figure 12.2   Autosomal dominant inheritance.

Table 12.2. *PGD for autosomal dominant diseases*

Marfan's syndrome
Familial adenomatous polyposis coli
Huntington's chorea
Myotonic dystrophy
Osteogensis imperfect

Table 12.3a. *PGD for X-linked diseases – sexing*

DMD
Becker's muscular dystrophy
Chronic granulomatosis
Hunter's syndrome
Haemophilia
Adrenoleucodystrophy
Barth syndrome
X-linked hydrocephalus
X-linked ataxia
XL retinitis pigmentosa
X-linked mental retardation
XL Wiscott Aldrich
XL Spastic paraplegia
Labers Optic Atrophy
Sensory Motorneurone Disease
Retinitis pigmentosa
Bruton's Disease
Menke's Disease

Table 12.3b. *PGD for X linked disease – specific diagnoses*

DMD
Haemophilia
Lesch Nyhan syndrome
Charcot Marie Tooth

involved has not been identified; in these cases prenatal sexing is offered. If the pregnancy is found to be male, there is a 50% chance that he will have the disease. Many couples will abort a male pregnancy rather than take the risk of transmitting the disease, but this scenario is not ideal. With PGD sexing can be performed at the cleavage embryo stage and female embryos selected for transfer.

X-linked diseases reported as diagnosed by embryo sexing are listed in Table 12.3a. Since X-linked diseases are single gene defects, the ideal way to perform the diagnosis would be to do a specific test for the mutation involved, but this can only be done if the mutation is known. The X-linked diseases where a specific diagnosis has been performed are listed in Table 12.3b.

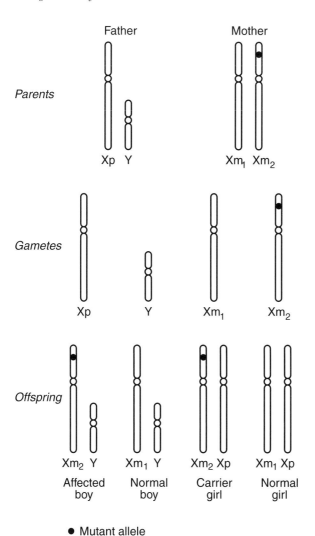

Figure 12.3   X-linked inheritance.

Triplet repeat disorders

A new class of genetic disorders was classified during the 1990s: the triplet repeat disorders are caused by the expansion of a triplet repeat of bases within a gene, and are usually associated with neurological disorders. Each disease has a range of repeats associated with a spectrum from normal individual to affected individuals. For example, for the triplet repeat responsible for Fragile X Syndrome, a normal individual will have from 6 to 54 triplet repeats; those having the 'premutation' will carry between 54 and 200 repeats, and those affected with Fragile X will have over 200 repeats.

Fragile X was originally thought to be an X-linked disease, as males are generally affected, but recently it has been reclassified as a triplet repeat disorder. It is caused by the unstable expansion of a CGG repeat in the 5′-untranslated region of the FMR1 gene, which is on the X chromosome. This triplet expansion results in mental retardation. Females carrying the premutation are at risk of transmitting the full mutation to their offspring, and, since males inherit the X chromosome from their mothers and have a single X chromosome, their male offspring are at a 50% risk of inheriting Fragile X. Females who inherit the expanded gene from their mothers will also inherit a normal X chromosome from their father, and show variable disease manifestations. Males carrying the premutation are at risk only of transmitting the premutation to their female offspring, who will be carrier females.

A number of cycles of PGD for Fragile X have been conducted; however, there is an additional problem, as many Fragile X carrier females experience premature menopause and do not respond very well to ovarian stimulation for IVF treatment.

Huntington's disease (HD) is a progressive neuropsychiatric disorder of late onset that is inherited in a dominant fashion. The gene is on chromosome 4, and involves a CAG triplet repeat where expansion beyond 36 results in HD. The age of onset is about 40 years and patients often die by their mid 50s. PGD has been performed for HD, but it draws some ethical discussion: many potential carriers of HD know that they have a 50% risk of being affected because one of their parents is affected, but they do not wish to know their own HD status. For prenatal testing, an exclusion test can be offered, where patients are given a risk factor without being told their actual status. PGD for HD has been developed and clinical cases performed. The option of offering an equivalent to the exclusion test by PGD has been discussed: patients who do not wish to know their HD status could undergo PGD and not be told if any affected embryos were detected. However, if all embryos were found to be affected, the patient's HD status would be obvious.

Myotonic dystrophy (DM) or Steinert's disease is a progressive muscular dystrophy. The gene is on chromosome 19 and DM is caused by expansion in a CTG repeat at the 3′-untranslated part of the DM kinase gene. Normal individuals have between 5 and 37 repeats, and affected individuals may have anything from 50 to several thousand repeats. Intermediate numbers of repeats can give rise to a premutation. PGD has been performed for DM.

Chromosomal abnormalities

Abnormalities which involve whole chromosomes are usually lethal. Those compatible with life are those which involve the sex chromosomes, such as Turner's syndrome (XO), Klinefelter's syndrome (XXY) or Down's syndrome (three copies of chromosome 21).

The most common chromosome abnormality is a chromosome translocation, where two chromosomes have broken and rejoined to the opposite chromosome. If the chromosomes are still balanced, i.e. all the genetic material is still present, the patient is described as having a balanced translocation. The majority of patients carrying a balanced translocation do not realize they have abnormal chromosomes until they try to reproduce. During meiosis, the segregation of the chromosomes becomes confused, and unbalanced chromosome complements are formed in the gametes, leading to the formation of an embryo with abnormal chromosomes (unbalanced translocation). Therefore patients carrying balanced translocations may experience infertility, repeated miscarriage or the birth of a child with abnormal chromosomes.

Robertsonian translocations involve breakages around the centromere of the 'acrocentric' chromosomes (13, 14, 15, 21, 22). These chromosomes contain a satellite region on their short arm, and loss of this area has no effect on phenotype. Since two of the acrocentric chromosomes join together, the patient has only 45 chromosomes. Robertsonian translocations are easier to diagnose using PGD, as only the number of chromosomes present needs to be identified; several cycles have been undertaken.

Reciprocal translocations involve breaks at any location on two chromosomes and thus can involve any chromosomes. The fact that every couple has different chromosome breakpoints makes PGD difficult.

Chromosome abnormalities can also be caused by chromosome inversions, insertions, deletions or rearrangements (such as ring chromosomes).

Age-related aneuploidy

Women over the age of 35 are known to be at increased risk of having a fetus with a chromosome abnormality. However, only 20% of Down's syndrome babies are born to women over the age of 35. Screening methods have been developed to help identify those pregnancies at risk, as the use of age alone as an indication for prenatal diagnosis of age-related aneuploidy will miss the majority of affected pregnancies. Biochemical (plasma alpha fetoprotein, hCG, unconjugated oestriol) and ultrasound screening methods are therefore used to determine which pregnancies are at risk. Patients found to be at risk undergo prenatal diagnosis, with a karyotype performed to ascertain the status of the fetus. The chromosomes most commonly involved in age-related aneuploidy are 13, 16, 18, 21, X and Y.

Serum screening

During the second trimester of pregnancy (16–17 weeks) a number of markers have been found to help identify pregnancies with chromosome abnormalities. Down's syndrome pregnancies show lower maternal serum alpha fetoprotein (AFP) and unconjugated oestriol, whereas human chorionic gonadotrophin (hCG) levels are two times higher than normal. Taking into account the patient's age, the use of the triple test to measure AFP, free β-hCG and unconjugated oestriol can increase the detection rate to 70%, thereby reducing the number of women who require invasive prenatal diagnosis.

Ongoing research is directed towards trying to identify first trimester markers for aneuploidy. Pregnancy associated plasma protein A (PAPP A) is reduced in Down's syndrome pregnancies; this, together with free β-hCG, is a promising marker.

Ultrasound

During the first trimester of pregnancy, ultrasound detection of nuchal translucency measuring greater than 3 mm may be associated with a chromosome abnormality. This is caused by fluid accumulation at the back of the fetal neck. In conjunction with maternal age, studies have shown this to give a detection rate of 86% with a false positive rate of 4.5%. When used in combination with second trimester serum screening, a detection rate of over 90% was reported.

In the second trimester, ultrasound markers such as cardiac malformations, duodenal atresia, hydrops, choroid plexus cysts, nuchal oedema, renal pyelectasis, omphalocoele, hypoplastic midphalanx of the 5th finger and short femur and humerus can be used to screen for aneuploidy.

Prenatal diagnosis of inherited disorders

Couples who have already had an affected pregnancy or child, or have a family member affected with the disease are aware that they are at risk of transmitting an inherited disease. Prenatal diagnosis is the main option open to such couples and to those who have a positive serum or ultrasound screen. Chorionic Villus Sampling (CVS) and amniocentesis are the methods of choice for prenatal diagnosis; techniques such as fetal blood sampling are rarely used.

Chorionic villus sampling (CVS)

CVS can be performed transcervically between 10–12 weeks of gestation, or from 12 weeks onwards by the transabdominal route. A sample of cells is removed from the placenta and used for diagnosis of chromosomal, metabolic and DNA analysis. The disadvantages of the procedure are that it can not be used for neural tube and other congenital abnormalities, and some studies have suggested a risk of limb reduction deformities if it is performed too early, or by inexperienced operators. There is also a 1–2% risk of miscarriage, which is a little higher than the risk after amniocentesis. In 1.5% of cases, the karyotype of the placenta is found to be different from that of the embryo (confined placental mosaicism).

Amniocentesis

This is the most common method used for prenatal diagnosis usually performed in the second trimester, from 15 weeks onwards. Under ultrasound guidance, 15–20 ml of amniotic fluid is aspirated; this can be used for the diagnosis of chromosome abnormalities, measurement of specific substances, detection of inborn errors of metabolism such as Tay-Sach's disease, measurement of enzyme activity and diagnosis of neural tube defects. Its disadvantages include the potential of causing fetal loss (1%) and rarely there may be continued leakage of the amniotic fluid. The main limitation of this technique is that results are available only very late in the pregnancy (17–20 weeks), so that a second trimester termination has to be induced. Early amniocentesis (11–14 weeks) is still under trial.

Fetal blood sampling, cordocentesis or PUBS (percutaneous umbilical blood sampling)

This is used less frequently than CVS or amniocentesis; samples can be taken from 18 weeks' gestation to term. Fetal blood is taken from the cord or intrahepatic umbilical vein and used for fetal karyotyping (quick result), evaluation of fetal status (if an infection is thought to be present) and haematological abnormalities (Rh or immune haemolytic disease). The most common indication is karyotyping for single or multiple congenital abnormalities and mosaicism.

Fetal tissue sampling

Using ultrasound guidance it is possible to biopsy skin, liver, muscle and fluid collections from the urinary tract, abdomen, thorax and cystic hygroma.

Diagnostic testing

Following CVS or amniocentesis, the sample must be diagnosed in order to identify the status of the fetus. Two tests are used: the polymerase chain reaction (PCR) or karyotyping. PCR is used for the detection of single gene defects, the triple repeat disorders, and identification of sex. A karyotype is performed for any diagnosis which involves chromosome identification, i.e. in those patients carrying chromosome abnormalities or who are at risk of age-related aneuploidy. In some situations, fluorescent in situ hybridization (FISH) is used to complement the karyotype result.

PCR

PCR is a technique whereby a portion of DNA is amplified thousands of times, and it is probably the most important technique used for genetic testing. For prenatal diagnosis, PCR can be used to detect the normal or mutated gene by amplifying the region around the mutation. This is achieved by using primers which have a complementary sequence to a region of the gene. Primers are selected which bind to either side of the mutation, they bind to their complementary sequence, and copies are generated for the region in between by a number of cycles of heating (to denature the DNA) and cooling (to allow synthesis). This is achieved with the use of an enzyme that can connect bases together and can also withstand the high temperatures needed for denaturation. The first such enzyme to be used for PCR was *Taq* polymerase.

Once the DNA sequence of interest has been copied, the PCR products are analysed by a number of different techniques. The simplest method, which can be used to detect an insertion or deletion, is to separate the PCR products by polyacrylamide gel electrophoresis; more recently techniques such as single stranded conformational polymorphism (SSCP), amplification refractory mutation system (ARMS) and heteroduplex analysis have been developed.

Using these techniques even just a single base change within a gene can be detected. PCR will be discussed in more detail in the section concerning PGD diagnosis.

Karyotyping

Karyotype analysis is the ideal method to examine the chromosomes of a cell. For prenatal diagnosis, the sample obtained by CVS or amniocentesis is cultured to increase the number of cells, and mitotic inhibitors are used to arrest some of the cells in metaphase. Agents which elongate the metaphase chromosomes are also used. Slide preparations of the nuclei are treated with Giemsa stain, which results in a specific banding pattern for each chromosome. Using this method, missing or extra chromosomes, translocations, inversions, etc. can be identified. Occasionally the results of a karyotype may be inconclusive, and FISH can be used to help elucidate the diagnosis.

Karyotyping is also used to check the number of chromosomes in diagnosis of age-related aneuploidy.

FISH

FISH uses DNA probes which bind to complementary sequences on specific chromosomes. There are three types of FISH probes:

1. Repeat sequences or alpha satellite probes which can be used in interphase and metaphase chromosomes. They bind to repeat sequences, usually to the centromeres (with the exception of chromosomes 9 and Y) and can be used directly labelled with fluorochromes. They require only 1 hour for hybridization and have been cloned in plasmids and cosmids. Probes for 13/21 and 14/22 cross hybridize
2. Locus specific probes can be used in interphase or metaphase chromosomes and bind to a unique sequence. They require 6–12 hours for hybridization and have been cloned in cosmids or YACs (yeast artifical chromosomes). These probes are still under development and are not yet avaliable for every part of every chromosome.
3. Chromosome paints can only be used in metaphase chromosomes, and they paint the entire chromosome.

There are several stages to the FISH technique.

1. Cell spreading.
2. Pepsin digestion. This is required to remove any protein from around the nuclei and is especially important for blastomeres.
3. Fixing. A paraformaldehyde fixative is used to ensure that the nuclei are stuck onto the slide.

4. Denaturation. This makes the nuclear and probe DNA single stranded.
5. Hybridization. Allows the probes to find and bind to the complementary sequence.
6. Posthybridization washes. Removes any unbound probe.
7. Detection – for use with indirect probes.
8. Visualization.

Preimplantation genetic diagnosis

PGD is comparable to prenatal diagnosis. The embryo biopsy is equivalent to the CVS or amniocentesis and the single cell diagnosis equates to the prenatal diagnosis. Since two techniques are involved, biopsy and diagnosis, a PGD team is made up of an IVF and a genetics team. The embryo biopsy technique should be performed by a trained embryologist, but the diagnosis must be performed by a genetics department.

Embryo biopsy

Cell biopsies can be taken from oocytes/embryos at three different stages:

1. Oocyte/zygote (polar body biopsy)
2. 6–10 cell cleavage stage embryo (cleavage stage biopsy)
3. Blastocyst stage embryos (blastocyst biopsy).

World-wide, cleavage stage biopsy is the most widely used procedure. Polar body biopsy examines only the maternal chromosomes.

Embryo biopsy can be performed using micromanipulation equipment used for ICSI, and all of the biopsy techniques involve two stages: zona drilling, and aspiration (or herniation in the case of blastocyst biopsy).

Zona drilling

Zona drilling can be achieved by using either acid Tyrode's solution or a laser beam, or by mechanical means. Zona drilling with acid Tyrode's uses a double pipette holder, or two manipulators on the same side, as different pipettes are used for the acid and for blastomere aspiration. A small hole is drilled in the zona pellucida using a small pipette (internal diameter 10 μm) containing acid Tyrode's solution (pH 2.2–2.4). The pipette is placed close to the zona pellucida and the Tyrode's solution gently expelled from the pipette until the zona thins and a hole is drilled (in some cases, the zona can be seen to 'pop' as a hole is made). The use of the same pipette for both zona drilling and blastomere aspiration has also been reported.

Acid Tyrode's drilling can be problematic, as some zonae are very sensitive and others very difficult to drill. The use of a laser gives more control over the size of the hole made, but this is still a relatively new technique. There are two types of laser: the one principally under current trial sends the beam up from the light source and drills a tunnel through the zona, so that the laser beam does not come into direct contact with the embryonic cells. The second method directs the beam directly onto the zona and would therefore transmit the beam through the embryo. A few centres use mechanical means for zona drilling, whereby the zona is ripped to enable access to the embryonic cells. When the hole has been drilled, the cells can be aspirated (polar body and cleavage stage biopsy) or herniated (blastocyst biopsy).

Polar body biopsy

The oocyte or zygote is immobilized and a hole drilled in the zona as above. A small pipette is used to gently aspirate the polar bodies.

Biopsy of the first polar body was developed in order to overcome ethical objections to embryo biopsy. Some individuals opt for PGD in order to avoid termination of pregnancy, and performing the test on the preimplantation embryo may be as objectionable as termination of pregnancy. Polar body biopsy was first used for the detection of CF, but due to crossing-over events the second polar body was required in some situations. More recently, biopsy of the first and second polar body has been used for PGD of age-related aneuploidy or in cases when the female carries a chromosome abnormality.

Cleavage stage biopsy

For the biopsy of human embryos, the embryo is immobilized using a fine-polished pipette (outer diameter 120 µm, internal diameter 30 µm) and applying gentle suction. Once the hole has been drilled, a finely polished 'sampling' pipette (internal diameter ranging from 30 to 40 µm) is used to aspirate the blastomere. The pipette is placed through the hole and close to the blastomere to be aspirated. By gentle suction, the blastomere is drawn into the pipette whilst the pipette is withdrawn from the hole. Once the blastomere is free from the rest of the embryo, it is gently expelled from the pipette.

Biopsies performed at earlier stages (4 cells) may alter the ratio of inner cell mass to trophectoderm cells, which may be detrimental to embryo development. Therefore, the main strategy used for embryo biopsy has been to biopsy embryos at the 6–10 cell stage, on Day 3 postinsemination.

Several difficulties arise from cleavage stage embryo biopsy: the first is that human embryonic cells are very fragile and easily lyse. If this occurs during the biopsy procedure, the nucleus may be lost and another cell will have to be removed. Compaction occurs between the 8-cell and morula stage, and during compaction the cells of the embryo can no longer be distinguished as they flatten out over each other to maximize intercellular contacts. If the biopsy is performed at this stage, it is very difficult to remove a blastomere, as it has established strong contacts with adjacent blastomeres. Trying to remove a cell from a compacted embryo may also result in lysis of the cell. The thickness and dynamics of the zona pellucida also vary between patients and can lead to some problems during the biopsy procedure. In many cases, numerous sperm are associated with the zona pellucida and therefore intracytoplasmic sperm injection (ICSI) should always be used with PCR techniques to reduce the risk of sperm contamination.

In the human, the cryopresevation of embryos in IVF treatment cycles is routine, and from frozen embryo replacement cycles up to 50% of blastomeres can be destroyed and the embryo is still capable of producing a viable fetus. No increase in fetal abnormalities has been reported following transfer of cryo-preserved embryos in which some cells have been destroyed by freezing/thaw-ing. Studies examining the effect of embryo biopsy have shown that at the 8-cell stage, removal of 2 cells was not detrimental to embryo metabolism or development and is an efficient process with more than 90% of the embryos surviving. Data from the ESHRE PGD consortium show that 97% of embryo biopsies were successful.

Two recent studies analysed the pregnancies obtained from biopsied em-bryos after PGD. Biochemical and ultrasound measurements showed that the pregnancies showed no significant developmental differences compared to controls. Deliveries, including infant birth weight and apghar scores, were considered to be normal.

Blastocyst biopsy

Blastocyst biopsy can be performed on Day 5 or 6 postinsemination. The best technique seems to be to stabilize the blastocyst by gentle suction through a holding pipette, and make an incision at the pole opposite to the inner cell mass using a 2 μm bevelled pipette. The pipette is pushed in and out through the zona and pulled upwards to make the incision. The blastocysts are then left for 6–24 hours until some trophectoderm herniates though the slit. When herniation involves about 25% of the blastocyst (20–30 cells), the herniated piece of trophectoderm is excised.

Blastocyst biopsy has the advantage that a larger number of cells can be removed from the outer trophectoderm layer without affecting the inner cell mass from which the fetus later develops. However, trophectoderm cells (TE) may have diverged genetically from the inner cell mass (ICM) as confined placental mosaicism is observed in at least 1% of conceptions, where the chromosome status of the embryo is different from the placenta. Recent studies have indicated that blastocysts may have high levels of chromosomal mosaicism. Preferential allocation of abnormal cells to the TE may be a mechanism of early development; in this case the TE would not be representative of the rest of the embryo, which would complicate and compromise PGD.

The main limitation of blastocyst biopsy is that a limited number of embryos will reach the blastocyst stage. In recent years improvements in culture conditions have been made which increased the success of blastocyst biopsy. However, for PGD to be successful a large number of embryos are required to ensure that normal embryos are available for transfer, which may not be the case when embryos are cultured to the blastocyst stage.

Single cell diagnosis

Cell(s) removed from the embryo after biopsy are used for diagnosis. Single cell diagnosis is a new field of diagnostic procedures. PCR is used for the single cell diagnosis of single gene defects, triplet repeat disorders, and embryo sexing. Karyotyping requires a metaphase spread of chromosomes, and therefore this cannot be used on single embryonic cells; these cells do not divide well in culture, and it is difficult to obtain metaphase spreads. In cases where a metaphase spread is obtained, the chromosomes are short and difficult to band. Therefore FISH is used to examine chromosomes in embryos for embryo sexing, chromosome abnormalities and age-related aneuploidy.

PCR diagnosis

PCR diagnosis from a single cell has been used for the diagnosis of single gene defects, triplet repeat disorders and embryo sex, but it is not an easy procedure. The two major problems encountered are contamination and allele dropout (see below) which both make PCR from a single cell a very difficult technique to perform. If a diagnosis is available on whole DNA, it should be possible to

make such a diagnosis sensitive at the single cell level. However, some modifications of the procedure may be required. A common method of making the
PCR procedure more sensitive is the use of nested PCR, where an inner set of
primers amplifies the original PCR product. Since amplification failure can
occur, it is essential that PGD does not rely on a negative result. To ensure that
a single cell PCR method is accurate and sensitive, a preliminary workup is
usually performed on single cells, such as buccal cells, from normal, carrier and
affected individuals. The analyses of PGD PCR products have been performed
by heteroduplex analysis, SSCP, ARMS and restriction endonuclease digestion. More recently, fluorescent PCR has been used which is a quantitative
PCR method. For the diagnosis of some diseases, such as Fragile X, polymorphic markers may be used which identify which chromosome the embryo has
inherited; i.e. the normal or at risk chromosome.

Contamination

Single cell PCR is so sensitive that it will amplify any DNA that may contami-
nate the PCR reaction, such as a stray cumulus or sperm cell that may have
been released from the zona during the biopsy, cells from the atmosphere or
DNA found in the air or medium. To reduce these problems to a minimum,
steps have to be taken to eliminate contamination. These include working in a
positive pressure PCR room, performing ICSI for all PCR diagnosis and
examining PCR products in a separate laboratory. Several misdiagnoses have
been reported after PGD, and these have probably arisen from contamination
of a PCR. These problems can be reduced with the use of a multiplex PCR with
markers which can identify all four parental alleles to ensure that the amplified
product is of embryonic origin.

Allele dropout

Allele dropout (ADO), or preferential amplification, refers to the situation
where one of the two alleles preferentially amplifies over the other. For
example, for a heterozygous cell, the normal allele may preferentially amplify
so that the diagnosis would only identify the normal allele – the embryo would
be diagnosed as normal instead of heterozygous. This would not cause a
problem for recessive conditions where both partners carry the same mutation,
but would create problems for dominant disorders, or in cases where the
couple carry different mutations for a recessive disorder, as affected embryos

could be diagnosed as normal. To reduce this problem, methods can be built into the diagnosis to ensure that both alleles can be identified.

FISH diagnosis

With the advent of fluorescent in situ hybridization (FISH), every nucleus within an embryo can be examined, but the number of chromosomes that can be analysed at one time is limited. Even with current technology, no more than 5 chromosomes can be analysed in one embryo. Repeat and locus-specific probes can be used for cleavage or blastocyst biopsies as the embryonic nuclei are in interphase, but chromosome paints can be used on polar bodies.

FISH has been used since 1991 to sex embryos for PGD of sex for X-linked disease. It has advantages over PCR sexing as the copy number is identified: the difference between XO and XX can be determined, and there is no risk of contamination. Usually, probes for chromosomes X, Y and 18 are used and only embryos showing normal female chromosomes are transferred.

With the development of a wider range of locus-specific probes, FISH can be used for the detection of chromosome imbalances in patients carrying chromosome abnormalities. In these situations, a normal and balanced chromosome pattern cannot be distinguished. If the female carries the translocation, polar body biopsy can be performed and chromosome paints used. For Robertsonian translocations, probes for any area of the chromosome involved can be used, but for Reciprocal translocations probes are used either side of the break points.

PGD of age-related aneuploidy

Women over 35 years who are undergoing IVF treatment may wish to have their oocytes or embryos screened in order to reduce the effects of age-related aneuploidy. Since chromosome abnormalities in embryos play a significant role in implantation failure and miscarriages, screening oocytes or embryos before implantation may increase delivery rate, and will reduce the need for prenatal diagnosis in these patients, who may not wish to undertake the 1% risk of miscarriage associated with these techniques. This can be achieved by the analysis of the first and second polar body, but cannot examine postzygotic events; cleavage stage biopsy may also be performed. In the studies performed to date, chromosomes 13, 18, 21, X and Y have been examined, but, interestingly, abnormalities of chromosomes 13, 18 and 21 account for less than 20% of trisomies, and the analysis of chromosome 16, which is the most common trisomy found in spontaneous miscarriages, would probably be more useful. Also, some of the larger chromosomes may be responsible for implantation failure.

Problems with PGD

Two phenomena cause problems for PGD: chromosomal mosaicism and allele dropout. The latter was discussed earlier in the section on PCR.

Chromosomal mosaicism

FISH has been used for the analysis of chromosome patterns in human preimplantation embryos which have been donated for research purposes. Studies on abnormally fertilized embryos (such as polyspermic embryos) have shown, as expected, that these embryos were highly abnormal, in agreement with the karyotype data obtained from such embryos. In the majority of cases, mosaicism was observed and, in some cases, normal diploid embryos were found from supposedly polyspermic embryos; this may have been due to misidentification of a vacuole as a pronucleus. Analysis of arrested embryos using three-colour FISH for chromosomes X, Y and 18 showed that 56.5% of embryos showed numerical aberrations (mostly polyploid or mosaics) suggesting that if more chromosomes were examined, extrapolation of the data would show very high levels of abnormalities in these embryos. As expected, embryos from older aged women show high levels of chromosome abnormalities.

Normally fertilized, normally developing embryos also show high levels of chromosomal abnormalities. In order to categorise these abnormalities, the patterns have been divided into four groups. Embryos are either:

(a) uniformly diploid for the probes examined,
(b) uniformly abnormal, such as Down's syndrome or Turner's,
(c) mosaic, where usually both diploid cells and aneuploid, haploid or polyploid nuclei are present or
(d) chaotic embryos, where every nucleus shows a different chromosome complement.

The data from FISH analysis show a higher rate of abnormalities than has previously been reported from karyotyping data. However, since mosaic and chaotic embryos are common, if only 1 or 2 cells are analysable from an embryo, then karyotyping would underestimate the level of chromosome abnormalities.

Normal, abnormal and mosaic embryos have all been observed in fetal development. It has been estimated that, in 1% of conceptions, the placenta has a different karyotype from the fetus (confined placental mosaicism – CPM). CPM was first detected when first trimester fetal karyotyping after chorionic villus sampling showed discrepancies between chorionic cells and the embryo proper. The presence of two cell lines could arise due to an abnormal chromosome arrangement caused by a postzygotic event, or the chromosome loss from a trisomic embryo, which restores the diploid state (trisomic rescue). Several mechanisms would indicate that these abnormal cells are more likely to be found in the trophectoderm, and hence the placenta. First, only four cells from a blastocyst give rise to the embryo and it would be unlikely that the abnormal cells would be found in the embryo; second, in most cases a fetus with abnormal chromosomes will not be compatible with life. Lastly, the embryo may preferentially allocate abnormal cells to the trophectoderm.

The chaotic group of embryos was an unexpected finding, as such embryos have not been observed in later stages of embryonic development, probably because these embryos would arrest and fail to implant.

Multinucleated blastomeres have been reported from both karyotyping and FISH analysis. The presence of such blastomeres may be more common in arrested embryos, and may occur more readily in some patients. Binucleate blastomeres have been observed in mouse embryos at the morula stage, and it has been suggested that these blastomeres might be the precursors for mural trophectoderm giant cells. However, in human embryos the binucleate cells appear at cleavage stages before trophectoderm differentiation. Binucleate cells may arise from asymmetrical cytokinesis so that one daughter cell contains two nuclei and the other is anucleate.

Embryos containing tetraploid cells may be a normal part of development of the trophectoderm as a precursor of syncitiotrophoblast formation. Such cells have also been found in cattle, pig and sheep.

Overall, extrapolation of this data would suggest that no embryo is completely chromosomally normal at early cleavage stage. However, various models for which there are experimental data may help to explain the observation that pregnancies following IVF do not result in an increased incidence of chromosomally abnormal infants. Firstly, few cells (possibly a single cell from an 8-cell embryo) differentiate to the embryo proper – the majority contribute to the cytotrophoblast and fetal membranes. Secondly, experimental production of tetraploid/diploid mouse conceptuses suggests that a mechanism exists to exclude chromosomally abnormal cells from the primitive ectoderm lineage (or they are selectively lost later). At 12 days of development, no tetraploid cells were detected in the fetus, and they rarely contributed to other derivatives of the primitive ectoderm and trophectoderm lineages. Data accumulated on the chromosomal constitution of surplus nontransferred embryos from PGD cycles have revealed that, despite the fact that these embryos are from women of proven fertility, the incidence of postzygotic chromosomal anomalies is similar to that in embryos from routine IVF patients. This finding may provide one explanation for the apparently poor success rate of IVF procedures; i.e. that, at best, only 1 embryo transfer in 5 results in an ongoing pregnancy. A second significant finding is that the incidence of the most bizarre type of anomaly, chaotically dividing embryos, is strongly patient-related. In repeated cycles, certain women regularly produced 'chaotic' embryos while others did not, although the frequency of diploid mosaics was similar in both groups.

All the studies performed in recent years to analyse chromosomes in embryos have been carried out using embryos generated by IVF, which may not be representative of in vivo development. However, the classic studies of Hertig (1956) showed that embryos from natural cycles also showed high levels of nuclear abnormalities, and from the studies of normally conceived pregnancies, we know that 60% of abortions are chromosomally abnormal.

Mosaicism and PGD

Chromosomal mosaicism may cause ·a problem in PGD for some diseases, namely dominant disorders and chromosome abnormalities. A misdiagnosis of embryo sex would be unlikely to occur as an XX cell would have to be found in an XY embryo. XO cells have been identified in male embryos, but XO embryos should never be considered for transfer; if the offspring have Turner's syndrome, they would have the same risk of suffering the X-linked disease as would a male. For recessive disorders, the presence of extra chromosomes or a haploid cell would not lead to a misdiagnosis. A carrier embryo with a haploid cell would be diagnosed as normal or affected depending on which gene was present in the cell: this would be the same situation if allele dropout had occurred. For dominant disorders, a haploid cell could lead to a misdiagnosis; if a cell from an affected embryo carried only the unaffected gene, the cell would be diagnosed as normal. Therefore the same precautions as for allele dropout would have to be applied. For chromosome abnormalities, mosaic embryos containing some normal and some abnormal cells have been identified, such as in cases where a few normal cells arise in an embryo which otherwise carried trisomy 21. If the normal cells are biopsied, the embryo would be diagnosed as normal, resulting in misdiagnosis. As with confined placental mosaicism, this problem cannot be solved. Patients undergoing PGD for chromosomal abnormalities have to be aware that chromosomal mosaicism can lead to a misdiagnosis, but that this is a rare event. The probability can be reduced if two cells are used for the diagnosis, but this is not always technically feasible.

Ethics and laws

The law governing PGD varies world-wide. Some countries have legislation regulating PGD, or PGD and embryo research, and others have no legislation. However, a few countries have banned PGD – which is astonishing in view of the fact that the aim of PGD is to eliminate termination of pregnancy. The main arguments against PGD are that it may be abused, as in the case of embryo sex selection for family balancing, or for choosing certain characteristics, the so-called 'Designer Baby'. Prenatal diagnosis has been abused for fetal sex selection in several countries for many years, but, as with all medical practices, the good should outweigh the bad: such practices should not be banned just because they could be abused. Legislation governing the use of PGD should eliminate such problems. In the UK, the Human Fertilisation and Embryology Authority (HFEA), which licences all IVF practices, has banned embryo sexing for family balancing and they licence all PGD centres. It must be remembered that it is no easy task to undergo PGD, mainly because the IVF procedure is so invasive and the pregnancy rate is low. If couples wished to design their baby, the cheaper and simpler route would be prenatal diagnosis, where many diseases could be diagnosed at one time.

The future of PGD

The development of PGD over the past 10 years has been slow to progress. It is not yet possible to diagnose CF and Down's syndrome from a single cell, and the list of diseases that have been diagnosed is very small. PGD is also more complicated than originally thought: the concept that a single cell would be representative of the rest of the embryo has been confused and compounded by the discovery of high levels of chromosomal mosaicism in human embryos. Unfortunately, a few misdiagnoses have also occurred, mainly due to chromosomal mosaicism, allele dropout or contamination (possible from cumulus or sperm cells). However, recent studies have shown that the risk of a CF misdiagnosis is 0.3–5.6% depending on whether 1 or 2 cells were analysed, and the risk would be reduced to 0.015–1.25% if only homozygous unaffected embryos were considered for transfer. The use of intragenic polymorphic markers, to ensure that the DNA amplified is of embryonic origin, should further reduce the risk of misdiagnosis.

Cost is also an important consideration, as some single cell diagnoses are expensive techniques. For example, the cost of FISH probes can equal the cost of an IVF treatment cycle, which makes PGD a very expensive technique. In the UK, some health authorities have paid for PGD cycles, and in other countries government or health insurance funds are available; if patients have to meet the cost they may opt for prenatal diagnosis.

Data from the ESHRE PGD consortium shows that the delivery rate per cycle for PGD is similar to that seen in IVF, even though PGD patients are normally fertile. Therefore, any centre or patient embarking on PGD has to be aware that the diagnosis may not be 100% accurate due to mosaicism and allele dropout, and that the chance of an unaffected baby after one cycle is low. The patients also have to decide whether undertaking an IVF cycle is more or less traumatic than natural conception and prenatal diagnosis. We have found that the natural pregnancy rate for patients registered for PGD is very high, as most of them have the alternative of prenatal diagnosis.

The most logical, and highly motivated group of patients to treat by PGD are those who are infertile or who have experienced repeated miscarriages. Patients who carry chromosome abnormalities are one of the most difficult groups of patients to treat, due to limitations of available probes and the high levels of abnormal embryos they produce.

Techniques under development for single cell diagnosis include whole genome amplification, where the whole genome is randomly amplified to allow several diagnoses to be performed on a single cell. This would allow examination of several mutations for a disease from one cell, and DNA fingerprinting could also be performed to ensure that the diagnosed DNA is embryonic. Products of whole genome amplification may also be used to examine chromosomes using a technique called comparative genomic hybridization (CGH). For CGH, embryonic DNA is labelled with a fluorochrome (for example red), and some control DNA is labelled with a green fluorochrome. Both samples are cohybridized onto a control metaphase plate and the ratio of red:green labelling indicates which chromosomes are in excess or missing from the embryo. For example, a Down's syndrome embryo will show more red than green on chromosome 21 as there will be an extra copy. The development of additional FISH probes and the use of fluorescent PCR or new FISH methods, such as multicolour FISH (M-FISH) will also increase the scope of single cell diagnosis.

Many couples around the world opt for PGD as an alternative to prenatal diagnosis, and at least 100 babies have been born. PGD is a very real alternative for these couples, and hopefully, with improvements in IVF and single cell diagnosis, the range of diseases that can be diagnosed at the single cell level and the number of patients who can be treated will increase.

Further reading

Prenatal Diagnosis – special issue, December 1998, **18(13)**. Issue dedicated to preimplantation genetics and diagnosis.

Index

Note: page numbers in *italics* refer to figures and tables

296